Clinical Cases in Tropical Medicine

T0127751

SECOND EDITION

Edited by

Camilla Rothe, MD, DTM&H

Head of Clinical Tropical Medicine
Division of Infectious Diseases and Tropical Medicine
LMU University Hospital
Munich, Germany

ELSEVIER

© 2022, Elsevier Limited. All rights reserved.

First edition 2015
Second edition 2022

The right of Camilla Rothe to be identified as editor of this work has been asserted by her in accordance with the Copyright, Designs and Patents Act 1988.

No part of this publication may be reproduced or transmitted in any form or by any means, electronic or mechanical, including photocopying, recording, or any information storage and retrieval system, without permission in writing from the publisher. Details on how to seek permission, further information about the Publisher's permissions policies and our arrangements with organizations such as the Copyright Clearance Center and the Copyright Licensing Agency, can be found at our website: www.elsevier.com/permissions

This book and the individual contributions contained in it are protected under copyright by the Publisher (other than as may be noted herein).

Notices

Practitioners and researchers must always rely on their own experience and knowledge in evaluating and using any information, methods, compounds or experiments described herein. Because of rapid advances in the medical sciences, in particular, independent verification of diagnoses and drug dosages should be made. To the fullest extent of the law, no responsibility is assumed by Elsevier, authors, editors or contributors for any injury and/or damage to persons or property as a matter of products liability, negligence or otherwise, or from any use or operation of any methods, products, instructions or ideas contained in the material herein.

ISBN: 978-0-7020-7879-8

Content Strategist: Lotta Kryhl
Content Development Specialist: Louise Cook
Project Manager: Andrew Riley
Design: Renee Duenow
Marketing Manager: Maria Moreno

Printed in the UK

Last digit is the print number: 9 8 7 6 5 4 3 2 1

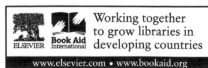

Clinical Cases in Tropical Medicine

Contents

Foreword

Twenty years following the launch of the Millennium Development Goals, malaria and neglected tropical diseases remain pervasive, especially among the world's poor. Information from the recently published Global Burden of Disease Study 2017 confirms that the world's major tropical infections, including malaria and the 20 major neglected tropical diseases (NTDs) identified by the World Health Organization, exert a horrific toll on human life[1,2]. Together these diseases kill an estimated 720,000,[1] while causing chronic and disabling effects measured in DALYs (disability-adjusted life years) that exceed almost any other cause of illness.[2] Tuberculosis and HIV/AIDS are also devastating infections that disproportionately occur in tropical developing countries.

Even beyond their adverse health impact, the leading tropical diseases are significant causes of economic underdevelopment. Indeed, malaria and the NTDs are probably the most common diseases of poor people and have been shown to thwart economic productivity through their negative effects on child health and the productivity of agricultural workers.[3] So far in 2020, we have also seen how a coronavirus, a zoonotic disease from bats, can profoundly affect the world's second largest economy – China. Yet another important effect – tropical infectious diseases also disproportionately devastate girls and women through their ability to damage the female urogenital tract or cause disfigurement and stigma.[4] Tropical diseases are the secret scourge of girls and women.

Despite their enormous global importance, there is a surprising lack of knowledge about tropical diseases among health care professionals including physicians. For example, recent studies from the United States Centers for Disease Control and Prevention indicate that very few US medical doctors know how to recognize and diagnose Chagas disease (American trypanosomiasis) even though it is now an important cause of heart disease in the US.[5,6] As a result, thousands of Chagas disease cases may go undiagnosed every year and patients inadvertently denied access to essential trypanocidal medicines. This finding emphasizes an emerging concept in tropical medicine that many parasitic and related infections occur outside of the poorest countries, with high levels of transmission also occurring in generally wealthy countries such as in the US or Eastern and Southern Europe.[7,8] The term 'blue marble health' has been coined to account for the finding that many of the world's neglected tropical diseases are found predominantly among the extreme poor living amidst wealth.[9] In other words, poverty has emerged as the overriding social determinant of neglected tropical diseases. But poverty is not the only social or physical determinant now driving 21st century diseases, as increasingly, we increasingly see how war or political collapse, urbanization, and climate change influence disease patterns[10-12].

Clinical Cases in Tropical Medicine ('*Clinical Cases*') is a key companion volume to the 23rd Edition of Manson's Tropical Diseases, but it will also be useful alongside other complete tropical medicine textbooks. An important role for *Clinical Cases* is to provide important practical applications and illustrative case reports in order to reinforce the material in these comprehensive texts. Comprised of over 100 detailed clinical cases from as many tropical medicine physicians across the world, *Clinical Cases* provides an excellent learning opportunity to reinforce concepts on practical approaches to the diagnosis, management, and treatment of the major tropical diseases endemic to Africa, Asia and the Americas. This new edition also contains important updates regarding emerging tropical diseases such as Zika virus infection and malaria caused by *Plasmodium knowlesi*, among other conditions. The book should be useful for trainees and practitioners working in disease-endemic developing countries, as well as those working in clinical settings that see immigrants or travelers from affected regions and now people living in poverty in North America and Europe who also suffer from these afflictions. *Clinical Cases* should serve as a powerful learning tool for years to come!

Peter Hotez MD PhD FAAP FASTMH*

References Cited

1. GBD 2017 Causes of Death Collaborators. Global, regional, and national age-sex specific mortality for 282 causes of death in 195 countries and territories, 1980-2017: a systematic analysis for the Global Burden of Disease Study 2017. Lancet 2018;392:1736-88.
2. GBD 2017 DALYs and HALE Collaborators. Global, regional, and national disability-adjusted life-years (DALYs) for 359

*Peter Hotez is Texas Children's Hospital Endowed Chair of Tropical Pediatrics, Professor of Pediatrics and Molecular Virology and Microbiology, and Dean of the National School of Tropical Medicine at Baylor College of Medicine in Houston, Texas.

diseases and injuries and healthy life expectancy (HALE) for 195 countries and territories, 1990-2017: a systematic analysis for the Global Burden of Disease Study 2017. Lancet 2018;392:1859–922.

3. Hotez PJ, Fenwick A, Savioli L, et al. Rescuing the bottom billion through control of neglected tropical diseases. Lancet 2009;373:1570–5.

4. Hotez PJ, Engels D, Gyapong M, et al. Female genital schistosomiasis. N Engl J Med 2019;381:2943–5.

5. Stimpert KK, Montgomery SP. Physician awareness of Chagas disease, USA. Emerg Infect Dis 2010;16:871–2.

6. Verani JR, Montgomery SP, Schulkin J, et al. Survey of obstetrician-gynecologists in the United States about Chagas disease. Am J Trop Med Hyg 2010;83:891–5.

7. Hotez PJ, Jackson Lee S. US Gulf Coast states: The rise of neglected tropical diseases in "flyover nation" PLoS Negl Trop Dis 2017;11(11):e0005744.

8. Hotez PJ. Southern Europe's Coming Plagues: Vector-Borne Neglected Tropical Diseases. PLoS Negl Trop Dis 2016;10(6):e0004243.

9. Hotez PJ. NTDs V.2.0: 'Blue marble health' – neglected tropical disease control and elimination in a shifting health policy landscape. PLOS Negl Trop Dis 2013;7:e2570.

10. Du RY, Stanaway JD, Hotez PJ. Could violent conflict derail the London Declaration on NTDs? PLoS Negl Trop Dis 2018;12(4):0006136.

11. Hotez PJ. Global urbanization and the neglected tropical diseases. PLoS Negl Trop Dis 2017;11(2):e0005308.

12. Blum AJ, Hotez PJ. Global "worming": Climate change and its projected general impact on human helminth infections. PLoS Negl Trop Dis 2018;12(7):e0006370.

Preface

Clinical Cases in Tropical Medicine was written for doctors and senior medical students who already have some background knowledge in tropical medicine which they wish to put into practice. It helps the reader prepare for an occupational stay in a tropical country and is equally useful for preparing for examinations, like the Diploma in Tropical Medicine and Hygiene (DTM&H) or a specialist examination. It can also just be used by anyone who takes pleasure in puzzling cases in tropical medicine for the mere fun of it! This book has been developed as a companion book to Manson's Tropical Diseases; however, it can be read alongside any other textbook of tropical medicine. It can also be used on its own since every case presentation closes with a 'summary box' providing a brief synopsis of the clinical problem discussed. The "summary box" is also meant to serve as a useful and compact tool for revision, e.g. before an exam.

The first edition of this book was a great success: Doctors and medical students around the world use it for self-study and teaching all over the world. This second edition of Clinical Cases in Tropical Medicine has been updated and extended and contains 30 new cases. Important "classical" tropical diseases missing in the first edition have now been added, such as African trypanosomiasis, chagas, leprosy and yaws. The world's epidemiological picture is rapidly changing: cases of newly emerging diseases have been included, such as Zika, Severe Fever with Thrombocytopenia Syndrome (SFTS) and Knowlesi malaria. In addition, migrant medicine has become of growing importance to clinicians in non-tropical countries. This novel trend is reflected by new cases in migrant medicine and contain decriptions eg. of louse-borne-relapsing fever, spinal brucellosis and hyperreactive malarial splenomegaly. On behalf of our team of authors from all over the world we hope you enjoy the second edition of this book.

List of Contributors

Charlotte Adamczick, MD, MIH, DTMH, PGDipPID
Consultant Paediatrician
Tropen- und Reisemedizin am Bellevue
Zürich, Switzerland

Cassandra Aldrich, BM BCh, PhD, DTMH
Division of Infectious Diseases and Tropical Medicine
University Hospital, LMU Munich
Munich, Germany

Koya Ariyoshi, MD, DTMH, MSc, PhD
Professor of Clinical Medicine
Department of Infectious Diseases
Nagasaki University Hospital
Nagasaki City, Nagasaki, Japan

Sudhir Babji, MD
Assistant Professor
The Wellcome Trust Research Laboratory
Division of Gastrointestinal Sciences
Christian Medical College
Vellore, India

Andrew Bastawrous, BSc (Hons), MBChB, MRCOphth, PGCTLCP, FHEA, PhD
Associate Professor
Clinical Research Department
London, School of Hygiene and Tropical Medicine
London, UK

M. Jane Bates, MBChB, MPhil, FRCGP
Family Physician
Department of Family Medicine
College of Medicine
Blantyre, Malawi

Daniel G. Bausch, MD, MPH&TM
Director
UK Public Health Rapid Support Team
Public Health England/London School of Hygiene and
    Tropical Medicine, London
London, UK;
Professor
Department of Disease Control
London, School of Hygiene and Tropical Medicine
London, UK

Nicholas A.V. Beare, MA, MB ChB, MD, FRCOphth
Consultant Ophthalmologist
St Paul's Eye Unit
Royal Liverpool University Hospital
Liverpool, UK

Cesar G. Berto, MD
Internal Medicine
Jacobi Medical Center
Bronx, NY, USA

Johannes Blum, Prof.
Prof. Dr. med.
Medical Department
Swiss Tropical and Public Health Institute
Basel, Switzerland

Marleen Boelaert, MD PhD
Professor
Department of Public Health
Institute of Tropical Medicine
Antwerp, Belgium

Gerd-Dieter Burchard, Prof. Dr. med.
Professor
Bernhard Nocht Institute for Tropical Medicine
Hamburg, Germany

Beatriz Bustamante, MD
Head of the Mycology Laboratory and Associate Researcher
Instituto de Medicina Tropical Alexander von Humboldt
Universidad Peruana Cayetano Heredia, Lima, Peru;
Assistant Physician
Department of Transmissible and Dermatological Diseases
Hospital Nacional Cayetano Heredia
Lima, Peru

Fátima Concha Velasco, MSc
Physician (Infectious Disease)
Medicine
Hospital Antonio Lorena
Cusco, Peru

Fernando Mejía Cordero, MD
Researcher
Instituto Medicina Tropical Alexander von Humboldt
Universidad Peruana Cayetano Heredia
Lima, Peru

Christina M. Coyle, MD, MS
Assistant Dean
Office of Faculty Development
Albert Einstein College of Medicine
New York, NY, USA

Bart J. Currie, MBBS, FRACP, FAFPHM, DTM+H
Professor in Medicine
Northern Territory Medical Program and Menzies School of
    Health Research
Royal Darwin Hospital,
Darwin, Northern Territory, Australia

David A.B. Dance, MB ChB, MSc, FRCPath
Clinical Research Microbiologist
Lao–Oxford–Mahosot Hospital–Wellcome Trust
    Research Unit
Microbiology Laboratory
Mahosot Hospital
Vientiane, Lao PDR and
Centre for Tropical Medicine
University of Oxford
Oxford, UK

Jeremy Day, MA, MB BChir, DTM&H, PhD, FRCP
Head, CNS and HIV Infections Research Group
Oxford University Clinical Research Unit
Ho Chi Minh City, Vietnam;
Professor of Infectious Diseases
Nuffield Department of Medicine
University of Oxford
Oxford, UK

Sebastian Dieckmann, MD
Senior Clinical Consultant
Charité Universitätsmedizin Berlin
Occupational Medicine
Berlin, Germany

Ivy Ekem, MB ChB, FWACP
Professor of Haematology
School of Medical Sciences
University of Cape Coast
Cape Coast, Ghana

Nadia El-Dib, PhD
Professor of Parasitology
Head of the Permanent Scientific Committee of Parasitology
    in Egyptian Universities
Department of Medical Parasitology
Faculty of Medicine
Cairo, Egypt

Viravong Douangnoulak, MD
Head, Department of Otorhinolaryngology
Mahosot Hospital
Vientiane, Laos PDR

Facundo M. Fernández, PhD
Associate Professor
School of Chemistry and Biochemistry
Georgia Institute of Technology
Atlanta, GA, USA

Arthur M. Friedlander, MD
Senior Scientist
Headquarters
U.S. Army Medical Research Institute of Infectious Diseases
    (USAMRIID)
Frederick, MD, USA;
Adjunct Professor of Medicine
School of Medicine
Uniformed Services University of the Health Sciences
Bethesda, MD, USA

Cristina Goens, MD, MScIH
Consultant in Internal Medicine
Medical School Academic
Department of Internal Medicine
Pontificia Universidad Católica de Chile
Santiago, Chile;
Consultant in Internal Medicine
Internal Medicine
Hospital La Florida
Santiago, Chile

Eduardo H. Gotuzzo, MD, FACP, FIDSA
Emeritus Professor
Instituto de Medicina Tropical Alexander von Humboldt
Universidad Peruana Cayetano Heredia
Lima, Peru;
Profesor Adscrito
Enfermedades Infecciosas y Tropicales
Hospital Nacional Cayetano Heredia
Lima, Peru

Michael D. Green, PhD
Research Chemist
Division of Parasitic Diseases and Malaria
US Centers for Disease Control and Prevention
Atlanta, GA, USA

Anthony D. Harries, MD, FRCP
Senior Advisor
Centre, for Operational Research
International Union Against TB and Lung Disease
Paris, France;
Honorary Professor
Infectious Diseases and Tropical Medicine
London, School of Hygiene and Tropical Medicine
London, UK

William P. Howlett, MB, DTM&H, FRCPI, PhD
Professor
Internal Medicine
Kilimanjaro Christian Medical Centre, Moshi
Kilimanjaro, Tanzania

Ralf Ignatius, MD
Prof. Dr.
Department of Microbiology
MVZ Laboratory
Berlin, Germany

Saythong Inthalad, MD
Luang Nam Tha Provincial Health Department
Luang Nam Tha Province
Lao PDR

Kentaro Ishida, MD, DTMH, FJSOG
Vice Director
Obstetrics and Gynecology
Nishijima Clinic
Fujimino, Saitama, Japan

Frederique Jacquerioz, MD
Physician
Division of Tropical and Humanitarian Medicine
HUG
Geneva, Switzerland

Benjamin Jeffs, FRCP
Medical Consultant
Acute Medicine
Bristol Royal Infirmary
Bristol, UK;
Physician
Médecins Sans Frontières
London, UK

Johannes Jochum, MD
Department of Medicine
University Medical Center
Hamburg-Eppendorf
Hamburg, Germany

Nick Jones, MBBS
Addenbrooke's Hospital
Department of Infectious Diseases
Cambridge University Hospitals NHS Foundation Trust
Cambridge, UK

Sabine Jordan, MD
Clinical Lecturer
I. Medical Clinic, Division of Tropical Medicine and
    Infectious Diseases
University Medical Center Hamburg-Eppendorf
Hamburg, Germany
Clinical Lecturer
Clinical Research Department
Bernhard Nocht Institute for Tropical Medicine
Hamburg, Germany

Gagandeep Kang, MD, PhD, FRCPath
Professor
Division of Gastrointestinal Sciences
Christian Medical College
Vellore, Tamil Nadu, India

Juri Katchanov, MD
Physician
Department of Internal Medicine
Klinikum Rechts der Isar
Munich, Germany

Valy Keoluangkhot, MD, MSc
Chief of Adult Infectious and Tropical Diseases Center
Senior Clinical Research
Mahosot Hospital;
Ministry of Health
Vientiane, Lao PDR;
Clinical Coordinator
Institut Francophone pour la Medicine Tropicale
Vientiane, Lao PDR

Guido Kluxen, Professor Dr. med.
Senior Clinical Research Fellow
Ophthalmological Regional Community Consulting and
    Clinic Wermelskirchen–Solingen–Remscheid
Wermelskirchen, Germany

Yoon Kong, MD, PhD
Professor
Molecular Parasitology
Sungkyunkwan University School of Medicine
Suwon, Gyeonggi-do, Republic of Korea

Esther Kuenzli, MD, MSc, DTM&H
Physician
Medical Department
Swiss Tropical and Public Health Institute
Basel, Switzerland

Saba M. Lambert, MBChB, Dip Trop Med, PhD
Clinical Research Fellow
Infectious and Tropical Diseases
London, School of Hygiene and Tropical Medicine
London, UK

Vatthanaphone Latthaphasavang, MD
Senior Clinical Research Fellow
Adult Infectious Disease Ward
Mahosot Hospital
Vientiane, Lao PDR

Alejandro Llanos-Cuentas, MD, MSc, PhD
Full Professor
School of Public Health
Universidad Peruana Cayetano Heredia
Lima, Peru

Pedro Legua, MD, MScCTM
Professor
Department of Medicine
Universidad Peruana Cayetano Heredia
Lima, Peru;
Attending Physician
Departamento de Enfermedades Infecciosas,
    Tropicales y Dermatológicas
Hospital Cayetano Heredia
Lima, Peru

Michael Libman, MD
Professor of Medicine
McGill University
Montreal, Quebec, Canada

**Elizabeth M. Molyneux, DSc Hc, FRCPCH,
    FRCEM, FRCP**
Honorary Professor of Paediatrics
Paediatric and Child Health
College of Medicine
Blantyre, Malawi

David C.W. Mabey, DM, FRCP
Professor of Communicable Diseases
Infectious and Tropical Diseases
London, School of Hygiene and Tropical Medicine
London, UK

Maria S. Mackroth, MD
I. Medical Clinic, Division of Tropical Medicine and
    Infectious Diseases
University Medical Center Hamburg-Eppendorf
Hamburg, Germany

Ciro Maguiña, MD
Principal Professor of Medicine
Instituto de Medicina Tropical Alexander von Humboldt
Universidad Peruana Cayetano Heredia
Lima, Peru

Reeta S. Mani, MD
Additional Professor
Neurovirology
National Institute of Mental Health and Neurosciences
    (NIMHANS)
Bangalore, India

Michael Marks, MRCP, PhD, DTM&H
Assistant Professor
Clinical Research Department
London, School of Hygiene and Tropical Medicine
London, UK

Dalila Martínez, MD, MSPH
Infectious Disease Physician
Departamento de Enfermedades Infecciosas,
    Tropicales y Dermatológicas
Hospital Cayetano Heredia
Lima, Peru;
Research Professor
Facultad de Medicina Alberto Hurtado
Universidad Peruana Cayetano Heredia
Lima, Peru
Associate Researcher
Instituto de Medicina Tropical Alexander von Humboldt
Universidad Peruana Cayetano Heredia
Lima, Peru

Haruhiko Maruyama, MD
Professor
Department of Infectious Diseases
University of Miyazaki
Faculty of Medicine
Miyazaki, Japan

Alice Mathuram, MBBS, MD, DTM&H
Professor
Department of Medicine
Christian Medical College
Vellore, India

Kohsuke Matsui, MD
Assistant Professor
Department of Infectious Diseases
Nagasaki University Hospital
Nagasaki City, Nagasaki, Japan

Mayfong Mayxay, MD, PhD
Associate Professor
Institute of Research and Education Development
University of Health Sciences, Vientiane
Lao PDR;
Head of Field Research
LOMWRU
Mahosot Hospital, Vientiane
Lao PDR

James McCarthy, FRACP
Professor of Tropical Medicine and Infectious Diseases
Infectious Diseases Program
QIMR Berghofer Medical Research Institute and
Department of Infectious Diseases
Royal Brisbane and Women's Hospital
Brisbane, QLD, Australia

Oriol Mitià, MD, PhD
Assistant Professor
Neglected Tropical Diseases
Barcelona, Institute for Global Health
Barcelona, Spain

Robert F. Miller, MBBS, FRCP
Professor
Institute for Global Health
University College London
London, UK

Israel Molina, MD, PhD
Head
Tropical Medicine and International Health
Vall d'Hebron University Hospital
Barcelona, Spain

Andreas J. Morguet, MD, PhD
Senior Cardiology Attending and Lecturer
Department of Cardiology
Campus Benjamin Franklin
Charité University Medicine Berlin
Berlin, Germany

Hiroyuki Nakase, MD
Department of Neurosurgery
Nara Medical University
Kashihara
Nara, Japan

Yukifumi Nawa, MD, PhD
Invited Professor
Tropical Diseases Research Center
Khon Kaen University, Khon Kaen
Muan Khon KLaen, Thailand;
Emeritus Professor
Infectious Diseases
University of Miyazaki
Miyazaki, Japan

Andreas Neumayr, MD, DTM&H, MCTM
Chief Medical Officer
Department of Medicine
Swiss Tropical and Public Health Institute
Basel, Switzerland

Paul N. Newton, BMBCh, DPhil, MRCP, DTMH&H
Professor
Lao-Oxford-Mahosot Hospital-Wellcome Research Unit
Mahosot Hospital, Vientiane
Lao PDR;
Professor
Centre for Tropical Medicine and Global Health
University of Oxford
Oxford, UK;
Professor
Infectious Diseases Data Observatory
University of Oxford
Oxford, UK

Thi Thuy Ngan Nguyen, MD
Clinician
Department of Tropical Diseases
Cho Ray Hospital
Ho Chi Minh, Vietnam;
PhD student
CNS/HIV group
Oxford University Clinical Research Unit
Ho Chi Minh, Vietnam

Caoimhe Nic Fhogartaigh, MRCP, FRCPath, MSc, DTMH
Consultant in Infectious Disease and Microbiology
Division of Infection
Barts Health
London, UK

Fumihiko Nishimura, MD, PhD
Department of Neurosurgery
Nara Medical University
Kashihara
Nara, Japan

Buachan Norindr, MD
Deputy, Department of Otorhinolaryngology
Mahosot Hospital
Vientiane, Lao PDR

Yukiteru Ouji
Department of Pathogen, Infection and Immunity
Nara Medical University
Kashihara
Nara, Japan

Gregor Pollach, Prof, Dr.
Professor of Anaesthesia and Intensive Care
University of Malawi
Blantyre, Malawi

Douglas G. Postels, MD, MS
Associate Professor
Pediatric Neurology
Children's National Medical Center
Washington, DC, USA;
Associate Professor
Pediatric Neurology
George Washington University
Washington, DC, USA

Ranjan Premaratna, MD
Professor in Medicine
Medicine
Faculty of Medicine, University of Kelaniya
Ragama, Sri Lanka

Sayaphet Rattanavong, MD
Research Clinician
Microbiology Laboratory
Mahosot Hospital, Vientiane Capital
Vientiane Capital
Lao PDR

Koert Ritmeijer, PhD, MPH, MSc
Coordinator Neglected Tropical Diseases
Medical Department
Médecins Sans Frontières
Amsterdam, The Netherlands

Hillary K. Rono, MB ChB, MMed (Ophthalmol), FEACO, MSc
Ophthalmologist
Kitale, District Hospital
Ministry of Health
Kirale, Kenya

Karen Roodnat, MD, MSc
Medical Doctor in Tropical Medicine and International
    Health
Rotterdam, The Netherlands;
Medical Doctor in Tropical Medicine and International
    Health
Médecins Sans Frontières
Amsterdam, Netherlands

Camilla Rothe, MD, DTM&H
Head of Clinical Tropical Medicine
Division of Infectious Diseases and Tropical Medicine
LMU University Hospital
Munich, Germany

Priscilla Rupali, MD, DTMH, FRCP
Professor
Infectious Diseases
Christian Medical College
Vellore, Tamil Nadu, India

Prakasit Sa-ngaimwibool
Department of Pathology
Faculty of Medicine
Khon Kaen University
Thailand

Thomas Schneider, Univ. Prof., PhD, MD
Head of Infectious Diseases
Charité – Universitätsmedizin Berlin
Berlin, Germany

Markus Schulze Schwering, Dr. med., FEBO
Dr. med.
Ophthalmology
University Eye Hospital
Tübingen, Germany

Carlos Seas, MD, MSc
Associate Professor
Department of Medicine
Universidad Peruana Cayetano Heredia
Lima, Peru;
Vice Director
Instituto de Medicina Tropical Alexander von Humboldt
Lima, Peru;
Attending Physician
Infectious and Tropical Medicine
Hospital Nacional Cayetano Heredia
Lima, Peru

Fredericka Sey, MB ChB
Principal Medical Officer
Sickle Cell Clinic
Ghana Institute of Clinical Genetics
Korle Bu
Accra, Ghana

Omar Siddiqi, MD, MPH
Assistant Professor
Neurology
Beth Israel Deaconess Medical Center
Boston, MA, USA;
Visiting Lecturer in Medicine
University of Zambia School of Medicine
Lusaka, Zambia

Eberhard Siebert, MD
Neuroradiologist
Department of Neuroradiology
Charité – Universitätsmedizin Berlin
Berlin, Germany

Siho Sisouphonh, MD
Senior Infectious Disease Clinician
Adult Infectious Disease Ward
Mahosot Hospital
Vientiane, Lao PDR

Günther Slesak, Dr. Med., DTM&H, MScIH
Dr
Tropical Medicine
Tropenklinik Paul-Lechler-Krankenhaus
Tübingen, Germany

Chris Smith, MBBCh, PhD
Professor
Clinical Medicine
Tropical Medicine and Global Health
Nagasaki University
Nagasaki-shi, Japan

Peter Sothmann, MD, DTM&H
Dr.
Division of Infectious Diseases and Tropical Medicine
LMU University Hospital
Munich, Germany

Douangdao Soukaloun
Lao-Oxford-Mahosot Hospital-Wellcome Trust Research
    Unit (LOMWRU), Microbiology
Laboratory, Mahosot Hospital, Vientiane, Lao PDR and
Paediatric Ward, Mahosot Hospital, Vientiane, Lao PDR

M. Leila Srour, MD, MPH, DTM&H
Pediatrician
Department of Pediatrics
Health Frontiers, Vientiane
Lao PDR

Cornelia Staehelin, MD, DTM&H, MIH
Physician
Department of Infectious Diseases
Inselspital, Bern University Hospital
Bern, Switzerland

Hartmut Stocker, MD
Head
St. Joseph Krankenhaus
Department of Infectious Diseases
Berlin, Germany

Marija Stojkovic, DTMH
Associate professor
Department of Infectious Diseases
Clinical Tropical Medicine
Heidelberg, Germany

Kensuke Takahashi, MD
Assistant Professor
Department of Infectious Diseases
Nagasaki University Hospital
Nagasaki City, Nagasaki, Japan

Hiroko Takamatsu
Takamatsu Hiroko Dermatology Clinic
Fukuoka, Japan

E. Tannich
Professor
Bernhard Nocht Institute for Tropical Medicine (BNITM)
Hamburg
Germany

Masaki Tomita, MD
Associate Professor
Department of Surgery II
University of Miyazaki
Miyasaki, Japan

Joep J. van Oosterhout, MD, PhD
Professor
Department of Medicine
University of Malawi College of Medicine
Blantyre, Malawi

Kristien Verdonck, MD, PhD
Research Fellow
Department of Public Health
Institute of Tropical Medicine
Antwerp, Belgium

Moritz Vogel, Dr. med.
Consultant Dr
Department of Pediatrics
Klinikum Mutterhaus
Trier, Rhineland-Palatine, Germany

Stephen L. Walker, MBChB, PhD, MRCP (UK), DTM&H
Consultant Dermatologist and Associate Professor
Department of Clinical Research
Faculty of Infectious and Tropical Diseases
London, School of Hygiene and Tropical Medicine
London, UK

Emma C. Wall, PhD
Clinical Lecturer
Infection and Immunity
University College London
London, UK

Thomas Weitzel, MD, DTM&P
Full Professor
Travel Medicine Program
Clínica Alemana
Universidad del Desarrollo
Santiago, Chile

Christopher J.M. Whitty, FRCP
Professor
Hospital for Tropical Diseases
University College London Hospitals
London, UK

Yohannes W. Woldeamanuel, MD
Physician Scientist
Neurology
Stanford University School of Medicine
Stanford, CA, USA;
Founder and Consultant
Advanced Clinical and Research Center
Addis Ababa, Ethiopia;
Founder and CEO
Propria Health Solutions
CA, USA

Mary E. Wright, MD, MPH
Medical Officer
Division of Clinical Research
National Institute of Allergy and Infectious Diseases
National Institutes of Health
Bethesda, MD, USA

Sophie Yacoub, BM, MRCP, MSc, PhD, DTM&H
Physician
Centre for Tropical Medicine
Oxford University Clinical Research Unit
Ho Chi Minh City, Vietnam

Masahide Yoshikawa, MD
Professor
Department of Pathogen, Infection and Immunity
Nara Medical University
Nara, Japan

Acknowledgements

I would like to thank the whole editorial team at Elsevier for their encouragement to go for the second edition of this book, for their tremendous support and patience. In particular I would like to thank content strategist Lotta Kryhl, content development specialist Louise Cook, and Andrew Riley as project manager.

I am very grateful to all authors who come from 6 different continents, for their great enthusiasm and uncomplicated cooperation. I am particularly obliged to all patients, whose cases are presented in this book, and some of whom sadly did not survive the diseases discussed.

Special thanks go out to Anthony D. Harries who's own wonderful case book, alas now out of print, inspired me to compile this current book. I am particularly happy that Tony is one of the contributors of this book. I would like to thank David Lalloo for bringing me into contact with Elsevier. I am also very grateful and honoured that Peter Hotez volunteered to write a very special foreword to this book.

1

A 20-Year-Old Woman from Sudan With Fever, Haemorrhage and Shock

DANIEL G. BAUSCH

Clinical Presentation

History

A 20-year-old housewife presents to a hospital in northern Uganda with a 2-day history of fever, severe asthenia, chest and abdominal pain, nausea, vomiting, diarrhoea and slight non-productive cough. The patient is a Sudanese refugee living in a camp in the region. She denies any contact with sick people.

Clinical Findings

The patient is prostrate and semiconscious on admission. Vital signs: temperature 39.6°C, (103.3°F) blood pressure 90/60 mmHg, pulse 90 bpm, and respiratory rate 24 cycles per minute. Physical examination revealed abdominal tenderness, especially in the right upper quadrant, hepatosplenomegaly and bleeding from the gums. The lungs were clear. No rash or lymphadenopathy was noted.

Questions

1. Is the patient's history and clinical presentation consistent with a haemorrhagic fever (HF) syndrome?
2. What degree of nursing precautions need to be implemented?

Discussion

This patient was seen during an outbreak of Ebola virus disease in northern Uganda, so the diagnosis was strongly suspected. She was admitted to the isolation ward that had been established as part of the international outbreak response. No clinical laboratory data were available because, for biosafety reasons, such testing was suspended. Although it is a reasonable precaution, the suspension of routine testing often causes difficulty in ruling out the many other febrile syndromes in the differential diagnosis and increases mortality from other non-Ebola disease. Fortunately, many clinical laboratory tests can now be safely performed with point-of-care

instruments, often brought into a specialized laboratory in the isolation ward, as long as the laboratory personnel are properly trained and equipped.

Answer to Question 1

Is the Patient's History and Clinical Presentation Consistent with an HF Syndrome?

The clinical presentation is indeed one of classic viral HF. However, most times the diagnosis is not so easy. Although some patients, such as this one, do progress to the classic syndrome with haemorrhage, multiple organ dysfunction syndrome and shock, haemorrhage is not invariably seen (and may even be noted in only a minority of cases with some virus species), and severe and fatal disease may still occur in its absence. The clinical presentation of viral HF is often very non-specific. Furthermore, haemorrhage may be seen in numerous other syndromes, such as complicated malaria, typhoid fever, bacterial gastroenteritis and leptospirosis, which are the primary differential diagnoses, depending on the region.

Answer to Question 2

What Degree of Nursing Precautions Needs to be Implemented?

The spread of Ebola virus between humans is through direct contact with blood or bodily fluids. Secondary attack rates are generally 15% to 20% during outbreaks in Africa, and much lower if proper universal precautions are maintained. Specialized viral HF precautions and personal protective equipment are warranted when there is a confirmed case or high index of suspicion, such as in this case.

The Case Continued. . .

Intravenous fluids, broad-spectrum antibiotics and analgesics were begun on admission. Nevertheless, the patient's condition rapidly worsened, with subconjunctival haemorrhage, copious bleeding from the mouth, nose and rectum

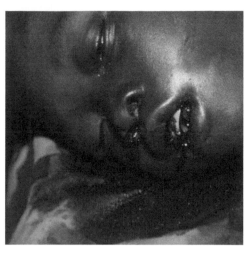

• **Fig. 1.1** Oral bleeding in Ebola virus disease. (Bausch, D.G., 2008. Viral hemorrhagic fevers. In: Schlossberg, D. (Ed.), Clinical Infectious Disease. Cambridge University Press, New York. Used with permission. Photo by Bausch, D.)

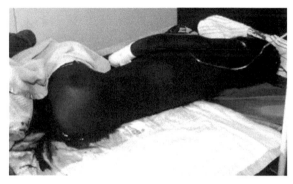

• **Fig. 1.2** Rectal bleeding in Ebola virus disease. (Bausch, D.G., 2008. Viral hemorrhagic fevers. In: Schlossberg, D. (Ed.), Clinical Infectious Disease. Cambridge University Press, New York. Used with permission. Photo by Bausch, D.)

(Figs. 1.1 and 1.2), dyspnoea and hypothermic shock (temperature 36.0°C, blood pressure = unreadable, pulse 150 bpm, respiratory rate 36 cycles per minute). She became comatose and died approximately 24 hours after admission. Laboratory testing at a specialized laboratory established as part of the outbreak response showed positive ELISA antigen and PCR tests for Ebola virus and a negative result for ELISA IgG antibody, confirming the diagnosis of Ebola virus disease.

SUMMARY BOX

Filoviral Diseases

Ebola and Marburg virus disease are the two syndromes caused by filoviruses. Microvascular instability with capillary leak and impaired haemostasis, often including disseminated intravascular coagulation, are the pathogenic hallmarks. There are four known pathogenic species of Ebola and one of Marburg virus, with relatively consistent case fatality associated with each species, ranging from 25% to 85%. Ebola and Marburg diseases are generally indistinguishable, both with non-specific presentations typically including fever, headache, asthenia, myalgias, abdominal pain, nausea, vomiting and diarrhoea. Conjunctival injection and subconjunctival haemorrhage are common. A fleeting maculopapular rash is occasionally seen. Typical laboratory findings include mild lymphopenia and thrombocytopenia, and elevated hepatic transaminases, with AST > ALT. Leucocytosis may be seen in late stages. The differential diagnosis is extremely broad, including almost all febrile diseases common in the tropics.

Ebola and Marburg virus diseases are endemic in sub-Saharan Africa, with Ebola virus typically found in tropical rainforests in the central and western parts of the continent and Marburg virus in the drier forest or savannah in the east. Evidence strongly implicates fruit bats as the filovirus reservoir, especially the Egyptian fruit bat *(Rousettus aegyptiacus)* as the reservoir for Marburg virus. Human infection likely occurs from inadvertent exposure to infected bat excreta or saliva. Male-to-female sexual transmission may occur months after infection because of the virus's persistence in the semen, although these events are relatively rare.

Miners, spelunkers, forestry workers and others with exposure in environments typically inhabited by bats are at risk, especially for Marburg virus disease. Non-human primates, especially gorillas and chimpanzees, and other wild animals may serve as intermediate hosts that transmit filoviruses to humans through contact with their blood and bodily fluids, usually associated with hunting and butchering. These wild animals are presumably also infected by exposure to bats and usually develop severe and fatal disease similar to human viral HF. Most outbreaks are thought to result from a single or very few human introductions from a zoonotic source followed by nosocomial amplification through person-to-person transmission in a setting of inadequate universal precautions, usually in rural areas of countries where civil unrest has decimated the healthcare infrastructure.

Because symptoms are generally non-specific and laboratory testing is not widely available, viral HF outbreaks are usually recognized only if a cluster of cases occurs, especially when healthcare workers are involved. Having been into caves or mines, and direct or indirect contact with wild animals or people with suspected viral HF, are key diagnostic clues, but these are not uniformly present. Outside consultation with experts in the field and testing of suspected cases should be rapidly undertaken and public health authorities must be alerted.

Contact tracing should be undertaken to identify all persons with direct unprotected exposure with the case patient, with surveillance of contacts for fever for 21 days (the maximum incubation period for Ebola and Marburg virus diseases). Any contact developing fever or showing other signs of viral HF should immediately be isolated and tested.

Treatment is supportive. Antimalarials and broad-spectrum antibiotics should be given until the diagnosis of viral HF is confirmed. Preliminary results from a clinical trial of experimental compounds conducted during an outbreak in the Democratic Republic of the Congo show very promising results, reducing case fatality to as low as 10% if treatment is administered early in the course of disease. Similarly, a clinical trial of an Ebola vaccine in the Democratic Republic of the Congo and during the massive 2013 to 2016 outbreak in West Africa showed protective efficacy of over 90%.

Further Reading

1. Blumberg L, Enria D, Bausch DG. Viral haemorrhagic fevers. In: Farrar J, editor. Manson's Tropical Diseases. 23rd ed. London: Elsevier; 2014 [chapter 16].
2. Vetter P, Fischer 2nd WA, Schibler M, et al. Ebola Virus Shedding and Transmission: Review of Current Evidence. J Infect Dis 2016;214(Suppl. 3):S177–84.

3. WHO. Interim Infection Prevention and Control Guidance for Care of Patients with Suspected or Confirmed Filovirus Haemorrhagic Fever in Health-Care Settings, with Focus on Ebola. Geneva: World Health Organization; 2014.

4. Lamontagne F, Fowler RA, Adhikari NK, et al. Evidence-based guidelines for supportive care of patients with Ebola virus disease. Lancet 2018;391(10121):700–8.

2

A 7-Year-Old Girl from Peru With a Chronic Skin Ulcer

DALILA MARTÍNEZ, KRISTIEN VERDONCK, MARLEEN BOELAERT AND ALEJANDRO LLANOS-CUENTAS

Clinical Presentation

History

A 7-year-old girl who lives in the Peruvian capital, Lima, is brought to a local clinic because of a chronic skin lesion on her nose. The lesion appeared 4 months ago as a small nodule and slowly turned into an ulcer. It is a bit itchy but not painful. There is no history of trauma. The girl is otherwise healthy. Six months ago, she travelled to a valley on the western slopes of the Andes.

Clinical Findings

The lesion is a localized ulcer on the nose (Fig. 2.1). The borders of the ulcer are indurated and there is a plaque-like infiltration of the surrounding skin. The whole lesion is about 2 cm in diameter. There are no palpable lymph nodes. She is afebrile and the rest of the physical examination is normal.

Questions

1. What are your differential diagnoses?
2. How would you approach this patient?

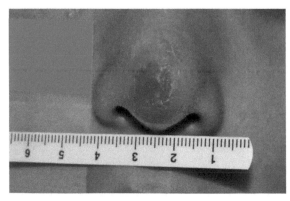

• **Fig. 2.1** Lesion at first consultation.

Discussion

A 7-year-old Peruvian girl presents with a painless ulcerative skin lesion on her nose, which has been present for the past 4 months. There are no systemic symptoms.

Answer to Question 1

What Are Your Differential Diagnoses?

Infectious diseases that can cause similar lesions in the face are cutaneous leishmaniasis, sporotrichosis, cutaneous tuberculosis and infection by *Balamuthia mandrillaris,* a free-living amoeba.

Although common bacterial infections of the skin that are partially treated or masked as a consequence of traditional remedies (e.g. chemical burns) are another possibility; this is less likely in our case given the chronic nature of the lesion. Cutaneous anthrax and tularaemia could be considered in the differential diagnosis of lesions located on the extremities, but the latter is endemic in the Northern hemisphere only, and the long duration without any further symptoms does not fit with either infection. In addtion, cutaneous anthrax tends to present with considerable localized oedema not seen in this case.

Cutaneous leishmaniasis is a common, vector-borne, parasitic disease that affects people living in or travelling to endemic areas. It typically begins as a small papule on air-exposed parts of the skin, progresses to a nodule or plaque and then turns into an ulcer with raised borders. The ulcer is painless unless there is bacterial superinfection. Patients may have several lesions.

Sporotrichosis is caused by *Sporothrix schenckii,* a dimorphic fungus that is found in soil and on plants. It enters the skin through direct inoculation (e.g. thorny plants or animal scratch). The disease usually starts with a papule that turns into a tender ulcer. Lesions can spread along draining lymphatic vessels. Sporotrichosis occurs throughout the world as a sporadic disease of farmers and gardeners. This disease is hyperendemic in parts of the Peruvian Andes, where it often affects children and typically produces facial lesions.

However, our patient did not travel to such a hyper-endemic place.

Cutaneous tuberculosis is an uncommon manifestation of tuberculosis. It occurs by direct inoculation of mycobacteria into the skin of non-sensitized individuals (e.g. children) or as a result of reactivation in persons with previous immunity against mycobacteria. As our patient lives in a poor neighbourhood with a high incidence of tuberculosis, we cannot rule out this diagnosis. Not only *Mycobacterium tuberculosis,* but also environmental mycobacteria, *Mycobacterium marinum* and *Mycobacterium leprae* can cause ulcerating skin lesions.

B. mandrillaris is a free-living amoeba that may cause a highly fatal disease. It usually starts as a painless plaque, often after local trauma. *Balamuthia* lesions are characterized by reddish or purplish infiltrations; ulceration is uncommon. The most frequent location of the initial lesion is the central face, over the nose. In a few months, it can progress to the brain causing granulomatous amoebic encephalitis. If this occurs, the survival time is usually less than 8 weeks.

The most likely diagnosis in our case is cutaneous leishmaniasis, because of the frequency of leishmaniasis in the valley our patient had travelled to and the characteristic presentation (localized painless ulcer with raised edges).

Answer to Question 2

How Would You Approach This Patient?

Gently clean the lesion with water, remove the scab and take a closer look at the process underneath. A definitive diagnosis of cutaneous leishmaniasis requires the demonstration of the parasite through microscopic examination, culture or molecular techniques.

The simplest approach is to scrape with a lancet under the edges of the lesion, and use the obtained material for a smear examination with Giemsa staining, looking for *Leishmania* amastigotes. The sensitivity of this technique is about 70%, decreasing as the duration of the lesion increases. The specificity is 100%.

Culture can be done on samples obtained by fine-needle aspiration or biopsy taken from the edge of a lesion. In reference centres, polymerase chain reaction (PCR) is used to confirm the presence of *Leishmania* and to identify the species.

The Montenegro or leishmanin skin test detects delayed immune response against *Leishmania* antigens and is sometimes used as a diagnostic aid. It can be negative in early stages of the disease and cannot distinguish current from past infection.

If leishmaniasis is ruled out, the following tests can be useful for the diagnosis of alternative causes of our patient's lesion: smear microscopy and culture in Sabouraud's medium (for sporotrichosis), a purified protein derivative (PPD) skin test (for tuberculosis) and, if necessary, a histopathological examination of a biopsy specimen.

The Case Continued…

The scab was removed revealing an ulcer with cobblestone-patterned bottom and raised edges, typical of cutaneous leishmaniasis. The microscopic examination of a sample obtained by scraping was negative. The leishmanin skin test was positive. PCR was also positive; and the infecting species was identified as *Leishmania (Viannia) peruviana.*

With a definitive diagnosis of cutaneous leishmaniasis, treatment was started with intravenous sodium stibogluconate (SSG, 20 mg/kg/day for 20 days) which is the first-line treatment of choice for cutaneous leishmaniasis caused by *L. (V.) braziliensis* or *L. (V.) peruviana* in Peru. In addition, the girl received topical imiquimod therapy, which was administered every other day for 20 days. Imiquimod, is an immune-modulating drug, which may be used as part of the therapy for facial lesions and relapses. The response after 20 days of treatment was good (see Fig. 2.2).

Treatment failure occurs in almost one quarter of patients after a first course of SSG monotherapy in Peruvian series, usually within 3 months. Follow-up is therefore recommended. Factors linked to treatment failure include young age and short stay in endemic area (as in this case) as well as recent onset of disease (≤5 weeks), multiple lesions, and *L. (V.) braziliensis* infection (not present in this case). At the third month of follow-up, our patient did not have any signs of relapse (Fig. 2.3).

The treatment of cutaneous leishmaniasis is challenging because SSG has a high failure rate and several side effects, including myalgia, arthralgia, loss of appetite, nausea, fever, increased levels of liver and pancreatic enzymes, reactivation of varicella zoster virus and cardiotoxicity, which can lead to

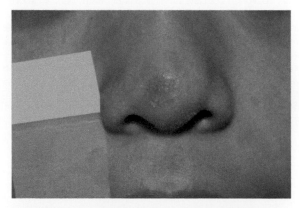

• **Fig. 2.2** Follow-up image after 20 days of treatment.

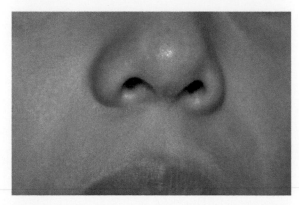

• **Fig. 2.3** Follow-up image of the scar 3 months after the end of treatment.

prolongation of QT-segment, severe arrhythmias and death. Information about the safety of this drug in children is limited. It is also unclear from the literature if there are safe and effective alternatives to SSG in children with *L. (V.) peruviana* infection. This is particularly relevant because, in endemic areas, cutaneous leishmaniasis often affects children.

SUMMARY BOX

Cutaneous Leishmaniasis

Cutaneous leishmaniasis (CL) is caused by protozoa of the genus *Leishmania*. Some 20 *Leishmania* species are associated with human disease. CL can be anthroponotic or zoonotic (reservoir: small mammals). The parasite is transmitted by sand flies of the genus *Lutzomyia* (New World) and *Phlebotomus* (Old World). Of the estimated 1.5 million annual cases, 90% occur in Afghanistan, Pakistan, Iran, Syria, Saudi Arabia, Algeria, Brazil, Colombia and Peru.

The incubation period between sand fly bite and appearance of skin lesions ranges from weeks to months. Clinical manifestations depend on characteristics of the parasite and the host immune response. Localized cutaneous leishmaniasis is the most common form. Some species of the *Leishmania Viannia*-complex can produce mucosal lesions resulting in disfiguring disease.

The lesions can heal spontaneously; this is more common in Old World (>50%) than in New World leishmaniasis (<20%). The aim of treatment is to accelerate healing, reduce scarring and decrease the risk of metastasis and recurrence. Topical therapy is recommended for Old World CL and for New World CL caused by species not belonging to the *Leishmania Viannia*-complex. This topical approach consists of intralesional pentavalent antimony, paromomycin cream and/or cryo- or thermotherapy. Systemic therapy is indicated for CL caused by species of the *Leishmania (Viannia)*-complex, which may lead to disfiguring mucocutaneous leishmaniasis. In addition, systemic treatment should be given when lesions are extensive or when topical treatment fails. Pentavalent antimonials are the first-line systemic treatment of choice for all New World forms except *L. guyanensis,* for which pentamidine is recommended. Miltefosine and azoles are alternatives.

Amphotericin B deoxycholate and liposomal amphotericin B are second-line drugs.

Further Reading

1. Boelaert M, Sundar S. Leishmaniasis. In: Farrar J, editor. Manson's Tropical Diseases. 23rd ed. London: Elsevier; 2013 [chapter 47].
2. Leishmaniasis, Epidemiological situation. World Health Organization; [cited 18 November 2019]. Available from: https://www.who.int/leishmaniasis/burden/en/.
3. Llanos-Cuentas A, Tulliano G, Araujo-Castillo R, et al. Clinical and parasite species risk factors for pentavalent antimonial treatment failure in cutaneous leishmaniasis in Peru. Clin Infect Dis 2008;46(2):223–31.
4. Reveiz L, Maia-Elkhoury AN, Nicholls RS, et al. Interventions for American cutaneous and mucocutaneous leishmaniasis: a systematic review update. PLoS One 2013;8(4):e61843.
5. Uribe-Restrepo A, Cossio A, Desai MM, Dávalos D, Castro MDM. Interventions to treat cutaneous leishmaniasis in children: a systematic review. PLoS Negl Trop Dis 2018;12:e0006986.

3

A 26-Year-Old Woman from Malawi with Headache, Confusion and Unilateral Ptosis

JURI KATCHANOV

Clinical Presentation

History

A 26-year-old Malawian woman is brought to the emergency department of a local central hospital by two relatives. She has been unwell for at least 1 week. She complained of a headache of insidious onset and has been confused for 2 days. One day before presentation the relatives ('guardians') noticed an eyelid drooping on the left side.

The guardians say her past medical history is unremarkable. The patient lives in an urban high-density area. She works as a businesswoman, selling vegetables. She has three healthy children, but another four of her children have died as toddlers. Her husband died a year ago of 'high fever.'

Clinical Findings

On examination she looks seriously unwell. Glasgow Coma Scale 14/15, temperature 38.4°C (101.1°F), blood pressure 115/75 mmHg, heart rate 86 bpm, respiratory rate 18 breath cycles per minute. There is no neck stiffness. The chest is clear. Figure 3.1 shows the examination of her eyes. The remainder of her neurological examination is normal.

Laboratory Results

Her blood results are shown in Table 3.1. A lumbar puncture is done. The opening pressure is markedly raised, at 32 cmH$_2$O (12–20 cmH$_2$O). The available CSF results are shown in Table 3.2.

Questions

1. What is the clinical syndrome and what is the differential diagnosis?
2. How would you manage this patient?

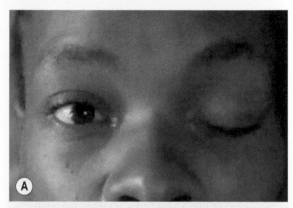

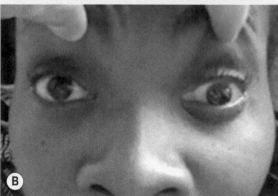

• **Fig. 3.1** (A) There is complete ptosis on the left. (B) On primary gaze, the left eye is in a 'down and out' position.

Discussion

A young Malawian widow presents with headache and confusion. She is febrile and has a unilateral third nerve palsy. The CSF examination reveals an inflammatory picture with low glucose.

TABLE 3.1 Blood Results on Admission

Parameter	Patient	Reference
WBC ($\times 10^9$/L)	3.2	4–10
Hb (g/dL)	10.2	12–14
Platelets ($\times 10^9$/L)	155	150–350
Serum glucose (mmol/L)	4.0	3.9–11.1
Thick film for malaria and trypanosomes	Negative	Negative

TABLE 3.2 CSF Results on Admission

Parameter	Patient	Reference
White cell count (/µL)	54	0–5
CSF protein (g/L)	3.0	0.25–0.55
CSF glucose (mmol/L)	1.3	2.0–2.64*

*½ to ⅔ of paired serum glucose sample.

Answer to Question 1

What Is the Clinical Syndrome and What Is the Differential Diagnosis?

The clinical syndrome is that of infectious meningitis. Infectious encephalitis should also be considered; however, the cranial nerve involvement makes this diagnosis less likely. Moreover, the main causes of infectious encephalitis are viral or – less commonly – protozoan (e.g. cerebral toxoplasmosis, human African trypanosomiasis), and the CSF findings of very high protein and very low glucose are not consistent with a viral or protozoan CNS infection. Cerebral malaria has to be considered in any patient with fever and impaired consciousness living in a malarious area. However, cerebral malaria would be an uncommonly severe manifestation in a most probably semi-immune adult residing in a holoendemic area. In addition, cranial nerve palsies are an unusual feature of cerebral malaria.

The differential diagnosis comprises bacterial, tuberculous and cryptococcal meningitis (Table 3.3). Neither the patient's clinical presentation nor her CSF results can help differentiate reliably between the three. Furthermore, onset, acuteness and duration of symptoms and signs may have to be interpreted with caution in many cultures, particularly when the history cannot be taken from the patients themselves.

Answer to Question 2

How Would You Manage This Patient?

The patient has a suspected CNS infection and is seriously ill with confusion, cranial nerve palsy and a high fever. Immediate action should be taken, and treatment should not be delayed whilst further test results are being awaited. Pragmatic treatment should cover bacterial, cryptococcal and tuberculous meningitis.

Gram-stain and bacterial culture should be done from the CSF. If available, an ultrasensitive PCR for *M. tuberculosis* (e.g. Xpert MTB/RIF Ultra) should be ordered. The sensitivity of Ziehl–Neelsen stain from the CSF is low in many settings. Cryptococcal antigen (CrAG) testing should be done from CSF and serum; additionally, India ink stain and fungal culture should be done for detection of *Cryptococcus neoformans*.

An HIV-serology study is crucial because cryptococcal meningitis is associated with immunosuppression. Tuberculous meningitis is also more common in HIV-positive than in uninfected persons.

The Case Continued. . .

The patient was started on ceftriaxone 2 g bid, fluconazole 1200 mg od (local protocol for cryptococcal meningitis in the absence of amphotericin B and flucytosin) and on treatment for presumptive TB-meningitis.

TABLE 3.3 Clinical and CSF Features of Acute Bacterial, Tuberculous and Cryptococcal Meningitis

	Bacterial Pathogen	Clinical Features	CSF Features
Acute Bacterial Meningitis	*Streptococcus pneumoniae, Neisseria meningitidis, Streptococcus suis* (Asia)	Often very rapid onset with high fever and meningism, cranial nerve involvement less common	Often cloudy, high leukocyte cell count, predominance of polymorphs, low glucose
Tuberculous Meningitis	*Mycobacterium tuberculosis*	Often a history of several days of illness, onset less abrupt, cranial nerve involvement common	Often clear, high CSF protein, low CSF glucose
Cryptococcal Meningitis	*Cryptococcus neoformans*	Often subacute onset, severe headache common, cranial nerve involvement common	CSF can be normal in at least 25% of cases

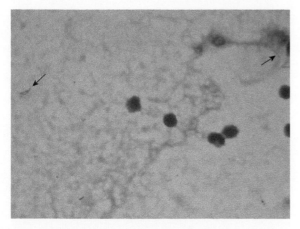

• **Fig. 3.2** Ziehl–Neelsen stain of CSF sample showing acid-fast bacilli *(arrows)*. (Courtesy Prof. Jeremy Day).

The HIV test came back reactive. India Ink stain, cryptococcal and bacterial culture were reported negative, but acid-fast bacilli were detected in the CSF (Fig. 3.2).

TABLE 3.4	The Four Pillars of Clinical Diagnosis of Tuberculous Meningitis
Clinical Criteria	Symptom duration >5 days Systemic symptoms suggestive of tuberculosis (one or more of the following): weight loss (or poor weight gain in children), night sweats, or persistent cough for more than 2 weeks History of close contact with an individual with pulmonary tuberculosis or a positive tuberculin skin test within the past year Focal neurological deficit Cranial nerve palsy Altered consciousness
CSF Criteria	Clear appearance Leukocytes: 10–500/μL Lymphocytic predominance (>50%) Protein concentration >1 g/L CSF to plasma-glucose ratio <50% or absolute CSF glucose concentration <2.2 mmol/L
Neuroimaging Criteria	Hydrocephalus Basal meningeal enhancement Tuberculoma Infarct Pre-contrast basal hyperdensity
Evidence of TB Elsewhere	Chest radiography suggestive of active TB Evidence for TB outside the CNS on CT, MRI or ultrasound AFB identified or *M. tuberculosis* cultured from another source (sputum, lymph node, gastric washing, urine, blood culture) Positive commercial *M. tuberculosis*-PCR from extraneural specimen

Footnote: Marais, S., Thwaites, G., Schoeman, J.F., et al., 2010. Tuberculous meningitis: a uniform case definition for use in clinical research. Lancet Infect Dis. 10, 803–812.

The diagnosis of tuberculous meningitis was established. A few days into treatment the patient slipped into a coma. An MRI scan of her brain revealed bilateral basal ganglia infarctions. She died in the hospital.

SUMMARY BOX

Tuberculous Meningitis

Tuberculous (TB) meningitis is the most dramatic form of tuberculosis. After the release of bacilli and granulomatous material into the subarachnoid space, a florid gelatinous exudate forms, which may impair CSF circulation and cause hydrocephalus, cranial nerve palsies and vasculitis. Vasculitis is the most serious complication of tuberculous meningitis and may lead to cerebrovascular accidents.

A definitive diagnosis of TB-meningitis is established when acid-fast bacilli are seen in the CSF or detected by a reliable molecular method such as PCR, or if *Mycobacterium tuberculosis* is cultured from the CSF. It is crucial to maintain a high index of suspicion in settings with high TB prevalence (Table 3.4). The WHO now recommends the use of Xpert MTB/RIF Ultra as the initial diagnostic test for suspected tuberculous meningitis. The Xpert is a cartridge-based fully automated PCR test that can easily be used, even in resource-limited settings.

TB-meningitis is an emergency. Treatment should be started without delay once the diagnosis is considered. The WHO recommends treatment with the same regimen as any form of tuberculosis starting with isoniazid, rifampicin, ethambutol and pyrazinamide. Usually, treatment is for 9 to 12 months. Corticosteroids seem to improve clinical outcomes and are currently recommended; however, their effects may vary in different clinical settings.

Further Reading

1. Thwaites G. Tuberculosis. In: Farrar J, editor. Manson's Tropical Diseases. 23rd ed. London: Elsevier; 2014 [chapter 40].
2. Bahr NC, Nuwagira E, Evans EE, et al. Diagnostic accuracy of Xpert MTB/RIF Ultra for tuberculous meningitis in HIV-infected adults: a prospective cohort study. Lancet Infect Dis 2018;18:68–75.
3. Marais S, Thwaites G, Schoeman JF, et al. Tuberculous meningitis: a uniform case definition for use in clinical research. Lancet Infect Dis 2010;10:803–12.
4. Thwaites G. Advances in the diagnosis and treatment of tuberculous meningitis. Curr Opin Neurol 2013;26:295–300.
5. Davis A, Mentjes G, Wilkinson RJ. Treatment of Tuberculous Meningitis and Its Complications in Adults. Curr Treat Options Neurol 2018;20:5–15.

A 4-Year-Old Girl from Uganda in a Coma

DOUGLAS G. POSTELS

Clinical Presentation

History

It is the rainy season in rural eastern Uganda. A 4-year-old girl, previously healthy, is carried into the Accident and Emergency (A&E) Department. Her father reports that she was well until yesterday. She had a bad headache in the early afternoon but later in the evening developed shaking chills. Believing this was yet another episode of malaria, a common problem in their village, the family planned to take her to the health centre in the morning. The child slept restlessly. At 5 a.m. today the family woke to find the girl was in the midst of a seizure, which lasted about ten minutes. It has taken 4 hours for the family to reach A&E and the little girl has not awoken. The child has not had any recent head trauma and the family knows of no other reason that the child might be ill.

Clinical Findings

Her temperature is 38.7°C (101.7°F), pulse 150 bpm, respiratory rate 36 breath cycles per minute and blood pressure 98/40 mmHg. She has no neck stiffness or jaundice. Capillary refill is normal. There is nasal flaring with respirations. Blantyre Coma Scale is 1/5. Pupils are 2 mm and reactive, and extraocular movements are normal by oculocephalic manoeuvres. She has no papilloedema on direct ophthalmoscopy. With stimulation there is decerebrate posturing that resolves spontaneously. On cardiac examination she has a gallop rhythm. Her liver is palpable 2 cm below the right costal margin and her spleen is 4 cm below the left costal margin. A rapid test for glucose is normal.

Laboratory Results

Laboratory results are given in Table 4.1.

Questions

1. What is the differential diagnosis?
2. What additional work-up should be performed?

TABLE 4.1 Laboratory Results on Admission

Parameter	Patient	Reference Range
Haematocrit (%)	17.6	≥30
Platelet count ×10⁹/L)	28	150–450
Malaria RDT	Positive	Negative

Discussion

A 4-year-old Ugandan girl is brought to the hospital unconscious with no neurological localizing signs, a supple neck, hepatosplenomegaly and a positive malaria rapid diagnostic test. Early laboratory testing reveals anaemia and thrombocytopenia.

Answer to Question 1
What Is the Differential Diagnosis?

The most important underlying aetiologies of coma to consider are cerebral malaria, acute bacterial meningitis, viral encephalitis and intoxication (particularly organophosphates). Metabolic abnormalities (hypoglycaemia, or renal or hepatic failure) and non-convulsive *status epilepticus* may be primary causes of coma or complicate these infectious and toxic aetiologies. Although there is no neck stiffness, she is deeply comatose, making this clinical finding less reliable; the absence of neck stiffness should not lower the clinician's suspicion of meningitis. Rapid testing shows that hypoglycaemia is not the cause of the child's abnormal mental status and it has been 4 hours since her last clinical seizure, making a post-ictal state unlikely.

The World Health Organization (WHO) defines cerebral malaria as an 'otherwise unexplained coma in a patient with malaria parasitaemia'. This clinical diagnosis is, however, non-specific because of high rates of asymptomatic parasitaemia in those geographical areas where malaria is most common and the abundance of differential diagnoses.

People living in an area of high malaria transmission (such as rural Uganda in the rainy season) may be frequently bitten by malaria-infected female anopheline mosquitoes. Initially, this produces clinical illness (either uncomplicated or complicated malaria); but with repeated infectious challenges, a state of asymptomatic parasitaemia may be attained. Therefore in African children in a coma, a positive malaria rapid diagnostic test (RDT) does not rule out an underlying non-malarial aetiology of acute illness. In parasitaemic African children in a coma, direct or indirect ophthalmoscopy may be useful in differentiating malarial from non-malarial aetiologies of coma (see Summary Box).

Answer to Question 2

What Additional Work-Up Should Be Performed?

Although the child has a positive malaria RDT, a lumbar puncture should be performed to rule out bacterial meningitis. If available, an electroencephalogram (EEG) may be useful to rule out non-convulsive status epilepticus as either a primary coma aetiology or a contributor to illness. More sophisticated laboratory evaluations (creatinine, electrolytes, bilirubin) may be useful but are seldom available in the geographical contexts where malaria is most prevalent.

An ophthalmoscopic examination to evaluate for malarial retinopathy may be helpful. The presence of one or more retinal findings (retinal whitening, haemorrhages or orange-white vessels with or without papilloedema) would lend support to a malarial aetiology of acute illness (Fig. 4.1). Children with retinopathy-negative cerebral malaria may be more likely to have a non-malarial aetiology for their coma. As both retinopathy-negative and retinopathy-positive cerebral malaria may be complicated by bacteraemia, bacterial meningitis, seizures and/or metabolic abnormalities,

a complete work-up for non-malarial coma aetiologies (including non-convulsive status epilepticus) is indicated in all patients presenting with WHO clinically defined cerebral malaria.

The Case Continued. . .

A lumbar puncture was performed. The CSF was clear and acellular; opening pressure was normal. Blood cultures were taken, and mydriatic drops instilled to perform ophthalmoscopy. This revealed white-centred haemorrhages in both eyes. A diagnosis of retinopathy-positive cerebral malaria was made.

After administration of artesunate 2.4 mg/kg IV in A&E, the child was admitted to the high-dependency section of the hospital's paediatric unit for frequent monitoring of vital signs and serum glucose. Artesunate was repeated at 12 and 24 hours and then once daily. An EEG showed diffuse slowing but no epileptiform activity. Twelve hours after admission the child had one short (1 minute) generalized seizure that spontaneously resolved and did not recur. Forty hours after admission her Blantyre Coma Score was 4/5. The child was discharged home on hospital day five, with a follow-up appointment in the neurology clinic scheduled after 4 weeks.

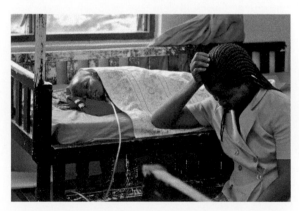

• **Fig. 4.2** Infant with cerebral malaria hospitalized at Queen Elizabeth Central Hospital, Blantyre, Malawi (Courtesy Mr James Peck).

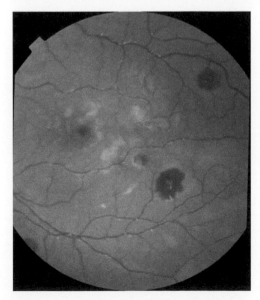

• **Fig. 4.1** White-centred haemorrhages and retinal whitening, both features of malaria retinopathy (Courtesy Dr Nicholas Beare).

SUMMARY BOX

Cerebral Malaria and Malarial Retinopathy

Cerebral malaria is defined as an otherwise unexplained coma in a patient with *Plasmodium falciparum* parasitaemia. Malaria kills almost 450 000 people per year, the vast majority of them children younger than 6 years old living in sub-Saharan Africa. Many of these children have cerebral malaria (Fig. 4.2).

In African children with parasitaemia in a coma, direct or indirect ophthalmoscopy may be useful in differentiating malarial from non-malarial aetiologies of coma. In autopsy studies, identification of malarial retinopathy during life was 95% sensitive and

100% specific for the post-mortem identification of sequestered parasitized erythrocytes in cerebral vasculature. Sequestered parasitized erythrocytes in the CNS are a pathological hallmark of cerebral malaria and likely indicate that acute malarial infection was responsible for the patient's illness and death. In these autopsy studies, children who fulfilled WHO clinical criteria for cerebral malaria but lacked malarial retinopathy (i.e. they had retinopathy-negative cerebral malaria) had other non-malarial aetiologies of death on autopsy, including systemic infections (pneumonia) and Reye syndrome. In contrast, an epidemiological modelling study in children with retinopathy-negative cerebral malaria showed that the attributable fraction of disease as a result of malaria infection itself is at least 85%. The proportion of children with retinopathy-negative (cerebral) malaria who have non-malarial etiologies of coma remains unknown.

The mainstay of therapy is antimalarials, intensive supportive care and diagnosis and treatment of non-malarial infectious and non-infectious contributors to illness. Even in specialized centres, the case fatality rate for cerebral malaria is 15% to 25%. One-third of survivors are left with neurological sequelae, including epilepsy, cognitive impairment, attention problems and behavioural disorders.

Further Reading

1. White NJ. Malaria. In: Farrar J, editor. Manson's Tropical Diseases. 23rd ed. London: Elsevier; 2013 [chapter 43].
2. MacCormick IJ, Beare NA, Taylor TE, et al. Cerebral malaria in children: using the retina to study the brain. Brain 2014;137(8): 2119–42.
3. Taylor TE, Fu WJ, Carr RA, et al. Differentiating the pathologies of cerebral malaria by postmortem parasite counts. Nat Med 2004; 10(2):143–5.
4. Small DS, Taylor TE, Postels DG, et al. Evidence from a natural experiment that malaria parasitemia is pathogenic in retinopathy-negative cerebral malaria. Elife 2017;6:e23699.
5. Taylor TE, Molyneux ME. The pathogenesis of pediatric cerebral malaria: eye exams, autopsies, and neuroimaging. Ann N Y Acad Sci 2015;1342:44–52.

5

A 4-Year-Old Boy from Laos With a Lesion of the Lip and Cheek

M. LEILA SROUR

Case Presentation

History

You are sent a picture of a 4-year-old boy taken by a visitor at a remote district hospital in Laos (Fig. 5.1). You receive a limited history and physical examination: Three days ago, the family noticed a dark sore on the child's cheek. The child's breath smells bad, he is not eating and he appears listless. The lesion progressed quickly from a sore to eat through the child's cheek. The child, who is unimmunized, had a fever and rash about 2 months ago and recovered. The family is very poor. The local doctors do not recognize this disease.

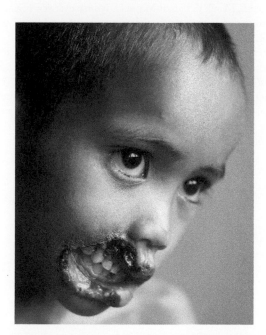

• **Fig. 5.1** A 4-year-old Lao boy with a necrotizing lesion on the right cheek.

Clinical Findings

The 4-year-old child appears small and quiet. He is stunted and thin. His mouth has a gangrenous lesion that has destroyed part of his upper and lower lips and cheek, exposing his teeth.

Questions

1. What is your differential diagnosis?
2. What should you recommend to help this child?

Discussion

This chronically malnourished child, living in a remote village of a poor developing country, has a rapidly advancing gangrenous lesion of the face.

Answer to Question 1
What Is Your Differential Diagnosis?

A few days earlier, when the child had a sore on the face and bad breath, you may have suspected a tooth abscess and cellulitis. The rapid destruction of tissue is typical of noma, an opportunistic infection that affects poor children whose immune systems are compromised by malnutrition and often other infections, commonly measles or malaria. Other ulcerating facial lesions such as oral cancer, syphilis and yaws are unlikely in a young child. Cutaneous leishmaniasis is unlikely to develop at such a rapid pace and be so destructive. Mucocutaneous leishmaniasis may lead to severe tissue destruction but it is non-endemic in Laos. There are no diagnostic laboratory tests because the diagnosis is made clinically.

Answer to Question 2

What Should You Recommend to Help This Child?

You recommend treating the child with penicillin and metronidazole to cover the suspected aerobic and anaerobic oropharyngeal bacteria. You emphasize the need for nutritional support, which can be challenging with a mouth lesion. Local foods, including eggs, milk, soy products and peanuts, can be liquefied and fed orally or enterally. Other diseases such as malaria, intestinal parasites, tuberculosis and vitamin deficiencies should be looked for and treated. Necrotic tissue can be removed. Physiotherapy will be needed to prevent contractures with healing. Reconstructive surgery should not be attempted for at least 1 year and be done only by an experienced surgical team. Improved nutrition before surgery may improve the outcome.

Survivors of noma suffer from disfigurement and functional problems with speech and eating. They may present as young adults seeking help. Their history reveals the illness as a child of younger than 10 years of age.

The Case Continued. . .

The child was treated successfully with antibiotics and nutritional support. His face healed with contractures, resulting in disfigurement and salivary incontinence. At age 9 years, he was referred for surgery by a visiting international surgical team. After two surgeries, his appearance was improved, and the salivary incontinence corrected (Fig. 5.2).

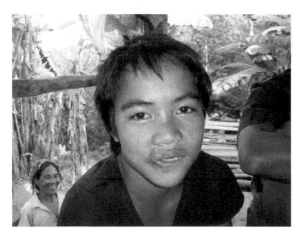

• **Fig. 5.2** At age 9 after two surgeries correcting facial contractures and salivary incontinence.

SUMMARY BOX

Noma

Noma is an opportunistic infection, primarily affecting children aged 1 to 7 years, whose immunity is compromised by malnutrition and vitamin deficiencies. Risk factors include extreme poverty, malnutrition, poor oral hygiene, viral infections (especially measles and HIV), poor sanitation and living in close proximity to livestock. The true aetiology of noma is unknown. The pathogenesis appears to be a complex combination of factors, including poverty, poor oral hygiene facilitating necrotizing ulcerative gingivitis, malnutrition and infectious diseases such as malaria and measles leading to impaired immunity.

Noma is a neglected and forgotten disease, because it primarily affects the poorest children living in remote areas of developing countries. Health workers throughout the world often do not recognize this disease, so it remains underreported and unknown. Case fatality rate if untreated is 70% to 90%. Treatment with antibiotics and nutritional support can prevent disease progression and save the child's life. Survivors suffer with disfigurement, functional impairment and psychosocial isolation.

Noma is an indicator of extreme poverty and inadequate public health systems. The elimination of extreme poverty, provision of prenatal care, promotion of exclusive breastfeeding, immunizations, food security and improved nutrition for the poorest children can lead to the eradication of this preventable childhood disease.

Further Reading

1. Srour L, Wong V, Wyllie S. Noma, actinomycosis and nocardia. In: Farrar J, editor. Manson's Tropical Diseases. 23rd ed. London: Elsevier; 2013 [chapter 29].
2. Srour L, Marck K, Baratti-Mayer D. Noma: overview of a neglected disease and human rights violation. Am J Trop Med Hyg 2017; 96(2):268–74.
3. WHO Regional Office for Africa. Information brochure for early detection and management of noma. 2016; http://www.who.int/iris/handle/10665/254579.
4. Bolivar I, Whiteson K, Stadelmann B, et al. Bacterial diversity in oral samples of children in Niger with acute noma, acute necrotizing gingivitis, and healthy controls. PLoS Negl Trop Dis 2012;6(3): e1556.

6

A 36-Year-Old Male Traveller Returning from Botswana With a Creeping Eruption

EMMA C. WALL

Clinical Presentation

History

A 36-year-old male restaurant owner presents to a travel clinic in Europe with a mobile itchy mass under his skin. Three weeks ago, he noted the mass in his groin for 4 days after which it subsided. He then noted an itchy, serpiginous rash tracking from his groin to his chest, which moved over the course of several days and then disappeared; he then noted the mass reappearing on his right shoulder, at which point he was referred for assessment. There is no history of fever or systemic illness.

Five weeks ago, he returned from a fishing holiday with four friends to the Okavango Delta in Botswana. He took malaria chemoprophylaxis, slept on the boat under a mosquito net and swam in fresh river water. He ate freshwater fish from the river.

He is married and denies sexual contact on the trip. Of the four friends who accompanied him, two also have the same complaint.

Clinical Findings

The patient is afebrile and organ system examination is normal. On his right upper deltoid is a firm mass with clear margins 3 × 8 cm in size. On further questioning this mass has recently migrated across his upper chest wall, and a serpiginous tract is visible (Fig. 6.1). There is no additional rash and no lymphadenopathy.

Laboratory Results

Total white cell count 8.9 ×10^9/L (reference range: 4–10), eosinophil count 0.9 × 10^9/L (<0.5), liver function tests, creatinine and electrolytes are normal. HIV antibodies are negative.

Questions

1. What is the likely diagnosis and what are your differentials?
2. What is the risk of this condition if untreated?

Discussion

A 36-year-old European presents because of a mobile migratory mass he has been noticing for the past 3 weeks. Five weeks ago, he returned from a fishing trip to the Okavango Delta. Two of his travel companions have the same symptoms. Full blood count shows eosinophilia.

Answer to Question 1

What Is the Likely Diagnosis and What Are Your Differentials?

This patient is systemically well, with a mobile itchy mass. The eosinophilia suggests a parasitic cause. The fact that

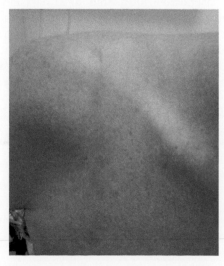

• **Fig. 6.1** Itchy serpiginous rash tracking up the right shoulder.

two of his travel companions are experiencing similar symptoms indicates a common exposure factor.

The presentation is classic for gnathostomiasis, even though his travel history appears uncommon. Gnathostomiasis is endemic in South-East Asia and Latin America, but only a few cases have been reported in Africa. It is a food-borne zoonotic nematode infection that classically presents with a mobile subcutaneous mass, intermittent creeping eruptions and eosinophilia. The infection is acquired by eating raw fish and other food items.

Intermittent migratory swellings are also typically seen in patients with *Loa loa* infection (calabar swelling), but *Loa loa* is not endemic in the Okavango Delta and the minimum incubation time is 5 months.

A very rare cause of migratory swellings and eosinophilia is sparganosis. It is caused by larvae ('spargana') of canine and feline tapeworms of the genus *Spirometra* and acquired by drinking water containing infected copepods or by eating raw or undercooked intermediate hosts such as amphibians or reptiles. It mainly occurs in East and South-East Asia, but cases have also been reported in East Africa.

Several other infections acquired in the tropics can be migratory and are associated with an itchy track-like rash. Such creeping eruptions are commonly caused by larvae of animal hookworms or *Strongyloides stercoralis* but these present with fine, serpiginous tracks and not with a large mobile mass, as seen in this patient. Very rare causes of creeping eruption are ectopic fascioliasis and migratory myiasis.

Answer to Question 2

What is the Risk of This Condition If Untreated?

Deaths from gnathostomiasis have occurred when the parasite has entered the brain or spinal cord, causing severe neurological sequelae.

The Case Continued. . .

The patient admitted that on their trip they had made sushi from fresh fish caught in the river. A clinical diagnosis of cutaneous gnathostomiasis was made and the patient was started on albendazole 400 mg bid for 21 days and ivermectin 200 µg/kg stat. Serology for *Gnathostoma* was negative. Over the next 6 days, the serpiginous lesion migrated over his shoulder and neck, disappeared for 24 hours, then reappeared between his eyebrows, moved to his forehead and face (Fig. 6.2), and then was felt inside his nose. On the sixth day

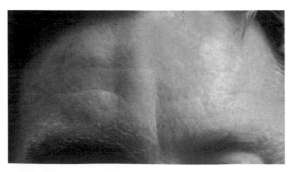

• **Fig. 6.2** A picture taken after treatment of the mass tracking down the patient's forehead.

of treatment he expressed a larva from his nostril, which was identified as *Gnathostoma spinigerum*. His two friends were also seen at the same institution and were given similar treatment with full resolution of their symptoms.

SUMMARY BOX

Gnathostomiasis

Gnathostomiasis is mostly caused by *Gnathostoma spinigerum*, a zoonotic nematode. Humans are accidental hosts. Gnathostomiasis is endemic throughout areas where large amounts of raw or undercooked freshwater fish and crustaceans are consumed, most importantly in East and South-East Asia and Central and South America. Case reports are emerging from Southern Africa.

Adult worms infect the gastrointestinal tract of feline and canine species. When eggs excreted through the faeces get into water, first-stage larvae hatch, which then infect small freshwater crustaceans. A large variety of animals can act as a second intermediate host. Humans become infected by eating raw or undercooked meat of intermediate hosts, such as freshwater fish, crabs, shrimps, frogs, snakes, fowl and pork. Gnathostomiasis commonly occurs in outbreaks.

Larvae penetrate the human intestinal wall and wander around the body. Initial symptoms are non-specific and may include fever, malaise, vomiting and diarrhoea lasting for 2 to 3 weeks. This is accompanied by marked eosinophilia. Within 1 month cutaneous infection may develop, manifesting as non-pitting oedematous migratory swellings that may be pruritic or painful and mainly affect the trunk and the proximal limbs. Visceral disease occurs when the larvae migrate through the internal organs such as the lungs, gut, genitourinary tract, eye and CNS. CNS invasion may manifest as eosinophilic meningoencephalitis, subarachnoid haemorrhages, cranial neuritis or painful radiculomyelitis as a result of invasion of the spinal cord. Diagnosis is suggested by eosinophilia, migratory swellings and a history of geographical and food exposure. Gnathostomiasis is confirmed when demonstration of the parasite is made microscopically, radiologically or on positive serological examination up to 3 months after presentation. Lumbar puncture and cranial imaging may be necessary in suspected CNS disease. CSF is often xanthochromic and may show eosinophilia. Imaging may reveal larval tracks within the brain and cord parenchyma. Treatment consists of albendazole 400 mg bid for 21 days and/or ivermectin 200 µg/kg on two consecutive days. For CNS infection, adjunctive corticosteroids are considered beneficial.

Further Reading

1. Heckmann JE, Bhigjee AI. Tropical Neurology. In: Farrar J, editor. Manson's Tropical Diseases. 23rd ed. London: Elsevier; 2013 [chapter 71].
2. Vega Lopez F, Ritchie S. Dermatological Problems. In: Farrar J, editor. Manson's Tropical Diseases. 23rd ed. London: Elsevier; 2013 [chapter 68].
3. Checkley AM, Chiodini PL, Dockrell DHm, et al. Eosinophilia in returning travellers and migrants from the tropics: UK recommendations for investigation and initial management. J Infect 2010;60(1):1–20.
4. Neumayr A (ed). Antiparasitic treatment recommendations. 2nd Ed. Tredition: Hamburg. 2018 (cf: https://tredition.de/autoren/andreas-neumayr-16821/antiparasitic-treatment-recommendations-paperback-104637/).

7

A 28-Year-Old Male Fisherman from Malawi With Shortness of Breath

CAMILLA ROTHE

Clinical Presentation

History

A 28-year-old Malawian man presents to a local hospital with progressive shortness of breath over the past 5 days. He reports orthopnoea and paroxysmal nocturnal dyspnoea. He has also developed bilateral flank pain in the past days, which is continuous and dull, and there is constant nausea. There is no cough and no fever.

He was diagnosed with arterial hypertension 2 years earlier and prescribed antihypertensive drugs, which he never took. No investigations were done at that time.

His medical history and family history are otherwise unremarkable. A recent HIV test was negative. The patient is a fisherman from a town on the southern shore of Lake Malawi.

Clinical Findings

The 28-year-old man is not looking chronically ill, but is in respiratory distress. His conjunctivae are notably pale. His blood pressure is 200/130 mmHg, pulse 66 bpm, temperature 36.8°C and respiratory rate 32 breath cycles per minute.

His apex beat is slightly displaced, but his heart sounds are clear and regular. The jugular venous pressure is not raised. There are bilateral fine crackles over the lung bases. The abdomen is flat and non-tender. There is bilateral renal angle tenderness, and the kidneys are ballottable. There is no peripheral oedema.

Laboratory Results

His laboratory results on admission are shown in Table 7.1.

Imaging

His chest radiograph on admission is shown in Figure 7.1.

TABLE 7.1	Laboratory Results on Admission		
Parameter		**Patient**	**Reference Range**
WBC (×10⁹/L)		3.8	4–10
Haemoglobin (mg/dL)		6.0	13–15
MCV (fL)		92	80–99
Platelets (×10⁹/L)		187	150–400
Creatinine (µmol/L)		1200	<120
BUN (mmol/L)		89.3	<17.9
K⁺ (mmol/l)		7.2	3.5–5.2

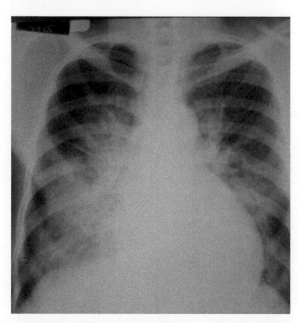

• **Fig. 7.1** Chest radiograph on admission.

Questions

1. What is your clinical impression?
2. What further investigations would you do to establish the diagnosis?

Discussion

A young Malawian fisherman presents with signs and symptoms of left ventricular heart failure, hypertension and anaemia. There is renal angle tenderness, and his kidneys appear enlarged. His creatinine is very high and he is hyperkalaemic.

Answer to Question 1

What Is Your Clinical Impression?

This young man presents with combined left-sided cardiac failure and renal failure. He was diagnosed with hypertension 2 years prior. It is unclear if his renal incompetence is a cause or the result of his raised blood pressure.

The reason for the enlargement of his kidneys could either be primary (e.g. polycystic kidneys) or secondary as a result of post-renal obstruction with hydronephrosis. In renal compromise secondary to hypertension, one would expect the kidneys to be small.

Being a fisherman, the patient has been in regular contact with *Schistosoma haematobium*–infested water in Lake Malawi. Chronic schistosomiasis with hydronephrosis is one of the top differential diagnoses to suspect.

Answer to Question 2

What Further Investigations Would You Like to Perform to Establish the Diagnosis?

The most useful investigation at this point is an ultrasound of the kidneys to differentiate between, primary renal pathological condition and a post-renal problem. If there was hydronephrosis, obstruction at the level of the bladder seems most likely because both kidneys appear enlarged.

On cystoscopy, endoscopists can macroscopically establish the diagnosis, but ideally, biopsies should be performed to look for evidence of granulomatous inflammation and *S. haematobium* ova in the tissue and to rule out neoplasia. In chronic infection, urine microscopy may be negative for ova of *S. haematobium*.

The Case Continued. . .

Despite high doses of furosemide, the patient remained oliguric. Glucose and insulin were administered for his hyperkalaemia.

Ultrasound showed bilateral hydronephrosis with massive dilatation of the renal pelvis and calyces. The remaining renal parenchyma was very thin in both kidneys.

Cystoscopy revealed a hyperaemic mucosa with multiple 'sandy patches' suggestive of granulomatous lesions in the mucosa. No tumour was seen. An endoscopic diagnosis of urogenital schistosomiasis was made. Histology was not available.

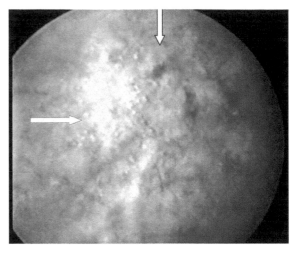

• **Fig. 7.2** Cystoscopy findings of a patient with urogenital schistosomiasis. The white arrows show 'sandy patches' (*left*) and hyperaemia of the bladder mucosa (*top*). (Courtesy Iran Mendonça da Silva.)

The next day the patient deteriorated. He became drowsy and vomited repeatedly. He got progressively bradycardic, and there was a new pericardial friction rub suggestive of uraemic pericarditis.

He was taken to theatre and a bilateral percutaneous nephrostomy was done. The patient was transferred to the intensive care unit and peritoneal dialysis (PD) was started (haemodialysis was not available).

The patient improved rapidly, vomiting and drowsiness ceased and his friction rub disappeared. He was discharged home on PD.

Two months later he was readmitted with fever and abdominal pain. He was treated for suspected bacterial peritonitis but sadly died 3 weeks later still in the hospital.

SUMMARY BOX

Genitourinary Schistosomiasis

Genitourinary schistosomiasis caused by *Schistosoma haematobium* is endemic in large parts of Africa and in the Middle East. Schistosomiasis is one of the most common tropical diseases in migrants from endemic countries and should actively be screened for.

About 50% of *Schistosoma* eggs are shed through urine, the other half remain trapped in the tissue causing granulomatous inflammation. Around 10% of people infected progress to chronic late-stage disease. Risk factors for disease progression are poorly understood and include intensity and duration of infection, host genetic factors and parasite strain differences.

Chronic infection leads to granulomatous inflammation of bladder wall and ureteral mucosa resulting in obstructive uropathy, hydronephrosis, recurrent bacterial pyelonephritis and end-stage renal disease. It is also suspected to contribute to the development of squamous cell carcinoma of the bladder. The pathological changes can long go unnoticed.

Egg deposition in the female genital tract may result in dyspareunia, chronic lower abdominal pain, ectopic pregnancy and infertility and has also been associated with an increased risk of HIV infection. Men may present with scrotal swelling, orchitis and prostatitis, haematospermia and oligospermia.

In advanced stages of schistosomiasis, the proof of *Schistosoma* eggs in the urine is challenging because the adult flukes may have long died and egg production may have stopped. Biopsy is often unavailable and serology is unhelpful in an endemic setting, because it can only detect exposure without indicating the activity, duration or quantum of infection. A promising point-of-care diagnostic tool may be circulating anodic antigen (CAA), which is under development.

The investigation of choice is ultrasound. Hydronephrosis and bladder wall abnormalities can easily be demonstrated.

On cystoscopy a hyperaemic mucosa with 'sandy patches' may be seen (Fig. 7.2). Sandy patches are raised, yellowish mucosal irregularities associated with heavy egg deposition surrounded by fibrous tissue pathognomonic for schistosomiasis.

Praziquantel may reverse the early stages of infection but has little role to play in advanced hydronephrosis. It may still be given to kill remaining adult flukes. Otherwise, late-stage urogenital schistosomiasis has to be managed symptomatically, which can be challenging in settings where renal replacement therapy is not an option.

Further Reading

1. Bustinduy AL, King CH. Schistosomiasis. In: Farrar J, editor. Manson's Tropical Diseases. 23rd ed. London: Elsevier; 2013 [chapter 52].
2. Colley DG, Bustinduy AL, Secor WE, King CH. Human schistosomiasis. Lancet 2014;383:2253–64.
3. Poggensee G, Feldmeier H. Female genital schistosomiasis: facts and hypotheses. Acta Trop 2001;79(3):193–210.
4. Asundi A, Belavsky A, Liu XJ, et al. Prevalence of strongyloidiasis and schistosomiasis among migrants: a systematic review and meta-analysis. Lancet Glob Health 2019;7:e236–48.

8

A 26-Year-Old Female Traveller Returning from Ghana With a Boil on the Leg

CAMILLA ROTHE

Clinical Presentation

History

A 26-year-old German student presents to the clinic because of a localized swelling on her left leg. She has just-returned from a 6-week trip to Ghana.

The swelling has developed slowly over the past 3 weeks. It is itchy, but not painful. There is no history of fever; no history of arthropod bites. The patient is otherwise fine.

Clinical Findings

There is localized swelling on the left leg, about 1.5 cm in diameter (Fig. 8.1). The skin surrounding the swelling is slightly hyperaemic. The boil is covered by a blackish scab. There is no lymphadenopathy. The patient is afebrile while the rest of the physical examination is normal.

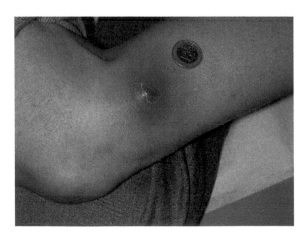

• **Fig. 8.1** Boil on the left leg covered with a dark scab. (Courtesy Dr Sebastian Dieckmann)

Questions

1. What are your most important differential diagnoses?
2. How would you approach this patient?

Discussion

A young traveller presents with a localized swelling on her leg after backpacking in Ghana. The swelling has been growing slowly and there are no systemic signs or symptoms.

Answer to Question 1

What Are Your Most Important Differential Diagnoses?

There is a localized swelling with a central scab. This lesion may look similar to an eschar seen in rickettsial disease or in cutaneous anthrax, yet the absence of systemic symptoms renders these differentials unlikely. The clinical presentation suggests a topical process.

Spider bites may cause lesions with an eschar-like central necrosis (e.g. the brown recluse spider); however, the slow growth of the lesion over several weeks makes this differential unlikely.

Localized bacterial skin and soft-tissue infections such as folliculitides, furuncles, carbuncles or abscesses are very common among backpacking travellers. A hot and humid tropical climate combined with low standards of hygiene favour bacterial and fungal skin infections. Itchy mosquito bites may serve as a portal of entry. Bacterial spread often occurs via scratching or contaminated items such as towels and shavers.

Another important differential diagnosis in this case is an infestation with fly maggots (myiasis). The slow growth of the boil, the absence of lymphadenopathy and systemic symptoms as well as the localized itch make myiasis the most likely differential diagnosis.

Answer to Question 2

How Would You Approach This Patient?

Gently remove the scab and take a closer look at the lesion using a magnifying glass.

The Case Continued...

The scab was removed and a whitish matter was detected underneath. Using a magnifying glass, one could see that the matter was not a pustular head but appeared to be pulsating and oozing transparent fluid. This appearance is typical of myiasis – the pulsating end of the larva seen contains the respiratory spiracles.

The lesion was covered with white petroleum jelly and bandaged. The patient returned 2 days later for review. The maggot of a Tumbu fly was easily removed with a pair of forceps. The remaining lesion looked clean and no further treatment was required.

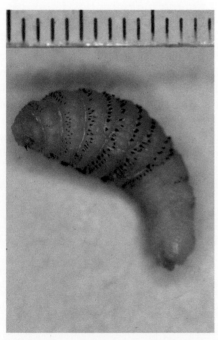

• **Fig. 8.2** Larva of a botfly (*Dermatobia hominis*). (Courtesy Dr Sebastian Dieckmann)

In sub-Saharan Africa, myiasis is usually caused by the larvae of *Cordylobia anthropophaga,* also known as Tumbu fly, Mango fly or Putzi fly. Adult female flies deposit their eggs on sandy ground or on damp laundry spread out on the ground or hung on a clothesline to dry. Normal hosts are dogs and rodents. Humans become infected when lying on the ground or wearing contaminated clothes without prior hot ironing. Larvae hatch and burrow into the skin. Over the following 2 to 3 weeks the developing larvae cause an itchy and at times painful 'blind boil.' Lesions are usually sterile because of bacteriostatic substances produced in the larvae's guts.

Treatment aims to deprive the larvae of oxygen, which prompts them to extrude from the skin. This can be achieved by applying white petroleum jelly or liquid paraffin on the lesion to block their respiratory spiracles. Immature larvae are best left to develop for a while because they are difficult to retrieve, and maceration of the larva can lead to inflammation and superinfection. Even untreated, cutaneous myiasis is self-limiting because the mature larva has to leave the host and pupate elsewhere.

In Central and South America, myiasis is caused by *Dermatobia hominis,* the human botfly (Fig. 8.2). Unlike the Tumbu fly, this species lays its eggs directly on exposed skin. Furthermore, it deposits its ova on blood-sucking insects such as mosquitoes, flies or ticks, which afterwards convey them to the human host, a technique called 'hitch-hiking.'

Removal of botfly larvae can be slightly challenging because of their shape, and the process may require local anaesthesia and cruciate incision.

Additional forms of myiasis exist whereby larvae may invade various body cavities such as nasal sinuses, ears, mouth, eye, vagina or anus (body cavity myiasis). Wounds can be infested as well.

Further Reading

1. Mumcuoglu KY. Other Ectoparasites: Leeches, Myiasis and Sand Fleas. In: Farrar J, editor. Manson's Tropical Diseases. 23rd ed. London: Elsevier; 2013 [chapter 60].
2. Solomon M, Lachish T, Schwartz E. Cutaneous myiasis. Curr Infect Dis Rep 2016;18(28):1–7.
3. Francesconi F, Lupi O. Myiasis. Clin Microbiol Rev 2012;25(1): 79–105.
4. Vasievich MP, Martinez Villarreal JD, Tomecki KJ. Got the travel bug? A review of common infections, infestations, bites and stings among returning travelers. Am J Clin Dermatol 2016;17: 451–62.

SUMMARY BOX

Myiasis

Myiasis is the infestation of live humans and vertebrate animals with larvae (maggots) of flies, which feed on the host's dead or living tissue, liquid body-substance or ingested food. It derives from the Greek word "myia" which means "fly." Cutaneous furuncular myiasis is one of the most common travel-associated skin disorders.

9

A 52-Year-Old Man from Vietnam With Evolving Shock

NICK JONES AND SOPHIE YACOUB

Clinical Presentation

History

A 52-year-old man is brought to an urban hospital in Ho Chi Minh City, Vietnam because of abdominal pain and vomiting. He describes 4 days of retro-orbital headache, lethargy, myalgia and fevers that had begun to improve over the last 24 hours. He has a history of type 2 diabetes mellitus and poorly controlled hypertension. His last travel outside the city was several years ago.

Examination findings

The patient is drowsy, but rousable. His Glasgow Coma Score (GCS) is 14/15, temperature 36.5°C, blood pressure 105/90 mmHg, heart rate 120 bpm, respiratory rate 28 breaths per minute and peripheral oxygen saturation 93% on air. He has a weak radial pulse, but normal heart sounds. Respiratory examination reveals a dull percussion note and reduced breath sounds at both lung bases. He has mild abdominal distension, with shifting dullness and a tender 3cm liver edge. Skin examination is unremarkable.

Laboratory results

See Table 9.1.

Questions

1. What are the main differential diagnoses to consider?
2. What are the priorities for management?

Discussion

The short duration of symptoms before presentation is suggestive of an acute infective process, and the relatively low CRP and absence of neutrophil leucocytosis make a viral aetiology likely. Clinical signs of shock are present: tachycardia, narrow pulse pressure (<20 mmHg), reduced GCS and raised serum lactate. The degree of thrombocytopenia and

presence of hepatic impairment are important markers of disease severity, and his raised haematocrit level is suggestive of haemoconcentration.

What are the main differential diagnoses to consider?

Having presented in a high-endemicity area, the clinical picture is typical of dengue infection with apparent progression to severe disease with vascular leak and compensated shock. Even without an eschar, rickettsial infections, such as scrub typhus, are the most important differential diagnoses. Malaria should also be considered, but there is no evidence of haemolysis to support this, and risk of malaria is very low in most urban areas of Vietnam. Many aspects of the presentation could be compatible with leptospirosis, but the absence of suspected rodent exposure makes this less likely.

TABLE 9.1	Laboratory Results on Admission	
Parameter	Patient	Reference Range
Haemoglobin (g/dL)	14.6	12.5–17.2
Haematocrit (%)	53.9	40–52
Platelets (×10^9/L)	58	160–370
WCC (×10^9/L)	2.1	3.6–10.5
Neutrophils (×10^9/L)	0.9	1.5–7.7
Lymphocytes (×10^9/L)	0.8	1.1–4.0
C-reactive protein (mg/L)	20	<4
Urea (mmol/L)	7.8	2.5–7.8
Creatinine (μmol/L)	114	62–115
Alanine aminotransferase (U/L)	812	7–40
Alkaline phosphatase (U/L)	260	30–130
Total bilirubin (μmol/L)	18	0–20
Lactate (mmol/L)	3.5	0.6–1.4

Another differential diagnosis to consider in a diabetic from South East Asia with possible sepsis is melioidosis.

What are the priorities for management?

With a diagnosis of severe dengue highly likely, supportive management of the patient's cardiovascular and respiratory systems should be prioritized. This involves careful fluid resuscitation, with thorough and frequent assessment for evidence of fluid overload. Ultrasound scans should be undertaken to ascertain the extent of pleural effusions and ascites; and if available, an echocardiogram could be considered to assess myocardial contractility and intravascular volume.

The case continued...

The patient is diagnosed with compensated shock and is admitted to a high-dependency unit for close observation and supportive care. Ultrasound scans confirm the presence of moderate bilateral pleural effusions and ascites, as well as mild hepatomegaly and a thickened gallbladder wall. He is infused with Ringer's lactate solution at a volume of 10mL/kg over 1 hour before his fluid status is reassessed. He remains tachycardic and oliguric with a haematocrit rise to 55.1%, therefore the rate of fluid therapy is increased to 15mL/kg/hr until sufficient haemodynamic improvement is shown. The rate of fluid delivery is subsequently reduced to 7mL/kg/hr for 2 hours and by a further 2mL/kg/hr every 2 hours until no longer required. Repeat clinical assessments are undertaken at two-hourly intervals throughout, with haematocrit checks every 6 hours. The patient is discharged from hospital 3 days later, after complete recovery. Reverse transcriptase PCR (RT-PCR) and a positive NS1 ELISA confirm dengue diagnosis.

progress to severe disease with organ impairment, bleeding, capillary leakage and distributive shock. Severe disease usually progresses through three phases: a febrile phase of 2 to 7 days' duration, characterized by high fever, headache, myalgia, thrombocytopenia and leukopenia; a critical phase with high risk of capillary leak, shock and occasionally bleeding at the point of defervescence; and a recovery phase, in which clinical improvement is accompanied by extravascular fluid resorption and organ recovery.

Dengue diagnosis is confirmed in the first 4 to 6 days of illness by detection of the NS1 antigen by RDTs or ELISA or detection of viral RNA using RT-PCR, after which the sensitivity of these methods declines because of the short viraemia in peripheral blood. Paired serology tests for IgM/IgG can also be performed, (at least 3 days apart) demonstrating seroconversion; however, cross-reaction with other flaviviruses remains a problem, especially in Zika endemic areas.

Warning signs for severe disease include abdominal pain or tenderness, persistent vomiting, fluid accumulation, mucosal bleeding, lethargy or restlessness, hepatomegaly, and increasing haematocrit with concurrent worsening of thrombocytopenia, six of which were present in this case. With no antiviral treatment available, cautious intravascular volume replacement and supportive treatment are the mainstays of management, accompanied by careful monitoring for signs of fluid overload. In many countries the epidemiology of dengue is changing in line with aging populations. Older patients often present with atypical features and have higher risk of complications and death as a result of difficulties in controlling haemodynamic status in the context of high-level comorbidity. Uncontrolled hypertension and diabetes, as in this case, have been shown to be risk factors for poor outcomes. Promising attempts at vaccine deployment have been thwarted by the fact that re-infection of immune-primed individuals is associated with greater risk of severe disease; therefore the searches for effective therapeutics and a pan-specific dengue vaccine continue.

SUMMARY BOX

Dengue

Dengue is the commonest arthropod-borne virus to infect humans, with an estimated annual incidence of 390 million infections worldwide. The virus is a member of the flavivirus family and has four closely related, but antigenically distinct serotypes. Transmission to humans is through *Aedes* mosquitoes; predominantly the daytime-biting *Aedes aegypti*. *Aedes albopictus* is a secondary vector in Asia, and its ability to survive temperate climates has allowed spread to many countries in Europe and North America. Although most clinically apparent infections result in a self-limiting febrile illness, a minority

Further reading

1. Yacoub S, Farra J. Dengue. In: Farrar J, editor. Manson's Tropical Diseases. 23rd ed. London: Elsevier; 2014 [chapter 15].
2. Bhatt S, Gething P, Brady O, et al. The global distribution and burden of dengue. Nature 2013;496(7446):504–7.
3. World Health Organisation. Dengue and severe dengue fact sheet. WHO.int. April 2019.
4. Lin R, Lee T, Leo Y. Dengue in the elderly: a review. Expert Rev Anti Infect Ther 2017;15(8) 729–5.
5. Diamond MS, Pierson TC. Molecular insight into Dengue virus pathogenesis and its implications for disease control. Cell 2015;162(3):488–2.

10

A 55-Year-Old Indigenous Woman from Australia With a Widespread Exfoliating Rash and Sepsis

BART J. CURRIE AND JAMES MCCARTHY

Clinical Presentation

History

You are working in a remote indigenous community in tropical northern Australia, and the community health worker asks you to visit a house to assess an elderly woman who has been living in the crowded back room. Her family are worried that she has become increasingly withdrawn and hasn't been getting out of the house much at all.

Clinical Findings

The patient is a 55-year-old indigenous Australian woman with a widespread exfoliative rash involving all limbs and especially the armpits, buttocks and thighs (Fig. 10.1). Many flakes of skin cover the mattress she is lying on. In addition, she has fissures over her wrists and knees. She also looks pale, is clammy and poorly responsive. Her temperature is 39.5°C (103.1°F), heart rate 110 bpm, respiratory rate 28 breath cycles per minute and blood pressure 85 mmHg systolic to radial pulsation. Oxygen saturation by pulse oximetry is 92% on room air.

Laboratory Results

You take blood cultures, full blood count, CRP and biochemistry. Samples are sent into the regional laboratory, with results expected the next day. You also take skin scrapings, which you can look at yourself using the community clinic microscope.

Questions

1. What is your provisional diagnosis?
2. What is your initial management?

Discussion

A 55-year-old indigenous Australian woman has a widespread exfoliating rash and is clearly systemically unwell with signs of sepsis.

Answer to Question 1

What is Your Provisional Diagnosis?

The exfoliating rash is classical for crusted scabies, which is uncommon but well recognized in remote indigenous communities where scabies remains endemic. Undiagnosed cases can be 'core transmitters' of scabies; and in this case many household members, and in particular the children, had multiple scabies lesions, some with secondary pyoderma. In addition, this woman has secondary sepsis which is likely to be from *Staphylococcus aureus* or *Streptococcus pyogenes* bacteraemia, with inoculation through her skin fissures. However, Gram-negative or polymicrobial sepsis is also occasionally seen in patients with crusted scabies.

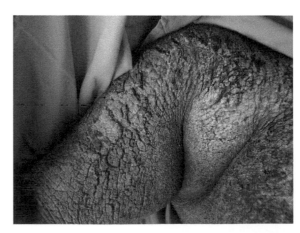

• **Fig. 10.1** Severe crusted scabies of the right axilla and chest wall.

Answer to Question 2

What is Your Initial Management?

She is transported to the community health centre where you put her on oxygen, insert a wide-bore cannula, take an additional set of blood cultures, give her 1 litre of normal saline over 30 minutes and commence her on intravenous (IV) ceftriaxone 2 g and gentamicin 320 mg (her weight is 62 kg).

The Case Continued...

After the IV fluids, her blood pressure rose to 95 mmHg systolic and her oxygen saturation was 97% with oxygen by nasal prongs. She was evacuated to the regional hospital. In the clinic, microscopy of her skin scrapings under low-power magnification confirmed the diagnosis, showing multiple scabies mites of varying maturity and multiple eggs. In the hospital, the patient was managed in a single room with enhanced contact precautions to prevent transmission of scabies to staff and visitors.

Treatment consisted of a five-dose course of ivermectin (200 µg/kg/dose) on days 0, 1, 7, 8 and 14, together with a topical scabicide (benzyl benzoate 25%) applied every second day for the first week; then twice weekly for the second week, with a keratolytic cream (lactic acid and urea in sorbolene cream) after bathing on the days the topical scabicide was not administered. Her blood cultures taken in the community grew *S. aureus* resistant to flucloxacillin and clindamycin, but sensitive to gentamicin, co-trimoxazole and doxycycline (i.e. community-acquired MRSA). She was therefore given 2 weeks of IV vancomycin. A transthoracic echocardiogram showed no features of endocarditis. Repeated blood cultures 48 hours after admission were negative, and by that stage she was afebrile, off oxygen and eating well. While she was in the hospital, all her family members were treated in the community with topical permethrin 5%, given as two doses 1 week apart, and the children with skin sores were each given a single dose of intramuscular benzathine penicillin, with excellent response.

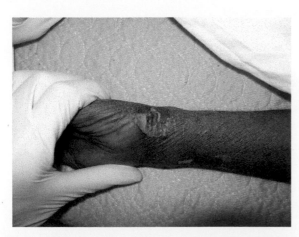

• Fig. 10.2 Fissure over the wrist with underlying less severe crusted scabies.

The household clothes, linen and furniture were put out in the sun for a day, and the rooms were treated with a commercial residual insecticide. The woman returned to the community after 3 weeks in the hospital, with her skin showing no residual hyperkeratosis or shedding. She and the family are followed up regularly by the health staff to allow early diagnosis and treatment should she again be infected with scabies.

SUMMARY BOX

Crusted Scabies

Although *Sarcoptes scabiei* infection and mite reproduction is usually self-limiting, hyperinfestation can develop in susceptible individuals. Crusted or Norwegian scabies was first described in patients with leprosy in Norway. Crusted scabies can occur after immunosuppressive therapy in transplantation, rheumatological conditions, chemotherapy for malignancy and in infection with HIV and HTLV-1. It can also occur in malnutrition, Down's syndrome and in the elderly and institutionalized, especially those with physical or cognitive disability who are unable to scratch. Patients with crusted scabies can have many thousands of mites in skin lesions and can serve as 'core transmitters' for continuing outbreaks of scabies in communities and nursing homes. Mites from crusted scabies cases are not genetically distinct, with ordinary scabies occurring in those infected from these cases.

Crusted scabies results from unfettered mite reproduction and host reaction, resulting in formation of hyperkeratotic skin crusts that may be loose and flaky or thick and adherent. Skin flakes with thousands of mites can be shed onto bed linen and floors. Although hands and feet are most commonly involved, the distribution is often extensive, including neck, face and scalp as well as axillae, trunk, buttocks and limbs, especially knees and elbows. Thick deposits of debris with mites accumulate beneath the nails, which are often thickened and dystrophic. Crusting can be limited to one or two limbs, hands or fingers. Unlike ordinary scabies, where itching is usually intense, the presence of itch is variable in crusted scabies. Fissuring and secondary bacterial infection are common (Fig. 10.2). A peripheral blood eosinophilia is common but not always present, and serum IgE levels are often extremely high. There is high mortality in crusted scabies cases from secondary bacterial sepsis, including with Gram-negative organisms such as *Pseudomonas aeruginosa* in addition to *S. pyogenes* and/or *S. aureus*.

The differential diagnoses of crusted scabies include psoriasis, extensive tinea corporis, skin malignancies such as the T-cell lymphomas mycosis fungoides and the Sézary syndrome, nutritional deficiencies such as pellagra, pemphigus, kava dermopathy, onchocerciasis, lepromatous leprosy and secondary syphilis.

Further Reading

1. Currie BJ, McCarthy JS. Scabies. In: Farrar J, editor. Manson's Tropical Diseases. 23rd ed. London: Elsevier; 2013 [chapter 58].
2. Currie BJ, McCarthy JS. Permethrin and ivermectin for scabies. N Engl J Med 2010;362(8):717–25.
3. Roberts LJ, Huffam SE, Walton SF, et al. Crusted scabies: clinical and immunological findings in seventy-eight patients and a review of the literature. J Infect 2005;50(5):375–81.

11

A 45-Year-Old Male Security Guard from Malawi With Difficulties in Walking and Back Pain

JURI KATCHANOV

Clinical Presentation

History

A 45-year-old security guard from Malawi is admitted to a local tertiary hospital because of back pain and progressive difficulty in walking.

His troubles started 1 year earlier with back pain and he presented to a local health centre. He was given paracetamol and sent home. The pain did not improve. Over the following weeks he also developed difficulty in walking and 'pins and needles' sensation in his legs.

Three months after the first visit he presented again to the same health centre. His temperature was slightly elevated (37.5°C, 99.5°F). He was given antimalarials, a single dose of praziquantel and paracetamol. He consulted a local traditional healer who applied tattoos to his chest and his back (Fig. 11.1A). Over the following 6 months his condition further deteriorated and he finally became bedridden.

The patient denies fever, night sweats and weight loss, and there is no chronic cough. There is neither haematuria nor diarrhoea and he is continent for stool and urine. There is no history of trauma or past tuberculosis (TB). He has never been tested for HIV.

He is a non-smoker, but drinks two paper cartons (about one litre) of Chibuku, a locally brewed beer, per day. He is married with three children, who are all well. He resides in an urban area and used to work as a security guard but has been unemployed for the last 6 months because of his illness.

Clinical Findings

He looks well and is afebrile with normal vital signs. There is tenderness over the lower thoracic spine and severe spasticity of both legs (Fig. 11.1B). The power in his legs is 1/5 (visible muscle flicker). Deep tendon reflexes of the lower limbs are exaggerated. The plantar reflexes are upgoing. There is a sensory level for pain and temperature sensation between T9 and T11, with diminished joint sense in his big toes bilaterally. The examination of his cranial nerves and the upper limbs is normal.

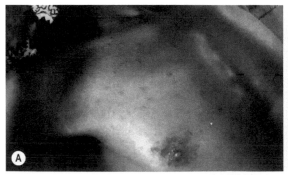
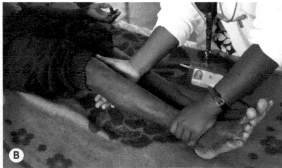

• **Fig. 11.1** Physical examination of a Malawian patient with back pain and difficulties walking. (A) Tattoos from a traditional healer on the chest of the patient. (B) Severe spasticity and contractures of both lower limbs.

Laboratory Results

His Full blood count results are normal.

Questions

1. What is the neuroanatomical syndrome and what is your differential diagnosis?
2. What further management should be carried out?

Discussion

A 45-year-old Malawian man presents with chronic back pain and slowly progressive spastic paraparesis. On examination there is tenderness over the lower thoracic spine and a thoracic sensory level. He denies any constitutional symptoms. His past medical history is unremarkable. His HIV status is unknown.

Answer to Question 1

What is the Neuroanatomical Syndrome and What is Your Differential Diagnosis?

The clinical signs – spastic paraparesis with hyperreflexia, upgoing plantar reflexes and thoracic sensory level – localize the lesion to the spinal cord. The bladder is usually involved in spinal cord disease, but the absence of bladder symptoms does not rule out spinal cord involvement, particularly in slowly progressive lesions, as in our case.

Spinal cord disease can be traumatic or non-traumatic. Nothing in the patient's history suggests trauma. Non-traumatic spinal cord disease can be compressive or non-compressive. Compressive disease is sometimes amenable to spinal surgery.

Common causes of adult non-traumatic compressive spinal cord disease in sub-Saharan Africa are spinal TB ('Pott's disease'), spinal metastases and degenerative spinal disease including slipped disc. Common causes of non-compressive spinal cord disease are schistosomiasis, autoimmune transverse myelitis and HIV-associated vacuolar myelopathy.

Answer to Question 2

What is the Further Management?

The diagnosis of spinal cord disease in resource-limited settings is often clinical (Table 11.1). Management should focus on diagnosis and treatment of the underlying aetiology and on prevention and treatment of the complications of spinal cord disease. Diagnostic clues and possible treatment regimens are summarized in Table 11.2.

All patients should be tested for HIV, ova of *Schistosoma* spp. in urine and stool and evidence of TB or neoplasia on chest- and spinal radiography. If available, ultrasound examination of the abdomen is very valuable in tumour-screening and TB work-up. CSF should be examined, which is of particular importance in immunosuppressed patients.

Realistically, most patients admitted to hospital with paraplegia because of spinal cord disease will leave the

TABLE 11.1 Important Causes of Spinal Cord Disease in the Tropics and Their Typical Clinical Features

	Typical Onset and Course	Clinical Features
Spinal tuberculosis	Insidious onset, chronically progressive over weeks, with months of back pain	Spasticity common, bladder may be spared, spinal deformity on examination
Spinal metastases	Subacute onset, chronically progressive over weeks	Spasticity or flaccidity, bladder may be spared
Transverse myelitis (incl. autoimmune)	Acute onset, often non-progressive	Bladder involvement common
Schistosomiasis	Acute (days) or subacute (a couple of weeks)	Often flaccid paresis, bladder involvement common

TABLE 11.2 Diagnostic Clues and Possible Treatment Regimens for Important Causes of Spinal Cord Disease in Resource-Limited Settings

	Diagnostic Clues	Treatment
Spinal tuberculosis	Typical spinal radiograph (see Box) Epidemiological evidence	Antituberculous treatment Spinal surgery if available and applicable (see Box)
Spinal metastases	Clinical evidence of the primary tumour (e.g. prostate, breast)	Very limited options: radiotherapy rarely available; corticosteroids to decrease oedema
Transverse myelitis (incl. autoimmune)	Young adults Inflammatory CSF	Corticosteroids
Schistosomiasis	Exposure to freshwater in endemic regions, young adults in endemic coutries or non-immune travellers; CSF eosinophilia; other manifestations of schistosomiasis may or may not be present.	Praziquantel, corticosteroids

TABLE 11.3	Common Complications of Spinal Cord Disease and Their Prevention and Management	
Complication	**Prevention/Management**	
Pressure sores	Nursing, training and counselling of guardians (two hourly turning)	
Urinary retention	Catheterization	
Contractures	Physiotherapy, training of guardians for home-based physiotherapy	
Pain	Pain relief by NSAID/opiates, involvement of local palliative care team	
Immobilization	If available, prescription of walking aids/ wheelchairs	
Depression	Spiritual and mental support, occupational therapy/community projects, pharmacotherapy, involvement of local palliative care team	

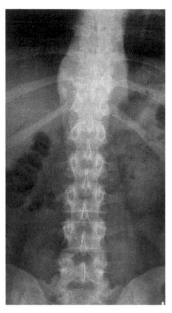

• **Fig. 11.2** AP radiograph demonstrating a paravertebral soft tissue mass in the lower dorsal region with collapse of the T11 vertebral body. (Waldman, S.D., Campbell, R.S.D., 2011. Imaging of Pain, 1st ed. Saunders, Amsterdam. pp. 147–8)

hospital paraplegic. The prognosis is overall poor, and often the secondary complications rather than the primary pathology dictate the further course of the disease. The prevention of complications of spinal cord disease is therefore of paramount importance. Health workers should work hand in hand with guardians, physiotherapists and the local palliative care team (Table 11.3).

The Case Continued…

The patient was found to be HIV-positive. His urine dipstick was normal and there were no ova of *Schistosoma* spp. detected in his urine and stool. The spinal radiograph showed a collapse of T11 vertebral body as well as soft tissue swelling around the spine (Fig. 11.2). Chest radiography and abdominal ultrasound examination were normal.

A presumed diagnosis of spinal TB was made and the patient was started on standard first-line antituberculous treatment. Vitamin B_6 was prescribed to prevent peripheral neuropathy. Physiotherapy and intensive guardian counselling were initiated at the hospital. The patient was reviewed by a spinal surgeon who did not recommend surgical intervention at that time, but suggested a review 3 months later. The patient was discharged home. The hospital palliative care team was involved and put him on their list for monthly home visits.

At 4 weeks he was followed up in the HIV outpatient clinic. His neurological deficits were unchanged. His CD4 count was 331 cells/μL and he was started on antiretroviral therapy.

At the 3-month follow-up by the palliative care team, the patient reported some subjective improvement in his gait. Clinically though, his deficits remained unchanged. He was taking his antituberculous and antiretroviral medication regularly and was still waiting for a wheelchair. He did not attend the neurosurgical outpatient clinic because of problems with transportation.

SUMMARY BOX

Spinal Tuberculosis (Pott's Disease)

Spinal TB is a collective term for spinal involvement in *Mycobacterium tuberculosis* infection. It comprises tuberculous spondylitis, tuberculous spondylodiscitis and tuberculous epidural and paraspinal abscess. Often, all manifestations occur together.

Spinal TB is the most common cause of tuberculous paraplegia and represents two-thirds of cases. Other causes are tuberculous radiculomyelitis (= arachnoiditis), tuberculous myelitis and intramedullary tuberculoma.

Constitutional symptoms are absent in more than half of patients, and simultaneous active pulmonary involvement is rather the exception than the rule. Inflammatory markers (ESR and CRP) are elevated in most cases and may be used as a screening method for patients from endemic regions presenting with back pain. Spinal radiographs may typically show focal areas of erosions and osseous destruction in the anterior corners of the vertebral bodies, involvement of the adjacent disc or vertebral body, 'wedging,' gibbus deformity or paraspinal abscess formation.

Compressive spinal cord involvement is a common and most feared complication caused by accumulation of epidural caseous debris or by vertebral collapse or dislocation.

CT-guided percutaneous vertebral or paravertebral biopsy and aspiration is the diagnostic gold standard. If biopsy is available, polymerase chain reaction (PCR)–based technology such as GeneXpert might expedite the diagnostic process and allow the early recognition of antibiotic resistance.

Antituberculous therapy is the same as for pulmonary TB; however, most national guidelines and centres recommend longer treatment for nine instead of 6 months.

Progression of bone destruction may continue for up to 1 year after effective antituberculous treatment has been initiated and should not be taken as a sign of treatment failure. Adjunctive corticosteroid treatment is not recommended for spinal TB. However, some centres use steroids in severe spinal cord compression to reduce oedematous swelling, which is a non-evidence-based approach. Surgery has been recommended for patients with (1) extensive extradural compression with features of spinal cord involvement, (2) no improvement or worsening of deficits after conservative treatment and (3) potentially unstable spine or kyphosis of more than 60 degrees. Surgical treatment relieves compression of the spinal cord, corrects kyphosis, may facilitate fusion and lead to faster pain relief.

Further Reading

1. Heckmann JE, Bhigjee AI. Tropical neurology. In: Farrar J, editor. Manson's Tropical Diseases. 23rd ed. London: Elsevier; 2013 [chapter 71].
2. Thwaites G. Tuberculosis. In: Farrar J, editor. Manson's Tropical Diseases. 23rd ed. London: Elsevier; 2013 [chapter 40].
3. Draulans N, Kiekens C, Roels E, et al. Etiology of spinal cord injuries in sub-Saharan Africa. Spinal Cord 2011;49:1148–54.
4. Jain AK. Tuberculosis of the spine: a fresh look at an old disease. J Bone Joint Surg Br 2010;92:905–13.
5. Dunn RN, Ben Husien M. Spinal tuberculosis: review of current management. Bone Joint J 2018;100-B(4):425–31.

12

A 29-Year-Old Man from The Gambia With Genital Ulceration

DAVID C.W. MABEY

Clinical Presentation

History

A 29-year-old man comes to your clinic in The Gambia complaining of painful sores involving his private parts for 7 days. He has been previously well. He admits to having had sex with a commercial sex worker 2 weeks ago, when he had not used a condom.

Clinical Findings

He is in considerable pain and is only able to walk with difficulty because of these sores. He is afebrile and well nourished. General examination is unremarkable. The only abnormality is the presence of numerous painful ulcers on his penis, scrotum and inner thigh (Fig. 12.1). The ulcers are tender, soft and bleed on contact. There is no inguinal lymphadenopathy.

Questions

1. What are the most important differential diagnoses?
2. How would you manage this patient?

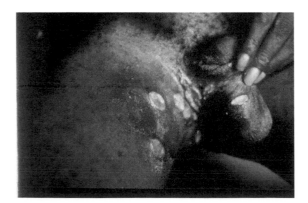

• **Fig. 12.1** Numerous painful ulcers on the penis, scrotum and inner thigh. The ulcers are soft, tender and bleed on contact.

Discussion

A 29-year-old Gambian man presents with genital ulcers which he has developed over the past week. He admits to having had unprotected sex with a commercial sex worker 2 weeks previously.

Answer to Question 1
What Are the Most Important Differential Diagnoses?

The three major causes of genital ulceration are *Herpes simplex,* syphilis and chancroid. Ulcers caused by *H. simplex* are self-limiting in immunocompetent individuals, and do not usually last longer than a few days. They can be severe and persistent in the immunocompromised. Ulcers caused by primary syphilis are usually painless, and it is unusual for there to be more than a single ulcer. Inguinal adenopathy is sometimes seen but is usually painless. Ulcers caused by chancroid are often multiple, and usually painful. In some 50% of cases painful inguinal lymphadenopathy is found. Inguinal buboes may be fluctuant and sometimes rupture, releasing large amounts of pus.

However, the clinical diagnosis of genital ulcer disease is unreliable. For this reason, the patient should be treated syndromically for both syphilis and chancroid. If he is HIV-positive, additional treatment for herpes should also be considered.

Answer to Question 2
How Would You Manage This Patient?

Treat him for syphilis with a single dose of IM benzathine penicillin 2.4 million units. Treat him for chancroid with a single dose of azithromycin 1 g PO or ciprofloxacin 500 mg bid for 3 days or erythromycin 500 mg qds for 7 days. If he is HIV-positive, consider adding aciclovir 400 mg tds for 7 days.

He is at high risk of HIV because he has acquired a genital ulcer from a commercial sex worker, so you should test him for HIV and start antiretroviral treatment if positive. Serology for syphilis will be helpful in guiding treatment for his sexual partners, but he should be treated for syphilis even if it is negative, because serology can be negative in early primary syphilis. He should be strongly encouraged to bring his sexual partners to the clinic for assessment and treatment.

The Case Continued...

The patient was treated with 2.4 million units of benzathine penicillin IM stat and given erythromycin 500 mg to take qds for 7 days. He was HIV-negative, his syphilis serology was positive (RPR and TPHA). A swab was taken for culture of *Haemophilus ducreyi,* and *H. ducreyi* was grown after three days' incubation at 33°C. Mixed infection are common in patients with sexually transmitted diseases (STIs), since for behavioural reasons patients with one STI are at increased risk of others. The patient returned for follow-up after 7 days. The pain had resolved and the ulcers were all healing (Fig. 12.2).

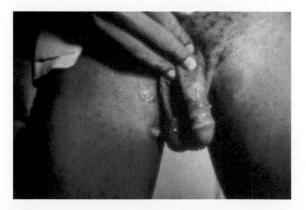

• **Fig. 12.2** Follow-up after 1 week of antibiotic therapy. The ulcers are healing and the pain has resolved.

SUMMARY BOX

Chancroid

Chancroid is a disease of core groups, principally sex workers and their clients. Unlike other STIs, asymptomatic infection is rare; most infected individuals have painful genital ulcers.

Laboratory diagnosis of chancroid is difficult. It depends on the identification of the causative agent, *H. ducreyi,* in material from lesions. Gram stain is neither sensitive nor specific. Nucleic acid amplification tests such as PCR have been used in research settings, but are not commercially available. Isolation is the gold standard. *H. ducreyi* is a fastidious organism, requiring an enriched culture medium that needs to be made selective by the addition of antibiotics to inhibit the growth of other organisms present in the ulcer. Unlike most bacteria, it grows best at 33°C.

Virtually all strains of *H. ducreyi* are resistant to penicillin, because of plasmids encoding various penicillin resistance genes. Most strains are also resistant to tetracyclines and sulphonamides. Treatment for chancroid is with azithromycin 1 g PO *or* ciprofloxacin 500 mg bid for 3 days *or* erythromycin 500 mg qds for 7 days.

It is important to treat all patients with genital ulcers for chancroid in regions where it is endemic (believed to be most parts of Africa, Asia and perhaps South America). Because it is difficult to diagnose, the incidence, prevalence and geographical distribution of chancroid are not well known; but it is thought to have become less common since the onset of the HIV/AIDS epidemic.

Further Reading

1. Richens J, Mayaud P, Mabey DCW. Sexually transmitted infections (excluding HIV). In: Farrar J, editor. Manson's Tropical Diseases. 23rd ed London: Elsevier; 2014 [chapter 23].
2. Mayaud P, Ndowa FJ, Richens J, et al. Sexually transmitted infections. In: Mabey D, et al, editors. Principles of Medicine in Africa. 4th ed Cambridge University Press, 2014 [Chapter 21].
3. Lewis DA, Ison CA. Chancroid. Sex Transm Infect 2006;82 (Suppl. 4): iv19–20.
4. Kemp M, Christensen JJ, Lautenschlager S, et al. European guideline for the management of chancroid, 2011. Int J STD AIDS 2011;22(5):241–4.
5. Kularatne RS, Muller EE, Maseko DV, et al. Trends in the relative prevalence of genital ulcer disease pathogens and association with HIV infection in Johannesburg, South Africa, 2007-2015. PLoS One 2018;13:e0194125. https://doi.org/10.1371/journal.pone.0194125.

13

A 16-Year-Old Girl from Malawi With Fever and Abdominal Pain

CAMILLA ROTHE

Clinical Presentation

History

A 16-year-old Malawian girl presents to the emergency room of a local hospital because of fever, generalized abdominal pain and frontal headache for the past 5 days.

She delivered a baby 5 months ago. An HIV test done in the antenatal clinic was negative. Her further past medical history is unremarkable.

She lives with her parents, her three siblings and her baby in an urban high-density area. There is no running water and no electricity in the house. The family fetch water from a community tap. The girl went to primary school but recently dropped out during her pregnancy.

Clinical Findings

16-year-old girl in a fair nutritional state. Temperature 38.1°C (100.6°F), blood pressure 110/60 mmHg, pulse 78 bpm, respiratory rate 20 breath cycles per minute, Glasgow Coma Scale 15/15. There is mild scleral jaundice, no neck stiffness. The examination of the abdomen shows diffuse tenderness but no guarding. The liver is not enlarged, the spleen is palpable at 2 cm below the left costal margin. The chest is clear and there is no lymphadenopathy. Pelvic examination is unremarkable and there is no vaginal discharge.

Investigations

Her laboratory results on admission are shown in Table 13.1. The blood film for malaria parasites is positive, parasitaemia is described as "low". Liver function tests are not available because reagents are out of stock.

Questions

What are your most important differential diagnoses?
How would you approach this patient?

Discussion

A 16-year-old girl presents with fever, abdominal pain and frontal headache. She has recently delivered a baby, otherwise her past medical history is unremarkable.

She is febrile, mildly jaundiced and there is diffuse abdominal tenderness with slight splenomegaly. There is mild normocytic anaemia. Malaria parasites are positive with low parasitaemia.

Answer to Question 1

What Are Your Most Important Differential Diagnoses?

Malaria could explain most of her signs and symptoms, even though her abdominal pain would be unusual. However, in a malaria-endemic area where large parts of the population are semi-immune, low parasitaemia is common and often subclinical. Nevertheless, malaria itself, particularly if combined with severe anaemia, is a predisposing factor for Gram-negative bacteraemia and sepsis.

Enteric fever (typhoid or paratyphoid) is another diagnosis to consider, particularly given her abdominal tenderness, her splenomegaly, her frontal headache and her relative bradycardia. Mild jaundice in enteric fever may be caused by hepatitis, cholangitis, cholecystitis or haemolysis.

TABLE 13.1 Laboratory Results on Admission

Parameter	Patient	Reference
WBC (×10⁹/L)	3.2	4–10
Haemoglobin (mg/dL)	10.9	12–14
MCV (fL)	90	80–99
Platelets (×10⁹/L)	164	150–400
Creatinine (µmol/L)	71	<80

In HIV-positive patients an infection with invasive non-typhoidal salmonellae (iNTS) should be considered.

Answer to Question 2

How Would You Approach This Patient?

Blood cultures should be taken in any febrile patient regardless of the malaria test result to rule out bacterial sepsis and enteric fever. Her HIV test should be repeated.

Since she is symptomatic and has malaria parasites in her blood, she should receive antimalarials according to the national guidelines and the local resistance profile. She should also be given broad-spectrum antibiotics to cover for Gram-negative and, less likely, Gram-positive bacteria. A urinary dipstick could quickly help rule out a urinary tract infection.

An abdominal ultrasound should be done to rule out posthepatic causes of jaundice and to assess texture and size of liver and spleen.

The Case Continued...

On admission the patient was started on artemether/lumefantrine PO and a broad-spectrum antibiotic (ceftriaxone 2 g IV od). A repeat HIV test was negative. Blood cultures grew *Salmonella Typhi*. The antibiotic therapy was switched to ciprofloxacin 500 mg bid. On day 5 of antibiotic treatment the patient's fever started to settle and she was feeling better. She was discharged on day 7. Ciprofloxacin was continued for a total of 10 days. The patient was also given one dose of praziquantel, because co-infection with schistosomiasis seems to favour chronic carriage of *S. Typhi* and relapse, and Malawi is a country highly endemic for schistosomiasis.

SUMMARY BOX

Typhoid Fever

Typhoid fever caused by *Salmonella Typhi* is an exclusively human disease and there is no animal reservoir. Typhoid is clinically indistinguishable from paratyphoid, caused by *S. Paratyphi* A, B and C.

The enteric fevers, typhoid and paratyphoid, are endemic all over the tropical world. Incidence appears to be highest on the Indian subcontinent (approx. 500:100 000 per year in urban slums).

In endemic countries, enteric fevers are most common in children and adolescents, whereas adults have acquired immunity through previous exposures. Typhoid is usually acquired through ingestion of food or water contaminated by faeces of a patient or carrier. Overcrowding and poor sanitation are major risk factors.

The incubation period of typhoid fever averages 10 to 20 days (range 3–56). It is shorter in paratyphoid (1–10 days).

Symptoms are nonspecific with fever, headache, dry cough and abdominal pain. Other than in malaria, fever starts insidiously and may go unnoticed by the patient for some time. Temperature typically rises in the evening hours and patients may be afebrile in the morning. Constipation is common, but foul-smelling diarrhoea may occur during the course of an untreated infection. Patients may become confused and apathetic and, if untreated, may die of myocarditis, overwhelming toxaemia, intestinal perforation or haemorrhage.

Full blood count typically shows leukopenia. Low-grade anaemia and thrombocytopenia as well as slightly elevated transaminases are also common, but non-specific.

The definitive diagnosis of typhoid requires proof of *S. Typhi* in blood cultures or bone marrow. Isolation from stool or urine indicates carrier state but does not prove disease. The serological Widal test lacks both sensitivity and specificity and should be abandoned altogether. Novel and more promising serological tests are under development. Meanwhile, blood culture remains the diagnostic gold standard. In many low-resource settings, blood culture testing is however unavailable.

Patients with suspected enteric fever should be started on empirical antibiotic therapy. Antibiotic resistance patterns vary considerably between endemic areas. In many countries, antibiotic resistance is on the rise. Fluoroquinolones are the drugs of choice in areas without antimicrobial resistance because they reach very high intracellular concentrations. Third-generation cephalosporins or azithromycin should be used in South Asia where fluoroquinolone resistance is common.

Duration of treatment is between 1 and 2 weeks depending on the drug used. Case fatality rate on antibiotic treatment is <1%.

Apart from public health measures to improve safe water supply and sanitation, targeted vaccination of high-risk populations seems to be a promising strategy to control typhoid fever. Typhoid conjugate vaccines which can also be applied to children <2 years of age seem to be promising.

Further Reading

1. Feasey NA, Gordon MA. Salmonella Infections. In: Farrar J, editor. Manson's Tropical Diseases. 23rd ed. London: Elsevier; 2013 [chapter 25].
2. Wain J, Hendriksen R, Mikoleit ML, et al. Typhoid fever. Lancet 2015;385:1136–1145.
3. Crump JA, Heydermann RS. A perspective on Invasive Salmonella Disease in Africa. Clin Infect Dis 2015;61(Suppl 4):S235–S239.
4. Hsiao A, Toy T, Seo HJ, et al. Interaction between Salmonella and Schistosomiasis: a Review. PlOS Pathog 2016;12(12):e1005928.
5. Andrews JR, Baker S, Marks F, et al. Typhoid conjugate vaccines: a new tool in the fight against antimicrobial resistance. Lancet Infect Dis 2019;19:e26–e30.

14

A 22-Year-Old Woman from Bangladesh With Profuse Watery Diarrhoea

GAGANDEEP KANG AND SUDHIR BABJI

Clinical Presentation

History

A 22-year-old woman from Ashulia near Dhaka, Bangladesh is brought to a local hospital with a history of passing 12 to 15 large-volume stools in the past day. The stools resemble diluted milk or rice water with white flakes. Her husband reports that she became unresponsive about an hour previously and he hired a rickshaw to bring her to the hospital. He says that she had not complained of pain and did not have fever.

The patient has recently attended a religious festival, where water was supplied in large metal containers. Her husband reports that there were five or six people who had attended the same event and were also ill with diarrhoea.

Clinical Findings

A thin young woman, who is stuporous and responds minimally to a painful stimulus (GCS 9/15). She is afebrile, with sunken eyes, dry mouth and a scaphoid abdomen. A skin pinch returns very slowly. Her pulse rate is 110 bpm, low volume, and her blood pressure is 90/50 mmHg. The remainder of her systemic examination is normal.

Laboratory Results

Laboratory results are given in Table 14.1

Stool Examination

Macroscopic: Liquid stool, rice-water appearance with no faecal matter. Hanging drop preparation shows small slender curved bacilli with darting motility. Motility is completely inhibited by using *Vibrio cholerae* antiserum O1. Stool culture grows *V. cholerae* (Fig. 14.1) and the organism is typed as *V. cholerae* O1, Serotype Ogawa, biotype El Tor.

TABLE 14.1	Laboratory Results on Admission	
Parameter	Patient	Reference Range
Sodium	143.8 mmol/L	(135-145 mmol/L
Potassium	3.0 mmol/L	(3.5-5.0 mmol/L)
Chloride	103.8 mmol/L	(98-108 mmol/L)
Bicarbonate	11.4 mmol/L	(23-28 mmol/L)
Lactic acid (venous)	4.1 mmol/L	(0.67-1.8 mmol/L)
Creatine	203 μmol/L	(62-115 μmol/L)
Blood Urea Nitrogen	8.6 mmol/L	(2.9-7.1 mmol/L)

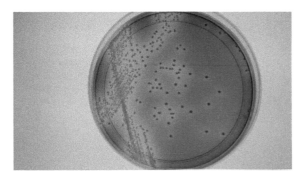

• **Fig. 14.1** Stool culture growing *Vibrio cholerae* which produces typical golden-yellow colonies on thiosulphate citrate bile salt sucrose (TCBS) agar.

Questions

1. How was the infection most likely acquired? Is there an outbreak?
2. How is dehydration assessed and managed?

Discussion

A 22-year-old Bengali woman who has recently visited a religious festival is brought into hospital in a stuporous condition with a history of rapid onset of severe, acute watery diarrhoea. There is no fever, vomiting or abdominal pain. She is severely dehydrated and her electrolytes are deranged. The microscopic examination of her stool indicates cholera which is confirmed on culture. A number of other people who attended the same festival have also fallen ill with diarrhoea.

Answer to Question 1

How Was the Infection Most Likely Acquired? Is There an Outbreak?

Cholera transmission is closely linked to inadequate environmental management. Typical at-risk areas include peri-urban slums where basic infrastructure is not available and rural and urban areas in endemic countries where sanitation is limited, including refugee camps. Additionally, natural disasters, as well as times of political and social unrest associated with a collapse of infrastructure, pose a risk of cholera.

An outbreak is defined as the occurrence of disease episodes in greater numbers than would be expected at a particular time and place.

In this case there seems to be a typical cholera outbreak. The source is most probably contaminated water consumed from the containers during the festival, with the likelihood that unless control measures for disease prevention and appropriate case management are instituted rapidly, there will be spread, significant morbidity and, possibly, mortality.

Answer to Question 2

How is Dehydration Assessed and Managed?

The WHO has recommended an assessment based on the general clinical condition of the patient (Table 14.2). Depending on their degree of fluid depletion, patients are assigned to rehydration at home, supervised oral rehydration or intravenous rehydration (Table 14.3).

Adequate fluid and electrolyte replacement are the cornerstones of cholera management and differ substantially from the approaches to patients with gastroenteritis of other aetiologies. Patients with severe cholera present with a higher

TABLE 14.2   Clinical Assessment of Dehydration in Patients with Suspected Cholera (After Harris J.B., et al.)

	No Dehydration (<5%)	Some Dehydration (5–10%)	Severe Dehydration (>10%)
General Appearance	Well, alert	Restless, irritable	Lethargic or unconscious
Eyes	Normal	Sunken	Sunken
Thirst	Drinks normally	Thirsty, drinks eagerly	Drinks poorly or is unable to drink
Skin Turgor	Instantaneous recoil	Non-instantaneous recoil	Very slow recoil (>2s)
Pulse	Normal	Rapid, low volume	Weak or absent

TABLE 14.3   Approach to Rehydration in Patients with Cholera Depending on the Degree of Clinical Dehydration (After Harris J.B., et al.)

	No Dehydration (<5%)	Some Dehydration (5–10%)	Severe Dehydration (>10%)
Requirement for Fluid Replacement	Ongoing losses only	75 mL/kg in the first 24 hours in addition to ongoing losses	>100 mL/kg in the first 24 hours in addition to ongoing losses
Preferred Route of Administration	Oral	Oral or intravenous	Intravenous
Timing	Usually guided by thirst	Replace fluids over 3–4 hours	As rapidly as possible until circulation is restored, then complete the remainder of fluids within 3 hours
Monitoring	Observe until ongoing losses can definitely be adequately replaced by ORS	Observe every 1–2 hours until all signs of dehydration resolve and patient urinates	Once circulation is established monitor every 1–2 hours

ORS = oral rehydration solution.

degree of initial dehydration, have more rapid continuing losses and proportionately greater electrolyte depletion than patients with other forms of gastroenteritis. The most common error is for clinicians to underestimate the speed and volume of fluids required for rehydration.

Up to 80% of sufferers can be treated successfully through prompt administration of oral rehydration salts (WHO/UNICEF ORS standard sachets). In adults, 2 to 4 litres of ORS may be required in the first 4 hours.

Patients with severe cholera typically require an average of 200 mL/kg of isotonic oral or IV fluids in the first 24 hours (Table 14.2). The initial fluid deficit should be replaced within 3 to 4 hours of initial presentation. 10 to 20 mL/kg bodyweight should be calculated for each diarrhoeal stool or episode of vomiting.

Antibiotic therapy in cholera is secondary; but in patients with severe disease, appropriate antibiotics diminish the duration of diarrhoea, reduce the volume of rehydration fluids needed and shorten the duration of *V. cholerae* excretion. In Bangladesh, resistance to furazolidone and tetracycline is increasing.

The Case Continued…

The patient was admitted immediately and started on intravenous rehydration with Ringer's lactate solution. After receiving 3 L in the first hour her pulse rate and blood pressure picked up to 84 bpm and 100/70 mmHg respectively. Over the next 3 hours she was given an additional 2 L and became alert and responsive. She was then started on oral rehydration and given a single dose of 300 mg doxycycline. She was discharged on the third day, by which time stool consistency had returned to normal.

The local health authorities identified an additional 44 cases of cholera. All were treated, health education carried out and the overhead tanks were chlorinated.

SUMMARY BOX

Cholera

Cholera, caused by *V. cholerae,* is a major cause of acute dehydrating diarrhoea, particularly in South and South-east Asia, where it is endemic; it also occurs as large-scale outbreaks in Africa and Latin America.

V. cholerae is an aerobic Gram-negative bacillus with typical darting motility. Man is the only natural host of *V. cholerae* and asymptomatic carriage is possible. The main source of transmission is from a contaminated water source. In some parts of the world, copepods are responsible for maintaining *Vibrio* spp. in a viable but non-cultivable state.

The incubation period ranges between 12 hours and 5 days. Patients are usually afebrile and do not have any abdominal pain. The major clinical challenge is dehydration, ranging from mild to severe, and electrolyte imbalance leading on to renal failure in severe cases.

In epidemics, the diagnosis of cholera may be presumptive on clinical and epidemiological grounds following the WHO clinical case definition. Laboratory confirmation may be required when sporadic cases occur or when an extensive outbreak requires confirmation and typing of the etiological agent.

Treatment typically involves isolation of the patient, correction of dehydration and antimicrobial treatment. In most cases oral replacement solutions may be used. Antimicrobial therapy is secondary; it is shown to decrease shedding of the bacteria and also hastens clinical resolution of illness. Tetracycline and doxycycline are the preferred drugs in adults, but ciprofloxacin or macrolides can also be used depending on availability and local resistance pattern.

Public health measures to improve water and sanitation are essential for long-term control. WHO has endorsed the inclusion of oral vaccines in cholera control programmes in endemic areas in conjunction with other preventive and control strategies.

Further Reading

1. Kang G, Hart CA, Shears P. Bacterial enteropathogens. In: Farrar J, editor. Manson's Tropical Diseases. 23rd ed. London: Elsevier; 2013 [chapter 24].
2. Clemens JD, Nair GB, Ahmed T, et al. Cholera. Lancet 2017;390 (10101):1539–49.
3. Holmgren J, Svennerholm AM. Vaccines against mucosal infections. Curr Opin Immunol 2012;24(3):343–53.
4. Klontz EH, Das SK, Ahmed D, et al. Long term comparison of antibiotic resistance in Vibrio cholerae 01 and Shigella species between urban and rural Bangladesh. Clin Infect Dis 2014;58 (9):e133–6.

15

A 3-Year-Old Boy from Laos With Right Suppurative Parotitis

SAYAPHET RATTANAVONG, VIRAVONG DOUANGNOULAK, BUACHAN NORINDR, PAUL N. NEWTON AND CAOIMHE NIC FHOGARTAIGH

Clinical Presentation

History

A 3-year-old rural Lao boy presents to the ENT clinic with a 10-day history of gradual, painful swelling of the right cheek with associated fever and poor appetite. Three days previously his mother noticed a purulent discharge from the ear. He has no cough, vomiting or diarrhoea. There is no history of previous ear infection or dental problems and no known history of trauma. The child is developing normally and is up to date with vaccinations. His parents are rice farmers.

Clinical Findings

The child looks unwell, with a fever of 39.5°C (103.1°F). There is a localized, fluctuant, hot, tender swelling below and anterior to the right ear, 6 to 8 cm in diameter, extending from the lower cheek to the submandibular region and consistent with a parotid mass (Fig. 15.1). Ear examination reveals a purulent discharge in the auditory canal and suspicion of a small fistula from which the pus is arising, with a right lower motor neuron facial nerve palsy. The oral cavity and throat are unremarkable. There is no lymphadenopathy and no hepatosplenomegaly. Heart sounds are normal and the chest is clear.

Laboratory Results

WBC 16.5×10^9/L (4–10 x10^9/L), 90% neutrophils. Hb 9.4 g/dL (13–15 g/dL), all other blood tests are normal.

Questions

1. What are your differential diagnoses?
2. What investigations would you perform?

Discussion

A 3-year-old boy from rural Laos presents to a local hospital because of high fever, unilateral parotid swelling and purulent discharge from his ear. The little boy has previously been well.

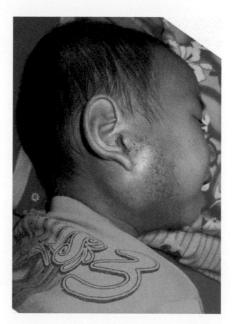

• **Fig. 15.1** A Lao boy with a unilateral parotid mass showing signs of local inflammation.

Answer to Question 1

What Are Your Differential Diagnoses?

Acute, suppurative, unilateral parotitis in children is usually bacterial. The most common pathogens are *Staphylococcus aureus, Streptococcus pyogenes* and *Haemophilus influenzae,* although the latter has declined because of widespread vaccination. Neonates are at risk of parotitis caused by Gram-negative bacteria, and *Streptococcus pneumoniae* parotitis may occur in HIV-infected children.

In an endemic area like Laos, *Burkholderia pseudomallei,* the causative agent of melioidosis, must also be considered. Studies in neighbouring countries have shown melioidosis to be the commonest cause of suppurative parotitis in children. Actinomycosis and cat-scratch disease (*Bartonella henselae*) are more unusual bacterial causes.

Mumps was the commonest cause of parotid swelling in children until the introduction of vaccination, which is still not commonly available in some countries, including Laos. Swelling is painful, but is non-suppurative and becomes bilateral in the majority of cases. Other less common viral agents causing parotitis include parainfluenza viruses, influenza A, cytomegalovirus, Epstein–Barr virus and enteroviruses, but these do not cause the degree of inflammation and suppuration seen here.

Granulomatous parotitis, caused by *Mycobacterium tuberculosis, Mycobacterium avium-intracellulare* and other mycobacteria, is rare and presents with a more chronic, painless, enlarging mass without surrounding inflammation. Salivary stones and malignancies are very rare in children.

Answer to Question 2
What Investigations Would You Perform?

Samples for bacterial culture before commencing antimicrobial therapy are crucial. Gram stain and bacterial culture of pus from the ear are quick and non-invasive. Blood cultures should be taken because the results have therapeutic and prognostic implications.

A throat swab may detect causative bacterial pathogens and has been used to diagnose melioidosis in children. Deep pus from incision and drainage of the parotid abscess is the most useful diagnostic material, and drainage may be necessary for management of the abscess. This may be performed under ultrasound guidance.

Full blood count may help differentiate between bacterial and viral causes. When melioidosis is suspected, chest radiograph and abdominal ultrasound should be requested to look for other foci of infection. In this patient a radiograph of the skull would be useful to detect any osteomyelitis.

The laboratory must be informed if melioidosis is suspected, because selective media are used to isolate *B. pseudomallei* from non-sterile sites, and suspected growth must be handled under containment level 3 conditions when available.

If melioidosis is confirmed, investigations should look for underlying predisposing conditions such as diabetes mellitus, although these are found less commonly in children with *B. pseudomallei* parotitis than in adults with melioidosis.

The Case Continued…

Pus culture from the right ear and parotid abscess isolated *B. pseudomallei*. Blood culture was negative. Chest radiography and abdominal ultrasound were normal.

The patient had incision and drainage of the parotid with removal of copious pus. Intravenous ceftazidime was administered for 10 days followed by oral co-amoxiclav for 16 weeks with good clinical response. No complications occurred, and no underlying disease was identified. Being from a rice farming family, the boy was likely to have been frequently exposed to soil and water containing *B. pseudomallei* in the paddy fields.

SUMMARY BOX

Melioidosis

Melioidosis is an infectious disease caused by *B. pseudomallei*, a saprophytic Gram-negative environmental bacterium endemic in South and South-east Asia, as well as in northern Australia. It is the third most common cause of death in north-east Thailand after HIV and tuberculosis. There is growing evidence that melioidosis is also of relevance in other parts of the tropics where its importance has long been underestimated.

In endemic areas *B. pseudomallei* is readily isolated from soil and surface water. The disease is highly seasonal and most cases present during the rainy season.

The clinical presentation ranges from mild localized infection to severe septicaemia. In endemic areas, 60–80% of children have evidence of seroconversion to *B. pseudomallei* by the age of 4 years and most paediatric infections are mild or asymptomatic.

Septicaemic melioidosis occurs in more than one-third of paediatric cases, with a similar clinical presentation as in adults. The lung is the most common organ involved, and septic shock is associated with a high mortality. Multiple organ involvement and disseminated infections are well described. Localized disease, however, accounts for the majority of paediatric melioidosis, with the parotid gland being the most common site involved. Skin and soft tissue abscesses are also common. Parotitis is uncommon in adults and has not been seen in children in Australia.

It is believed that ingestion of water contaminated with *B. pseudomallei* may cause colonization of the oropharynx and ascending infection to the parotid gland, particularly where drinking water is obtained from boreholes. Less than 10% of children have a predisposing condition. The prognosis is usually favourable, although complications include spontaneous rupture into the auditory canal, facial nerve palsy, septicaemia and osteomyelitis.

The aims of treatment are to reduce mortality and morbidity, prevent recurrence and drain abscesses. Referral to a surgeon for consideration for drainage should be arranged; however, such surgery risks damage to the facial nerve. There is little evidence to inform the choice and duration of antimicrobial treatment for localized melioidosis in children. The authors recommend precautionary intravenous ceftazidime, meropenem or imipenem for the acute phase (10–14 days); however, parenteral therapy is very expensive. This is followed by co-trimoxazole monotherapy for the eradication phase (12–20 weeks), which has been shown to be non-inferior to dual therapy with co-trimoxazole and doxycycline and avoids adverse effects of doxycycline in children. Amoxicillin-clavulanate is an alternative for patients with sulfa allergy or resistance and in pregnancy.

Further Reading

1. Dance DAB. Melioidosis. In: Farrar J, editor. Manson's Tropical Diseases. 23rd ed. London: Elsevier; 2013 [chapter 34].
2. Lumbiganon P, Viengnondha S. Clinical manifestations of melioidosis in children. Pediatr Infect Dis J 1995;14(2):136–40.

3. Stoesser N, Pocock J, Moore CE, et al. Paediatric suppurative parotitis in Cambodia between 2007 and 2011. Paediatr Infect Dis J 2012;31(8):865–8.

4. Phetsouvanh R, Phongmany S, Newton P, et al. Melioidosis and Pandora's box in the Lao People's Democratic Republic. Clin Infect Dis 2001;32(4):653–4.

5. Chetchotisakd P, Chierakul W, Chaowagul W, et al. Trimethoprim-sulphamethoxazole versus trimethoprim-sulphamethoxazole plus doxycycline as oral eradicative treatment for melioidosis (MERTH): A multicentre, double-blind, non-inferiority, randomised controlled trial. Lancet 2014;383:807–14. https://doi.org/10.1016/S0140-6736(13)61951-0.

16

A 25-Year-Old Female School Teacher from Malawi With Abrupt Onset of Fever and Confusion

EMMA C. WALL

Clinical Presentation

History

A 25-year-old Malawian primary school teacher presents to a local central hospital. She was reported to be well at 8 a.m., confused by 10 a.m. and drowsy with a high fever and convulsions on admission at 11 a.m.

She is HIV-positive and has been on first-line antiretroviral therapy (ART) with tenofovir, lamivudine and efavirenz for 6 months with good adherence. Her CD4 count on starting ART was 320 cells/µL. She completed treatment for pulmonary tuberculosis 2 months ago.

Clinical Findings

The patient is restless and agitated; Glasgow Coma Scale 10/15. Pupils are equal and reactive with photophobia; the neck is stiff and there is no rash. Plantar responses are down-going, Kernig's sign is positive. Chest and abdominal examinations are unremarkable. Temperature 40°C (104°F), pulse 125 bpm, blood pressure 125/68 mmHg, oxygen saturation 93% on room air. During the physical examination she suffers a renewed seizure.

Laboratory Results

Her blood results are shown in Table 16.1. A spinal tap is done. The CSF appears hazy; CSF results are shown in Table 16.2. Rapid antigen test for *Plasmodium falciparum* is negative.

Questions

1. What are your treatment priorities for this woman?
2. What adjunctive interventions should be used in this setting?

TABLE 16.1 Blood Results on Admission

Parameter	Patient	Reference
WBC ($\times 10^9$/L)	10.5	4–10
Neutrophil count ($\times 10^9$/L)	8.9	2.5–6
Haemoglobin (g/dL)	8.9	12–14
MCV (fL)	85	78–90
Platelets ($\times 10^9$/L)	255	150–400
Creatinine (µmol/L)	106	35–106
Random blood glucose (mmol/L)	5.6	3.9–7.8

TABLE 16.2 Results on Admission

Parameter	Patient	Reference
Leukocytes (cells/µL)	35 (60% neutrophils)	0–5/µL
Protein (g/L)	2.6	0.15–0.42
Glucose (mmol/L)	1.2	2.5–5

Discussion

A 25-year-old Malawian woman, known to be HIV-positive and on ART, presents with acute severe symptoms including a high fever, a rapid decline in consciousness and new onset convulsions, suggesting a severe neurological infection. Her CSF is hazy and shows a neutrophilic pleocytosis, as well as a high CSF-protein and low glucose.

Bacterial meningitis is the most likely diagnosis; tuberculous meningitis and cryptococcal meningitis are possibilities, though much less likely, since they tend to present in a subacute manner.

Answer to Question 1

What Are Your Treatment Priorities for This Woman?

The suspected diagnosis is acute bacterial meningitis. In Africa *Streptococcus pneumoniae* is the most common cause of meningitis in adults and children. Additionally, in the meningitis belt, seasonal outbreaks of bacterial meningitis caused by *Neisseria meningitis* occur during the dry season. Case numbers have dropped considerably after the introduction of large-scale vaccination programmes.

The immediate treatment priority is emergency resuscitation, including rapid administration of antibiotics. A third-generation cephalosporin such as ceftriaxone at a high dose to penetrate the CSF is appropriate; where this is not available, high dose benzylpenicillin plus chloramphenicol is a suitable alternative. Resistance rates of *S. pneumoniae* to both penicillins and chloramphenicol are rising, hence local advice about resistance patterns should be sought. Data to guide resuscitation in adults are limited, but airway support and seizure control are indicated. Public health services are required for case management to ensure that appropriate vaccination programmes and case notification for outbreak monitoring are done.

Answer to Question 2

What Adjunctive Interventions Should be Used in This Setting and What Are Your Differential Diagnoses?

Several meta-analyses suggest that while in well-resourced countries dexamethasone should be given to adults and children presenting to hospital with meningitis, steroids should not be used in resource-limited hospitals in Africa given their lack of efficacy. Glycerol has been tested in paediatric meningitis with mixed results but was shown to be harmful in adults with meningitis in Malawi. No other adjuncts have been tested in clinical trials to date; adjunctive treatment is not indicated.

In cases of suspected meningitis, a lumbar puncture (LP) must be undertaken to obtain a diagnosis. Despite clinical contraindications to lumbar puncture in this patient (seizures and altered conscious level), the risk of causing harm by doing an LP is low. LP should not be delayed by attempts to obtain cerebral imaging unless obvious signs of a space-occupying lesion are present. CT scan of the brain is of limited value in bacterial meningitis. Administration of antibiotics should not be delayed while the LP is undertaken, particularly in resource-limited settings.

The main differential diagnoses for this patient are cryptococcal meningitis (CCM) and TB meningitis (TBM). However, her CD4 count is too high for CCM and her recent completion of TB treatment makes TBM less likely. In addition, both of these infections classically have a more chronic course.

She is not pregnant, therefore meningitis caused by *Listeria monocytogenes* is very unlikely. Bacterial pathogens that cause meningitis in HIV-infected adults include *S. pneumoniae,* group A streptococci, *Staphylococcus aureus,* invasive non-typhoidal salmonellae, *Salmonella typhi, Escherichia coli* and *Haemophilus influenzae;* all will be treated with a third-generation cephalosporin. European guidelines recommend 14 days of antibiotics in HIV-infected adults with bacterial meningitis. However, in sub-Saharan Africa often shorter courses are given, determined by the patient's recovery rate, local guidelines and availability of antibiotics for long courses. In children with bacterial meningitis in Malawi, 5 days of ceftriaxone was shown to be non-inferior to ten days, with substantial savings shown, and shorter courses are now commonly used.

The Case Continued...

In the emergency department the patient received ceftriaxone 2 g IV, 10 mg of diazepam IV and 600 mg of phenobarbitone IV. Her oxygen saturation improved with resuscitation. She received 10 days of IV ceftriaxone and recovered consciousness by day 3. CSF culture grew *S. pneumoniae.* Audiometry revealed a minor hearing loss in her right ear. No further neurological impairment or seizures were noted; anticonvulsants were weaned by day 3.

SUMMARY BOX

Acute Bacterial Meningitis

In resource-rich settings, acute bacterial meningitis in adults and children is declining in incidence because of successful vaccination campaigns, but sporadic cases continue to occur. In contrast, many countries with high HIV prevalence have reported an increase in patients presenting with acute bacterial meningitis (ABM) since the start of the HIV epidemic.

Case fatality rates in resource-rich settings have declined from 45–50% to 11–25% over the past 50 years, associated with early administration of broad-spectrum antibiotics and better supportive care. In contrast, adult ABM lethality rates in sub-Saharan Africa are reported to vary between 50 and 70% without any change over time, and survivors experience higher rates of neurological disabilities.

Adjunctive treatments have failed to reduce lethality in large randomized controlled trials in Africa despite efficacy elsewhere. In well-resourced settings, important risk factors for poor outcome include advanced age, hyperglycaemia and immunosuppression. In Africa, coma, seizures, anaemia and delayed presentation to hospital are poor prognostic features. Antibiotic treatment depends on local sensitivities. A third-generation cephalosporin at high dose given as early as possible is the treatment of choice.

Further Reading

1. Heckmann JE, Bhigjee AI. Tropical neurology. In: Farrar J, editor. Manson's Tropical Diseases. 23rd ed. London: Elsevier; 2013 [chapter 71].

2. van de Beek D, Cabellos C, Dzupova O, et al. ESCMID guideline: diagnosis and treatment of acute bacterial meningitis. Clin Microbiol Infect 2016;22(Suppl 3):S37–S62.

3. Wall EC, Mukaka M, Denis B, et al. Goal directed therapy for suspected acute bacterial meningitis in adults and adolescents in sub-Saharan Africa. PloS One 2017;12(10)e0186687.

4. van de Beek D, Farrar JJ, de Gans J, et al. Adjunctive dexamethasone in bacterial meningitis: a meta-analysis of individual patient data. Lancet Neurol 2010;9(3):254–263.

5. Global Burden of Diseases Study Collaborators. Global, regional, and national burden of meningitis, 1990-2016: a systematic analysis for the Global Burden of Disease Study 2016. Lancet Neurol 2018;17(12):1061–1082.

17

A 34-Year-Old Man from Thailand With Fever and a Papular Rash

JURI KATCHANOV AND HARTMUT STOCKER

Clinical Presentation

History

A 34-year-old man from Phuket, Thailand presents to a hospital in Germany with a 2-week history of fever. He has also noticed a papular rash affecting his whole body, particularly his face and trunk. When asked, he reports weight loss (7 kg in the last 3 months).

He lives in Thailand and arrived in Germany only 3 days previously to visit friends.

Clinical Findings

On examination, the patient is febrile with a temperature of 38.2°C (100.76°F). His conjunctivae are pale. He is very wasted, with a body mass index of 14 kg/m².

The patient has a generalized non-pruritic rash, predominantly on his face and trunk, which consists of small umbilicated papules (Fig. 17.1). There is generalized lymphadenopathy with visibly swollen lymph nodes in the left supraclavicular region; his inguinal and axillary lymph nodes are also enlarged. On abdominal examination, the spleen is palpable at two fingers below the left costal margin. The liver span is 15cm in the midclavicular line.

Laboratory Results

Full blood count: WBC 2.1 ×10⁹/L (reference range 4–10), haemoglobin 9.8 g/dL (13–16), platelets 110 ×10⁹/L (150–350). C-reactive protein 150 mg/L (<5).

Questions

1. What is the single most important test to be done in this patient?
2. What is your differential diagnosis?

Discussion

A 34-year-old man from Thailand presents with a 2-week history of fever and a 3-month history of wasting. On examination, he has mild hepatosplenomegaly, generalized lymphadenopathy and a papular rash. The laboratory results reveal pancytopenia and an elevated C-reactive protein.

Answer to Question 1
What is the Single Most Important Test to be Done in This Patient?

The most important test to be done is an HIV serology. The patient presents with fever, unexplained weight loss, lymphadenopathy and a papular rash; his blood results show pancytopenia. Each of these conditions alone should warrant HIV testing.

Answer to Question 2
What is Your Differential Diagnosis?

Common causes of fever, generalized lymphadenopathy and hepatosplenomegaly are infectious diseases and neoplasms.

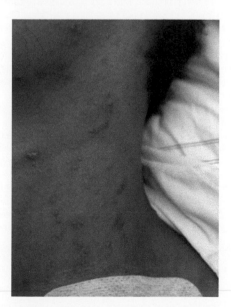

• **Fig. 17.1** Multiple umbilicated papular skin lesions on the neck.

Apart from HIV, CMV and EBV infection should be considered. All three of these viral infections may present with fever, hepatosplenomegaly and a rash, but umbilicated papular lesions are not part of the clinical picture. However, in HIV-infected individuals, mollusca contagiosa are common, which resemble the lesions seen in this patient.

Disseminated tuberculosis and infections with atypical mycobacteria are important differential diagnoses. Both can also present with cutaneous manifestations. An infection that resembles mycobacterioses in many ways is melioidosis. Melioidosis is one of the leading causes of community-acquired septicaemia in Thailand. It may present with lymphadenitis and disseminated papular skin lesions.

Bartonella spp. (*B. henselae, B. quintana*) cause bacillary angiomatosis in immunosuppressed individuals. Bacillary angiomatosis presents with non-specific systemic symptoms and umbilicated papular skin lesions. However, these papules are usually erythematous.

Fungal infections to consider in this patient are cryptococcosis, histoplasmosis and talaromycosis (previously penicilliosis), which are all commonly associated with immunosuppression but may also rarely occur in non-immunosuppressed individuals. All three may also present with umbilicated, papular skin lesions. Visceral leishmaniasis causes fever, wasting, hepatosplenomegaly and pancytopenia. It does however not cause a papular rash. It has been reported from Thailand, but appears to be uncommon.

Neoplasms to consider include lymphomas and non-malignant neoplastic conditions such as HHV-8-associated Castleman's disease.

The Case Continued...

The HIV test came back positive. The patient was found to be highly immunosuppressed, with a CD4 cell count of $2/\mu L$ (normal range: $500–1000/\mu L$).

Blood cultures were taken. A fine needle aspirate of the lymph node and a skin biopsy were performed, and the material was sent for microbiological and pathological work-up. Histopathology of the lymph node biopsy showed multiple yeast-like structures (Fig. 17.2). There were no acid-fast bacilli seen. The blood culture and cultures from the skin biopsy and lymph node all grew *Talaromyces (Penicillium) marneffei.*

The diagnosis of talaromycosis was made and the patient was started on a 2-week course of intravenous liposomal amphotericin B followed by oral itraconazole. On 3-week follow-up he was afebrile and gaining weight. Antiretroviral therapy (ART) was initiated.

Six months later the patient presented with a recurrence of his cervical lymphadenopathy. A talaromycosis relapse was suspected. However, this time an infection with atypical mycobacteria was found. His CD4 count had come up to

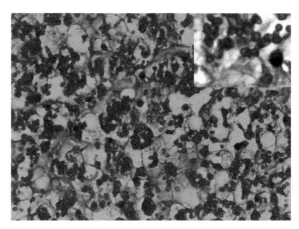

• **Fig. 17.2** Histology of the supraclavicular lymph node showing multiple round-shaped yeast-like structures (PAS stain, × 400). *Inset:* Prominent septal wall ('septation') as a result of reproduction by fission. (Courtesy U. Zimmermann, M. Grünbaum and H. Herbst.)

$102/\mu L$ and the viral load was suppressed. This second infection within 6 months after starting ART was interpreted as an immune reconstitution inflammatory syndrome (IRIS) of the unmasking type.

SUMMARY BOX

Talaromycosis (Penicilliosis)

Talaromycosis (previously penicilliosis) is caused by *Talaromyces (Penicillium) marneffei*, a dimorphic fungus endemic to East and South-east Asia. Incidence of talaromycosis has increased in parallel with the AIDS pandemic. It is the third commonest AIDS-related opportunistic infection in Thailand and Vietnam after tuberculosis and cryptococcosis. Talaromycosis has also been reported in immunosuppressed travellers to endemic areas. Acquisition and transmission of talaromycosis, either by inhalation or by direct inoculation, have not been fully understood; the only known hosts are humans and bamboo rats.

Talaromycosis usually affects severely immunocompromised individuals who frequently have other concurrent opportunistic infections. Patients present with non-specific symptoms such as prolonged fever, fatigue, weight loss and diarrhoea. Clinical signs are lymphadenopathy, hepatosplenomegaly and anaemia. Generalized umbilicated papular skin lesions can help the clinician narrow down the differential diagnosis. The papules are often located on the face, on the chest and on the extremities. Lung involvement is common and chest radiography may reveal diffuse reticulonodular or alveolar infiltrates.

Diagnosis is made by identification of the fungus by microscopy and culture. Blood, bronchoalveolar lavage fluid, or biopsies of skin, lymph nodes or bone marrow are appropriate clinical specimens. Microscopical examination reveals extracellular and intracellular yeasts. The extracellular forms often have a transverse septum as a result of binary fission.

Treatment is with intravenous amphotericin B for 2 weeks followed by oral itraconazole. Secondary prophylaxis in HIV-infected patients with itraconazole (200 mg od) has been suggested until a CD4-count of ≥ 100 cells/μL has been maintained for at least 6 months.

Further Reading

1. Wood R. Clinical features and management of HIV/AIDS. In: Farrar J, editor. Manson's Tropical Diseases. 23rd ed. London: Elsevier; 2014 [chapter 10].

2. Hay RJ. Fungal infections. In: Farrar J, editor. Manson's Tropical Diseases. 23rd ed. London: Elsevier; 2013 [chapter 38].

3. Chakrabarti A, Slavin MA. Endemic fungal infections in the Asia–Pacific region. Med Mycol 2011;49(4):337–344.

4. Chastain DB, Henao-Martínez AF, Franco-Paredes C. Opportunistic Invasive Mycoses in AIDS: Cryptococcosis, Histoplasmosis, Coccidiodomycosis, and Talaromycosis. Curr Infect Dis Rep 2017;19(10):36.

5. Le T, Kinh NV, Cuc NTK, et al. A Trial of Itraconazole or Amphotericin B for HIV-Associated Talaromycosis. N Engl J Med 2017;376(24):2329–2340.

18

A 56-Year-Old Man Returning from a Trip to Thailand With Eosinophilia

SEBASTIAN DIECKMANN AND RALF IGNATIUS

Clinical Presentation

History

A 56-year-old European man is referred to a local specialist clinic for further work-up of peripheral eosinophilia. Clinically, he suffers from fatigue and back pain. The patient returned from a 3-week round trip to Thailand 4 months ago.

He is known to have mild hypertension and suffered a transient ischaemic attack (TIA) 5 years ago. He has never experienced any allergic reactions. The patient has taken aspirin since suffering the TIA and an angiotensin receptor blocker (sartan) for 1 year.

Clinical Findings

The vital signs are normal, he is afebrile. His physical examination does not reveal any pathological findings.

Laboratory Results

The patient's full blood count is shown in Table 18.1.

Questions

1. How is eosinophilia defined and what is the differential diagnosis?
2. How do you narrow down your differential diagnosis in a traveller with eosinophilia?

Discussion

A 56-year-old European man presents with non-specific symptoms and pronounced peripheral blood eosinophilia. He has recently travelled to Thailand. He is on medications with low-dose aspirin and an angiotensin receptor blocker. His physical examination is unremarkable and he is afebrile.

TABLE 18.1 Full Blood Count Results on Admission

Parameter	Patient	Reference
WBC ($\times 10^9$/L)	8.6	4–10
Haemoglobin (g/dL)	14	12–15
Platelets ($\times 10^9$/L)	400	150–450
Basophils (%)	2	0–2
Eosinophils (%)	32	0–6
Total eosinophil count ($\times 10^9$/L)	2.75	<0.45
Neutrophils (%)	38	20–50
Band neutrophils (%)	0	0–5
Lymphocytes (%)	21	20–40
Monocytes (%)	7	0–10

Answer to Question 1

How is Eosinophilia Defined and What is the Differential Diagnosis?

Eosinophilia is usually defined as a total peripheral blood eosinophil count $>0.45 \times 10^9$/L. It can be caused by a whole variety of aetiologies (Table 18.2) and the differential diagnosis is wide.

In travellers or migrants from tropical and subtropical areas, the most common identifiable cause of eosinophilia is helminth infection. Ectoparasitic diseases such as scabies and myiasis may also cause eosinophilia, which usually is mild. Protozoal infections usually do not cause eosinophilia, with the exception of *Isospora belli* and *Sarcocystis* species infections, which may be accompanied by a mostly mild eosinophilia.

Bacterial, viral and fungal infections may cause eosinopaenia. One important exception is HIV infection, where immune dysregulation can lead to eosinophilia. Endemic

TABLE 18.2	Causes of Eosinophilia

Infections, in particular infections with tissue-invasive
  helminths
Convalescence from any infection
Allergies
Drug-induced
Connective tissue diseases
Idiopathic hypereosinophilic syndromes
Leukaemias and lymphomas
Paraneoplastic

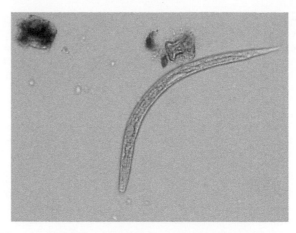

• **Fig. 18.1** Rhabditiform larva of *Strongyloides stercoralis* in a stool preparation (ether-based concentration, magnification 100 ×).

fungal infections associated with eosinophilia are coccidioidomycosis and paracoccidioidomycosis.

Answer to Question 2

How Do You Narrow Down Your Differential Diagnosis in a Traveller With Eosinophilia?

It is crucial to get a detailed history of possible exposures and concomitant symptoms. The travel history should include recent and past travel, because some causes of eosinophilia such as *Strongyloides stercoralis* infection or schistosomiasis may present after years, even decades.

Exposure to food items (e.g., salads, watercress, crabs, raw fish, snails and frogs) should be explicitly enquired. Patients should be asked about freshwater exposure (schistosomiasis) and contact with sand or soil (soil-transmitted helminths). However, negative exposure history does not rule out risk, because many patients simply do not recall their exposure.

Concomitant symptoms may also help narrow down the differential diagnosis. However, eosinophilia is asymptomatic in up to one-third of returning travellers and migrants. Common causes of asymptomatic eosinophilia include intestinal helminths (after migration through tissues), in particular hookworm infection and strongyloidiasis, and schistosomiasis.

The Case Continued...

Serology revealed antibodies against *Ascaris lumbricoides* while the serological tests for other helminth infections, including *S. stercoralis,* remained negative. However, larvae of *S. stercoralis* were detected in sediments of stool samples (Fig. 18.1). Upon single-dose treatment with ivermectin, the absolute eosinophil count (AEC) declined and the *A. lumbricoides* serology (most likely cross-reactive antibodies against *S. stercoralis*) turned negative.

The backpain, however, did not settle, and it was later discovered that it was caused by a slipped disc.

SUMMARY BOX

Strongyloidiasis

S. stercoralis is a human nematode without an animal reservoir. It is usually acquired by invasion of the intact skin or by auto-infection via the intestinal mucosa or perianal skin. Faecal-oral transmission is also possible.

Upon invasion, larvae of *S. stercoralis* migrate along the bloodstream, exit the blood vessels in the pulmonary alveoli and enter the airways where they are coughed up and swallowed to eventually reach the small intestine where they complete their life cycle.

Only female adults live in the small intestine and reproduce asexually by parthenogenesis (i.e. production of fertile eggs without fertilizing males). They release eggs from which non-infectious rhabditiform larvae hatch that are excreted in the stool. Eggs are rarely seen in stool specimens; the normal finding is live larvae.

Outside of the human host, larvae either mature into free-living male and female adult worms, which reproduce sexually, or transform into infectious filariform larvae ready to invade another host.

Alternatively, auto-infection is possible: in the gastrointestinal tract some larvae moult into infective filariform larvae and penetrate the gut wall or the perianal skin to enter the circulation. Auto-infection may result in decades of ongoing disease.

Strongyloidiasis may cause non-specific gastrointestinal symptoms, and sometimes swiftly moving cutaneous eruptions are noticed, especially on the trunk, which correspond to subcutaneously migrating larvae, a phenomenon called 'larva currens'. In the majority of patients, however, strongyloidiasis is asymptomatic.

In severely immunocompromised hosts, e.g. in association with steroid therapy, malignancies, chemotherapy or infection with HTLV-I, strongyloidiasis may disseminate and cause overwhelming life-threatening disease ('hyperinfection syndrome'). In advanced HIV infection, strongyloides hyperinfection syndrome has been described but seems to be uncommon.

Definitive diagnosis is made by detection of larvae in stool specimens using various techniques; however, false-negative results often occur because of intermittent larval excretion and low infectious burden. Indirect evidence may be provided by serology, but false-negative results are possible, as seen in our case. Furthermore, most serological tests become positive only 4 to 12 weeks post infection and may be negative when eosinophilia is first detected. False-positive serological results may occur because of cross-reacting antibodies against other helminths, particularly other nematodes.

The diagnosis is supported by clinical signs, such as 'larva currens', and eosinophilia, although the latter is not always present during chronic infection.

Treatment of choice is ivermectin (200µg/kg stat). Patients with *Strongyloides* infection returning from West or Central Africa and who might be co-infected with *L. loa* should be screened for microfilaraemia before receiving ivermectin. In patients unable to receive ivermectin, albendazole 400mg bd for 3 days is an alternative.

Because the diagnosis of strongyloidiasis is difficult, presumptive treatment with ivermectin or albendazole may be justified in individuals with eosinophilia, larva currens or a positive serology and a possible exposure to *S. stercoralis*.

Further Reading

1. Brooker S, Bundy DAP. Soil-transmitted helminths (Geohelminths). In: Farrar J, editor. Manson's Tropical Diseases. 23rd ed. London: Elsevier; 2013 [chapter 55].
2. Ming DK, Armstrong M, Lowe P, et al. Clinical and diagnostic features of 413 patients treated for imported Strongyloidiasis at the Hospital for Tropical Diseases, London. Am J Trop Med Hyg 2019;101(2):428–31.
3. Checkley AM, Chiodini PL, Dockrell DH, et al. Eosinophilia in returning travellers and migrants from the tropics: UK recommendations for investigation and initial management. J Infect 2010;60:1–20.
4. Afshar K, Vucinic V, Sharma OP. Eosinophil cell: pray tell us what you do!. Curr Opin Pulm Med 2007;13:414–21.
5. Puthiyakunnon S, Bossu S, Li Y, et al. Strongyloidiasis – an insight into its global prevalence and management. PLoS Negl Trop Dis 2014;8(8):e3018.

19

A 40-Year-Old Man from Togo With Subcutaneous Nodules and Corneal Opacities

GUIDO KLUXEN

Clinical Presentation

History

A 40-year-old man from Togo presents to a local clinic. He has noticed changes in both of his eyes over the past 4 years. There are no visual disturbances, but he is worried: In his village there are adults in each family who have turned completely blind after their eyes had shown features very similar to the changes he has noticed in his own eyes.

He has also observed some painless bumps under his skin which have developed over the past two decades. The patient also complains of suffering from intense itching of his skin that keeps him awake at night.

The patient has always lived in a village in the savannah near a fast-flowing river. He reports that small biting flies are common near the river.

Clinical Findings

There are opacities in the cornea of both eyes. The patient's left eye is shown in Figure 19.1.

The skin appears atrophic in some areas (thinning with loss of elasticity), and there are multiple scratch marks. Subcutaneous nodules are palpable in various regions of his body, especially over bony prominences like the ribs (Fig. 19.2), iliac crest, femoral trochanters and on the head. The nodules are firm, non-tender and measure 1 to 3 cm in diameter.

Questions

1. What is your most important differential diagnosis?
2. What investigations would you like to carry out?

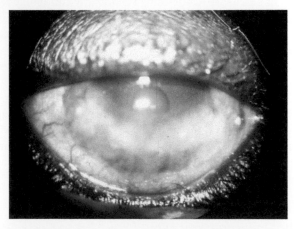

• **Fig. 19.1** The patient's left eye showing corneal opacities. (Courtesy H. Trojan)

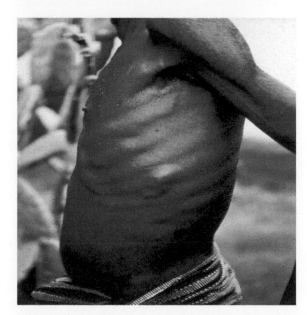

• **Fig. 19.2** Subcutaneous nodule over the costal arch. (Courtesy H. Trojan)

Discussion

The patient presents with a triad of corneal opacities, skin changes and subcutaneous nodules. He comes from a village in the North of Togo, located close to a rapidly flowing river. Many adults in the village are blind.

Answer to Question 1

What is Your Most Important Differential Diagnosis?

The clinical triad of ocular changes, itchy dermatitis with atrophy of the skin and subcutaneous nodules in a patient from rural Togo makes onchocerciasis (river blindness) the most likely differential diagnosis. A fast-flowing river is the preferred breeding site for *Simulium* blackflies, which transmit the disease.

The picture of his left eye shows keratitis semilunaris, a form of band-shaped sclerosing keratopathy commonly seen in onchocerciasis. The central and upper parts of the cornea are initially clear, but may become affected as the disease progresses.

Subcutaneous nodules can resemble lipomas and cysticerci of *Taenia solium*.

Pruritic dermatitis may also be caused by scabies or be seen in papular pruritic eruptions associated with HIV infection. In patients from West Africa, infection with *Mansonella streptocerca* can also cause pruritus. Chronic dermatitis can also be seen in yaws, leprosy, mycotic infections and eczema.

Answer to Question 2

What Investigations Would You Like to Carry Out?

The patient's presentation appears very typical for onchocerciasis. In an endemic, resource-limited setting his diagnosis would most probably be made on clinical grounds alone. Skin snips taken from the vicinity of a subcutaneous nodule may show microfilariae of *Onchocerca volvulus*.

Slit-lamp examination of the eyes may reveal microfilariae in the anterior chamber of the eye and in the cornea. Nodulectomy of subcutaneous nodules may show adults of *O. volvulus*, but this is not routinely done.

Serological tests were less useful in patients from endemic areas in the past, because antibody test results lacked specificity and were not clearly linked to clinical disease.

However, serological tests which detect IgG4 responses to *O. volvulus* antigen (OvAg) and the recombinant Ov16 antigen are recommended by WHO. In case of a positive result it is recommended to continue ivermectin therapy.

The lifespan of the adult worms is about 12 years. After 10 years, usually no further treatment with ivermectin is required after therapy with a combination of ivermectin and doxycycline, if ivermectin was administered 2 to 3 times every year and if serological tests have turned negative. However, in onchocerciasis-endemic areas new infections are possible. To calculate the probability of a reinfection through an individual black fly with *O. volvulus*,

worm-specific DNA (Ov150) is tested by poolscreen in vector samples (black flies) using polymerase chain reaction.

The Case Continued…

The patient was treated with ivermectin (150 µg/kg) STAT which was repeated after 3 months and after 1 year. He also received doxycycline 100 mg/d for 6 weeks (see Summary Box).

SUMMARY BOX

Onchocerciasis

Onchocerciasis ('river blindness') is caused by *O. volvulus,* a filarial nematode. It is transmitted by biting *Simulium* species blackflies, which breed in rapidly flowing freshwater. Adult females of *O. volvulus* lodge in human subcutaneous tissue and shed live microfilariae. Microfilariae migrate through the skin and often into the eyes. Most pathology is caused by immune reactions to dead and dying microfilariae and perhaps to their endosymbiotic *Wolbachia* bacteria. Typical clinical features of onchocerciasis are:

1. Non-tender subcutaneous nodules located mainly over bony prominences
2. Dermatitis, depigmentation of the skin ('leopard skin'), lichenification and thickening of the skin ('lizard skin'), and skin atrophy at times leading to 'hanging groins'. The skin changes may be stigmatizing and the unrelenting itch may cause sleep disturbances, depression and even lead to suicide
3. Ocular changes may present as pear-shaped pupil, punctate subepithelial stromal keratopathy, sclerosing keratitis, iritis, uveitis, 'flecked retina' or scarred choroidoretinal fundus (Hissette–Ridley fundus). Optic nerve atrophy may occur.

Ivermectin is now the drug of choice for individual and mass treatment of onchocerciasis. Ivermectin kills microfilariae but has little effect on adult worms apart from reducing embryogenesis. It has to be given repeatedly throughout the lifespan of the adult worm (10–14 years). For individual treatment, ivermectin is provided as a single dose of 150 µg/kg PO. Treatment should be repeated in 3- to 6-month intervals. In mass treatment programmes it is usually provided annually. Ivermectin should not be given to patients with heavy *Loa loa* infections and microfilarial counts greater than 30,000/mL, because this may result in fatal encephalitis. Ivermectin can also cause significant adverse events in patients with lower microfilarial counts. For regions co-endemic of onchocerciasis and *L. loa*, a mobile phone-based, point-of-care microscopy tool – the LoaScope – has proven helpful to easily identify patients with high parasitaemia of *L. loa* and to exempt them from mass treatment with ivermectin. This technology has increased the acceptance of ivermectin MDA for onchocerciasis and lymphatic filariasis in *L. loa* co-endemic areas.

Ivermectin is contraindicated in pregnancy and in children below the age of five or below a height of 90 cm.

Doxycycline at a dosage of 100 to 200 mg/d for 4 to 6 weeks kills the *Wolbachia* endosymbionts, permanently sterilizes adult worms, blocks embryogenesis and slowly kills approximately 60% of adult worms.

A major breakthrough in the battle against onchocerciasis was the ivermectin-donation programme initiated by the producing company Merck. Large control programmes implementing mass drug administration (MDA) of ivermectin in endemic areas in Africa and South America lead to interruption of transmission of onchocerciasis in many countries.

Elimination of the disease is still on the agenda.

Further Reading

1. Simonsen P, Fischer PU, Hoerauf A, et al. The filariases. In: Farrar J, editor. Manson's Tropical Diseases. 23rd ed. London: Elsevier; 2013 [chapter 54].

2. D'Ambrosio MV, Bakalar M, Bennuru S, et al. Point-of-care quantification of blood-borne filarial parasites with a mobile phone microscope. Sci Transl Med 2015;7(286):1–10.

3. Cantey PT, Roy SL, Boakye D, Mwingira U, Ottesen EA, Hopkins AD, Sodahlon YK. Transitioning from river blindness control to elimination: steps towards stopping treatment. Int Health 2018;10:i7–i13. https://doi.org/10.1093/inthealth/ihx049.

4. WHO. 2017 Onchocerciasis guidelines for stopping mass drug administration and verifying the elimination of human onchocerciasis, Available from: http://apps.who.int/iris/bitstream/handle/10665/204180/9789241510011_eng.pdf?sequence=1.

5. Lawrence J, Sodahlon YK. Onchocerciasis: the beginning of the end. Int Health 2018;10:i1–i2. https://doi.org/10.1093/inthealth/ihx070.

20

A 43-Year-Old Male Traveller Returning from Mozambique With Fever and Eosinophilia

GERD-DIETER BURCHARD

Clinical Presentation

History

A 43-year-old German man presents to a local travel clinic on 21 May because of fever. He had been in Mozambique from 16 April to 30 April, and travelled to Chile afterwards from 30 April to 17 May. He did not take any malaria chemoprophylaxis in Mozambique and reports self-treatment for malaria with atovaquone/proguanil because of fever (27 April to 29 April). He is now complaining of recurrent fever for the past 3 days. The day before presentation his temperature was as high as 39.8°C (103.6°F). He also has some headache and diarrhoea.

He reports freshwater contact in a small lake near Maputo. His past medical history is unremarkable.

Clinical Findings

43-year-old male, febrile, with a temperature of 39.2°C (102.6°F). The rest of the physical examination is normal and there is no rash, no hepatomegaly, no splenomegaly and no lymphadenopathy.

Laboratory Results

The relevant laboratory results on admission are shown in Table 20.1.

Further Investigations

Electrocardiogram is normal. Chest radiography reveals some nodular lesions ranging in size from 2 to 5 mm in the periphery of the lower lung zones bilaterally (Fig. 20.1); this finding is confirmed by a CT scan of his chest.

TABLE 20.1	Laboratory Results on Admission		
Parameter		**Patient**	**Reference**
WBC (×10⁹/L)		9.0	4–11.3
Eosinophils (×10⁹/L)		2.1	<0.5
LDH (U/L)		422	135–225
Creatinine (µmol/L)		88.4	53–106
AST/GOT (U/L)		106	10–50
ALT/GPT (U/L)		179	10–50
GGT (U/L)		186	<65
C-reactive protein (mg/L)		57.9	<5

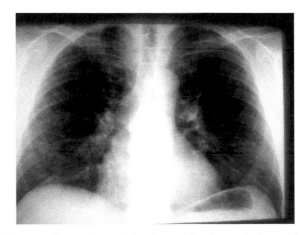

• **Fig. 20.1** Chest radiograph showing nodular changes in the periphery of both lungs.

Questions

1. What are your differential diagnoses and which investigations would you like to do?
2. What is the significance of eosinophilia in returning travellers?

Discussion

A 43-year-old man presents with of a 3-day history of high fever. He has recently returned from a 5-week trip to Mozambique and Chile. He did not take any malarial chemoprophylaxis, but he took standby emergency treatment for presumed malaria when feeling febrile about 3 weeks ago. He reports freshwater contact in Mozambique. On examination he is febrile. His FBC shows eosinophilia with a normal total white cell count. His liver enzymes, lactate dehydrogenase (LDH) and C-reactive protein (CRP) are slightly raised. Chest radiography and CT show small, nodular changes in the periphery of both lungs.

Answer to Question 1

What Are Your Differential Diagnoses and Which Investigations Would You Like to Do?

The patient has travelled in Mozambique without taking any antimalarial chemoprophylaxis. Thus first of all malaria has to be excluded – irrespective of any other symptoms or laboratory results.

The differential diagnosis of pyrexia in a returned traveller is long, but typhoid fever and amoebic liver abscess should always be excluded because they are common and potentially life-threatening diseases. Therefore blood cultures should be taken and an abdominal ultrasound should be done. In contrast to what was seen in this patient though, typhoid fever usually causes eosinopaenia.

The further differential diagnosis of fever after a stay in tropical areas relies on the precise itinerary, the activities indulged in during travel, the presence of focal symptoms, signs and laboratory results.

The patient has slightly elevated liver enzymes. The differential diagnosis of acute infections involving the liver includes viral hepatitis, including hepatitis E.

EBV and CMV infections may also cause fever, elevated liver enzymes and a rise in LDH. They are important differentials of fever in returned travellers. However, EBV and CMV cause lymphocytosis with atypical lymphocytes, rather than eosinophilia. Splenomegaly is usually part of the clinical picture of mononucleosis and lymphadenopathy, even though the latter can be less prominent in acute CMV infection.

Leptospirosis, rickettsioses and Q-fever are bacterial infections to consider, as well as brucellosis, secondary syphilis and relapsing fever. Yet none of these infections as such would explain the patient's pronounced eosinophilia.

Answer to Question 2

What is the Significance of Eosinophilia in Returning Travellers?

In any patient returning from the tropics with eosinophilia, a helminth infection should be ruled out. The most relevant differential diagnosis in this patient who presents with eosinophilia and fever reporting freshwater contact is acute schistosomiasis, also known as Katayama syndrome. Another rare cause of fever, eosinophilia and elevated liver transaminases is acute fascioliasis.

The Case Continued…

Thick films for *Plasmodium* species were negative. Microscopy of stool and urine samples for *Schistosoma* eggs were three times negative.

The patient was tested for antischistosomal antibodies using an enzyme-immunoassay and an immunofluorescence assay (IFA); both came back negative.

Four weeks later antischistosomal antibodies could be detected (IFA 1:1280, cercarial- and egg-ELISA positive). *S. mansoni* ova were found in the stool and a diagnosis of schistosomiasis was established. The patient was treated with praziquantel.

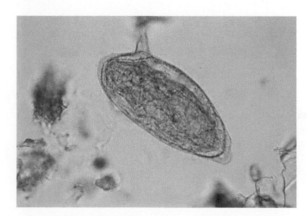

• **Fig. 20.2** Schistosoma mansoni egg.

SUMMARY BOX

Acute Schistosomiasis (Katayama Syndrome)

Acute schistosomiasis (Katayama syndrome) is an acute hypersensitivity reaction caused by newly expressed antigens on developing worms. It is named after the Katayama region in Japan, where it was first described.

Katayama syndrome usually occurs 2 to 12 weeks after *Schistosoma* infection. It is characterized by fever, urticaria and a dry cough sometimes accompanied by a wheeze. Patchy pulmonary infiltrates or micronodular changes in the lower lung zones may be present on chest radiograph. Full blood count in the majority of cases shows eosinophilia, but of note, eosinophilia can occur with a delay of several weeks after the onset of symptoms and may be missed. Most patients recover spontaneously after 2 to 10 weeks. Rarely, neurological complications can occur, e.g. transverse myelitis, conus medullaris or cauda equina syndrome.

Diagnosis of acute schistosomiasis can be challenging. *Schistosoma* ova (Fig. 20.2) may still be absent from urine or stool at this early stage and serological tests can take up to 3 months to become positive. As a consequence, these investigations have to be repeated several times after the diagnosis has been clinically suspected. PCR-based methods are promising for the diagnosis of acute *Schistosoma* infection in recently primarily exposed populations such as travellers.

Praziquantel has a lack of activity against immature flukes and severe reactions have been reported after praziquantel treatment during the acute phase. Therefore antiparasitic treatment should be delayed until the flukes are adult, i.e. until eggs can be detected in stool or urine.

Under certain circumstances, such as severe symptoms and in particular neurological complications, supportive steroid therapy may be useful in Katayama syndrome.

Of note, different stages of the parasite life cycle may overlap in a patient who is infected with many schistosomules. Therefore control examinations after several months are necessary and treatment with praziquantel may have to be repeated.

Further Reading

1. Bustinduy AL, King CH. Schistosomiasis. In: Farrar J, editor. Manson's Tropical Diseases. 23rd ed. London: Elsevier; 2014 [chapter 52].
2. Langenberg MCC, Hoogerwerf MA, Janse JJ, et al. Katayama syndrome without *Schistosoma mansoni* eggs. Ann Intern Med 2019;170(10):732–3.
3. Checkley AM, Chiodini PL, Dockrell DH, et al. Eosinophilia in returning travellers and migrants from the tropics: UK recommendations for investigation and initial management. J Infect 2010; 60(1):1–20.
4. Logan S, Armstrong M, Moore E, et al. Acute schistosomiasis in travelers: 14 years' experience at the Hospital for Tropical Diseases, London. Am J Trop Med Hyg 2013;88(6):1032–4.
5. Bonneford S, Cnops L, Duvignaud A, et al. Early complicated schistosomiasis in a returning traveller: Key contribution of new molecular diagnostic methods. Intern J Inf Dis 2019;79:72–4.

21

A 35-Year-Old American Man With Fatigue and a Neck Lesion

MARY E. WRIGHT AND ARTHUR M. FRIEDLANDER

Clinical Presentation

History

A 35-year-old Caucasian male presents to a clinic in the United States with fatigue and a rash on his neck that started as a papule 2 days earlier. The lesion is non-pruritic, but it is associated with significant non-painful swelling and a pressure sensation in the neck. There is no history of fever, but the patient reports at least one episode of diaphoresis with mild confusion and headache.

The patient recalls a break in the skin at the site of the lesion 3 days before while shaving and is sure that he has not been bitten by an insect. He has had no contact with animals and no foreign travel within the previous year.

He had come to the clinic 24 hours earlier with similar symptoms. After blood cultures were obtained, he was given one dose of a first-generation cephalosporin and discharged on a ten-day oral course. He returns because of worsening malaise and neck swelling associated with mild difficulty breathing.

The past medical history is unremarkable. The patient is a postal worker by profession.

Clinical Findings

Examination reveals a 2cm irregularly shaped, indurated non-tender patch on the left anterior neck with mild overlying erythema and several 2 to 3 mm vesicles. The main lesion has a 6 mm shallow ulceration. There is massive neck oedema making lymph nodes difficult to assess (see Fig. 21.1). His neck circumference had increased from 57 cm at baseline to a peak of 81 cm. Temperature is 36.9°C (98.4°F), pulse 118 bpm, blood pressure 138/90 mmHg and respiratory rate 20 breath cycles per minute. The remainder of the initial physical examination is normal.

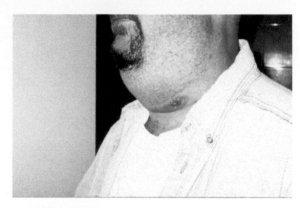

• **Fig. 21.1** Papulovesicular lesion with extensive neck oedema 2 days after the onset of a small papule.

Investigations

Full blood count, Na⁺, K⁺, Cl⁻ HCO₃, BUN, creatinine and random glucose are normal except for a mildly elevated haemoglobin at 18.7 g/dL (reference range: 13.0–18.0 g/dL).

Questions

1. What are the distinguishing features of this lesion that help narrow down your differential diagnosis?
2. What investigations need to be performed to establish early diagnosis and appropriate treatment?

Discussion

A 35-year-old male postal worker presents to a clinic in the United States with a papulovesicular lesion on his neck associated with massive neck swelling. There is no fever but diaphoresis is present. The patient's condition is worsening despite antibiotic therapy with an oral cephalosporin.

Answer to Question 1

What Are the Distinguishing Features of This Lesion that Help Narrow Down Your Differential Diagnosis?

The differential diagnosis of an ulcerative skin lesion with concomitant massive soft tissue swelling and systemic symptoms depends on the epidemiological setting and the individual exposure; it includes bacterial ecthyma *(Streptococcus pyogenes, Staphylococcus aureus)*, rickettsial diseases, necrotic arachnidism (bite by brown recluse spider), rat-bite fevers *Streptococcus moniliformis* and *(Spirillum minus)*, ulceroglandular tularaemia and bubonic plague.

At the time of the patient's presentation, the United States was in the process of investigating a possible event of bioterrorism. Therefore the most important, though overall rare, diagnosis to consider was cutaneous anthrax.

There may be few distinguishing features at the time of presentation, depending on the age of the lesion. Although it is commonly known that cutaneous anthrax is manifested by a central black eschar, this is not seen until approximately a week after inoculation. The anthrax lesion begins as a painless papule that lasts 1 to 2 days before becoming a vesicle that later ruptures. It then develops the classic necrotic central ulcer and may be surrounded by smaller peripheral vesicles. Therefore a patient may present with a non-specific localized papulovesicular eruption. Key associated findings include a preceding history of a break in the skin at the affected site, the presence of systemic symptoms such as malaise and headache and extensive, non-tender oedema. Fever and leukocytosis may not be present. In parts of the world where anthrax is endemic, zoonotic exposure to infected animals or contaminated animal products is important to establish, whereas exposure from a bioterrorism act may not be immediately apparent.

Answer to Question 2

What Investigations Need to be Performed to Establish Early Diagnosis and Appropriate Treatment?

Aspirate of fluid from the skin lesion should be sent for Gram stain, culture and susceptibilities along with blood cultures in patients with systemic symptoms regardless of fever status. In the absence of preceding antimicrobial therapy, numerous Gram-positive rods in high concentration will grow within 24 hours. Empirical antibacterial treatment with a quinolone or doxycycline should be instituted while awaiting microbiological results. Because negative cultures do not exclude anthrax, full-thickness punch biopsy from the vesicle and the eschar should be obtained, fixed in 10% buffered formalin and sent to a specialized laboratory for nucleic acid amplification and immunohistochemical (IHC) staining to detect *Bacillus anthracis* antigens. Serum should also be tested for antibodies to the protective antigen at baseline and 4 weeks later.

The Case Continued...

Blood cultures taken at the first clinic visit grew gram-positive rods. Gram stain and culture of the skin lesion obtained at the second visit were negative for *B. anthracis*. The patient was admitted and received intravenous levofloxacin and ampicillin-sulbactam and recovered. Stains for bacteria and IHC of the skin biopsy performed at a reference laboratory showed abundant bacilli in the dermis and the presence of *B. anthracis* antigens, respectively. Serology revealed that antibody to protective antigen was present in convalescent serum.

The patient was exposed during his occupation as a postal worker, handling contaminated mail. Overall, 22 cases were identified, of which 11 presented with cutaneous anthrax, and a further 11 fell ill with the inhalational form. Five people died; all deaths occurred secondary to inhalational anthrax.

SUMMARY BOX

Anthrax

Anthrax is caused by *B. anthracis,* a Gram-positive rod that forms spores under certain environmental conditions. It is primarily a zoonotic disease affecting domestic and wild herbivores. Anthrax remains endemic in animals worldwide, most importantly in Asia, Africa and South-eastern Australia, as well as parts of the southern and western United States. Humans usually acquire the infection when they are exposed to infected animals or animal products, but anthrax has also been used as an agent of bioterrorism. In the developed world, cases usually tend to be sporadic. In resource-limited countries anthrax remains a relevant public health problem and large outbreaks can occasionally occur.

Depending on the route of entry, *B. anthracis* can cause cutaneous, gastrointestinal or inhalational disease. Cutaneous anthrax is the most common form worldwide, accounting for 95% of all human cases. Although only a small percentage develop systemic disease, it can be lethal if not treated quickly.

The clinical marker lesion is a painless central ulcer with vesicles and extensive surrounding oedema, but the initial lesion will appear as a non-specific papulovesicular eruption.

History includes recent exposure to infected animals or contaminated animal products, unless the setting is a bioterrorism event, a previous break in the skin at the affected site and the presence of systemic symptoms in disseminated disease. A high index of suspicion is critical to the diagnosis. Differential diagnosis of cutaneous anthrax depends on the setting and the individual exposures; it includes bacterial ecthyma, rickettsial diseases, rat-bite fevers, necrotic arachnidism, ulceroglandular tularaemia and bubonic plague.

Gram stain and culture of affected fluids (blood, skin lesion aspirate, pleural fluid) and paired serological testing for antibodies to protective antigen remain the cornerstone of diagnosis. However, negative cultures do not exclude anthrax. In cutaneous anthrax, full-thickness punch biopsy from the vesicle and eschar should be fixed and sent to a specialized laboratory for PCR and immunohistochemical staining. Empirical antibacterial treatment with a quinolone or doxycycline should be instituted while awaiting results for limited cutaneous infection. When disseminated infection or other forms of anthrax are suspected, multi-drug therapy that includes those with CNS penetration should be used.

Although 7 to 10 days of antibiotic treatment are usually sufficient in cutaneous anthrax, up to 60 days of antibiotics are needed in inhalational disease because of the possibility of retained ungerminated spores in the lungs. Prevention of anthrax involves either prevention of exposure in occupational settings or immunization. In the setting of a suspected bioterrorism event, those at risk of exposure should receive a 60-day course of postexposure prophylaxis with oral antibiotics.

Further Reading

1. Eitzen E. Anthrax. In: Farrar J, editor. Manson's Tropical Diseases. 23rd ed. London: Elsevier; 2013 [chapter 31].

2. Carlson CJ, Kracalik IT, Ross N, et al. The global distribution of *Bacillus anthracis* and associated anthrax risk to humans, livestock and wildlife. Nat Microbiol 2019;4:1337–43.

3. Gold H. Anthrax: a report of one hundred seventeen cases. AMA Arch Intern Med 1955;96(3):387–96.

4. Shieh WJ, Guarner J, Paddock C, et al. The critical role of pathology in the investigation of bioterrorism-related cutaneous anthrax. Am J Pathol 2003;163(5):1901–10.

5. Hendricks KA, Wright ME, Shadomy SV, et al. Centers for Disease Control and Prevention expert panel meetings on prevention and treatment of anthrax in adults. Emerg Infect Dis 2014;20(2). https://doi.org/10.3201/eid2002.130687.

22

32-Year-Old Woman from Nigeria With Jaundice and Confusion

CHRISTOPHER J.M. WHITTY

Clinical Presentation

History

A 32-year-old, previously fit woman of African descent born in Europe, travelled to rural Jos in Nigeria to visit relatives. According to her husband, 18 days after her return to Europe she developed a fever, and 3 days later became very unwell with abnormal behaviour.

Clinical Findings

On examination she has a temperature of 37.5°C (99.5°F), is mildly jaundiced and confused; her Glasgow Coma Scale is 14/15. She has no rash or palpable lymph nodes, and throat and sclerae are not injected. She has some fine crepitations at the lung bases.

Laboratory Results

The laboratory refuses to undertake tests because of recent rural exposure in an area known to have viral haemorrhagic fever (Lassa).

Questions

1. What is the differential diagnosis?
2. Is viral haemorrhagic fever (VHF) a real risk, and which single test is the most important?

Discussion

A young woman presents with a fever, jaundice and confusion almost 3 weeks after returning from a visit to rural Nigeria. The patient is of African ethnicity but was born in Europe.

Answer to Question 1
What is the Differential Diagnosis?

The differential diagnosis is wide, but by some distance the most common cause of fever and jaundice or fever and confusion in West Africa is severe falciparum malaria. The fact that the patient had a low-grade fever at presentation is not a

reason to exclude malaria, because the temperature swings in malaria and a significant proportion of cases are apyrexial at presentation. A common misdiagnosis is acute viral hepatitis; there, fever precedes the jaundice, and this rapid fulminant course would not be typical. Other causes of acute fever and jaundice include typhoid fever, leptospirosis and ascending cholangitis. Patients with advanced HIV disease and Gram-negative sepsis can also present like this.

People returning from visiting friends and relatives constitute a large proportion of imported malaria and are at high risk of not taking antimalarial prophylaxis. A woman born in Europe would be unlikely to have any immunity to malaria.

Answer to Question 2
Is Viral Haemorrhagic Fever (VHF) a Real Risk, and which Single Test is Most Important?

The laboratory is right to raise VHF as a possible diagnosis, but VHF is very rare and 18 days (or more) since leaving the high-risk area is on the outer limit of the incubation period of Lassa fever and other VHF (generally up to 21 days). The absence of injected sclerae or rash is also against the diagnosis. A malaria blood film would be mandatory in this case. If it is positive, the woman could be treated as malaria and other tests taken with standard universal precautions.

The Case Continued...

The patient was found to have a *Plasmodium falciparum* parasite count of 18% and a plasma creatinine of 430 μmol/L (reference range 45–90 μmol/L), demonstrating acute kidney injury. Urine output failed to respond to fluid challenges, therefore pre-renal failure could be ruled out. She was treated with intravenous artesunate and the parasite count dropped to 5% but she lapsed into deep coma. Renal function deteriorated and she needed haemofiltration. After the parasites had cleared on day 5, her consciousness level began to improve, but she developed laboured breathing. The chest radiography findings were suggestive of ARDS, and she required prolonged respiratory support. She eventually made a full recovery.

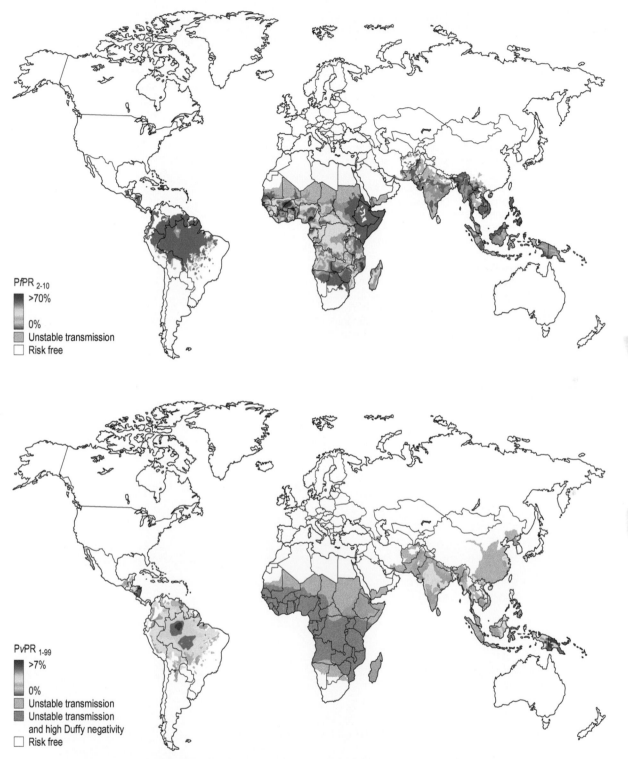

• **Fig. 22.1 Global distribution of *Plasmodium falciparum* and *Plasmodium vivax* malaria.** Upper panel shows the model-based geostatistical point (MBG) estimates of the *Plasmodium falciparum* annual mean parasite rate PfPR2–10 (defined as the predicted proportion of 2–10-year-olds with patent parasitaemia) for 2010 within the spatial limits of stable *P. falciparum* malaria transmission. Lower panel shows equivalent estimates of the *Plasmodium vivax* annual mean parasite rate (PvPR1–99). Note this prediction is for all age groups (1–99). Areas in which the Duffy negativity gene frequency is predicted to exceed 90% are shown in hatching. (Reproduced from Farrar, J. et al., 2013. Manson's Tropical Diseases, 23rd ed. Elsevier, London. Fig. 43.1.)

SUMMARY BOX

Malaria

Malaria is the most common life-threatening infection in patients who have recently arrived from Africa. It is also common, but much less so, from South and South-east Asia (Fig. 22.1).

A history of fever is usual in non-immune patients, but other features of the presentation are non-specific and overlap with many other infections, with headache and malaise. Malaria should always be high on the list of differential diagnoses for any unwell patient from the tropics, because there are many misleading presentations.

The only way to exclude malaria is a malaria blood test. Diagnosed early before complications begin, falciparum malaria is relatively easily treated with antimalarial drug combinations. In patients with severe malaria, artesunate is the drug of choice; if this is not available locally, artemether or quinine are the alternatives.

In adults, cerebral malaria (for practical purposes altered consciousness, seizures), acute renal failure and pulmonary oedema or ARDS are the most common manifestations of severity, and may occur together or in any combination. Renal failure, and in particular ARDS, often presents later in treatment, and may first become apparent after all parasites have cleared. Disseminated intravascular coagulation and shock (often with co-existing bacteraemia) are rare complications. Elderly patients have a high mortality. Various adjunctive treatments for malaria complications have been tried but to date none shows survival advantage. The key to malaria management is to diagnose it early and get effective antimalarial drugs into the patient as soon as possible.

Further Reading

1. White NJ. Malaria. In: Farrar J, editor. Manson's Tropical Diaseses. 23rd ed. London: Elsevier; 2013 [chapter 43].
2. Checkley AM, Smith A, Smith V, et al. Risk factors for mortality from imported falciparum malaria in the United Kingdom over 20 years: an observational study. BMJ 2012;344:e2116.
3. WHO Global Malaria Programme. Management of Severe Malaria – A Practical Handbook. 3rd ed. Geneva: WHO; 2013.
4. Ashley EA, Phyo AP, Woodrow CJ. Malaria. Lancet 2018;391:1608–21.

23

A 31-Year-Old HIV-Positive Business Traveller With Cough, Shortness of Breath and Night Sweats

ROBERT F. MILLER

Clinical Presentation

History

A 31-year-old HIV-positive man presents to the Emergency Department of a London hospital. He has a 6-week history of increasing shortness of breath on exertion, dry cough, and drenching night sweats. He also reports general fatigue and a weight loss of about 10 kg over the past 5 months.

He travels extensively for business and in the past 6 months has had work trips to Europe, China, Korea, Japan, Singapore and the United States. He lives with his male partner, denies any recreational drug use and has never smoked tobacco. He was diagnosed with HIV 6 years ago. He says that 1 month ago his CD4 was 280/µL. He is not yet on antiretroviral therapy (ART), nor on co-trimoxazole prophylaxis or any other regular medications. There is no other significant past medical history.

Clinical Findings

He is alert, short of breath at rest but able to complete full sentences. Temperature 39.2°C (102.6°F), blood pressure 120/70 mmHg, pulse 100 bpm, respiratory rate 26 breaths per minute, sO$_2$ 87% on air, and 97% on 15 L O$_2$. Chest is clear on auscultation. The rest of the physical examination is unremarkable.

Laboratory results

His arterial blood gases on air are shown in Table 23.1.

His FBC is normal. CRP is 6.7 mg/dL (<5). Creatinine, urea, bilirubin, ALT, AP and albumin are normal. CD4 150/µL, HIV viral load 1 500 000 copies/mL (fully sensitive on resistance testing).

TABLE 23.1 Arterial Blood Gases on Ambient Air

Parameter	Patient	Reference Range
pH	7.44	7.35–7.45
Pao$_2$ (kPa)	7.6	10.67–13.33
Paco$_2$ (kPa)	3	4.67–6.00
HCO$_3$ (mmol/L)	19	22–26
Base excess (mmol/L)	-3.8	± 2
Lactate (mmol/L)	1.6	0.5–1.6

Chest Radiography

His chest radiograph is shown in Figure 23.1.

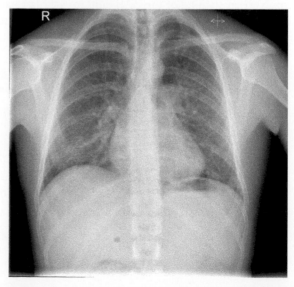

• **Fig. 23.1** Chest radiograph on admission, showing bilateral perihilar infiltrates.

Questions

1. What further investigations would you perform in order to confirm the diagnosis?
2. What is your immediate management of the patient?

Discussion

An HIV-positive man who is not yet on ART presents with progressive shortness of breath, dry cough and drenching night sweats, with associated significant weight loss. He has a history of extensive work-related travel. He is febrile with type 1 respiratory failure and bilateral perihilar infiltrates seen on chest radiography. Routine laboratory tests are normal, except for a very slightly elevated CRP, his CD4-count is low.

Answer to Question 1

What Further Investigations Would You Perform to Confirm the Diagnosis?

Pneumocystis pneumonia (PCP) should be high up in the differential of any ART-naïve, HIV-positive patient with a low CD4 count, who presents with progressive shortness of breath on exertion and dry cough, with patchy perihilar infiltrates on the chest radiograph. Tuberculosis, atypical bacterial pneumonia, cryptococcosis or histoplasmosis should also be considered. Serum 1,3 β-D-glucan (β-glucan) is frequently elevated in patients with PCP. Although the β-glucan assay has a high sensitivity for PCP, the specificity of an elevated β-glucan for PCP diagnosis is low because other fungal infections, such as histoplasmosis, some drugs including amoxicillin-clavulanate or piperacillin-tazobactam, and cellulose membranes used for haemodialysis can elevate β-glucan levels. Bronchoscopy and immunofluorescence or Grocott methenamine silver staining of bronchoalveolar lavage (BAL) specimens are the diagnostic tests of choice. Ziehl–Neelsen staining of the BAL fluid for acid-fast bacilli (AFB) should also be requested. Similar staining of induced sputum is a less sensitive alternative. Polymerase chain reaction (PCR) is highly sensitive and specific for detecting *Pneumocystis* in BAL fluid or induced sputum. However, PCR cannot reliably distinguish colonization from active disease, although higher organism loads, as determined by quantitative PCR, likely represent clinically significant disease. CD4 count should be requested as well.

Answer to Question 2

What is Your Immediate Management of the Patient?

Correction of hypoxia aiming for oxygen saturation greater than 95% is top priority. Some patients will require CPAP or ventilatory support in addition to oxygen therapy. High-dose co-trimoxazole is first-line treatment for PCP; this may be given IV in severe respiratory failure or if the patient is unable to tolerate oral therapy. In moderate to severe PCP (Table 23.2) corticosteroids should be added. Standard starting dose is prednisolone 40 mg bid or methylprednisolone 30 mg bid, IV if unable to tolerate PO.

The Case continued…

The patient was treated with high-flow oxygen and started on high-dose co-trimoxazole plus prednisolone combined with a proton-pump inhibitor. His tachycardia settled with reversal of his hypoxia and he remained otherwise stable. In view of his multiple recent long-haul flights a computed tomography (CT)-pulmonary angiogram was performed to rule out pulmonary embolism (Fig. 23.2). This showed extensive "ground-glass" infiltrates in both lungs, especially in the lower lobes, but no evidence of pulmonary emboli or cavitations. Serum β-glucan was >500 pg/mL (<80pg/mL).

Bronchoscopy was macroscopically normal. Grocott staining of BAL fluid revealed *Pneumocystis jirovecii* cystic forms, and PCR was strongly positive for *P. jirovecii* DNA. Oxygen was gradually weaned and the patient was discharged on oral co-trimoxazole to complete a 21-day total course. Ten days into PCP treatment, the patient commenced antiretroviral therapy with tenofovir, emtricitabine and

TABLE 23.2	Grading of Severity of *Pneumocystis* Pneumonia		
	Mild	**Moderate**	**Severe**
Clinical features	Increasing exertional dyspnoea ± cough and sweats	Dyspnoea on minimal exertion, occasional dyspnoea at rest, fever + sweats	Dyspnoea at rest, tachypnoea at rest, persistent fever, cough
Arterial blood gas (room air)	Pao_2 normal, Sao_2 falling on exercise	$PaO_2 = 8.1–11\,kPa$	$PaO_2 < 8.0\,kPa$
Chest radiography	Normal or minor perihilar infiltrates	Diffuse interstitial shadowing	Extensive interstitial shadowing ± diffuse alveolar shadowing ('white out'), sparing costophrenic angles and apices

Source: Farrar, J. et al., 2013. Pneumocystis jirovecii infection, In: Farrar, J., ed. Manson's Tropical Diseases, 23rd ed. Elsevier, London. Ch. 39.

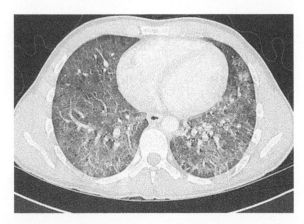

• **Fig. 23.2** CT scan of the chest showing bilateral ground-glass infiltrates, but no pulmonary emboli.

efavirenz. Two weeks into PCP treatment, he developed a widespread pruritic maculopapular rash most likely attributable to either co-trimoxazole or efavirenz. As a result, co-trimoxazole was changed to clindamycin and primaquine for the final week of treatment and efavirenz was replaced by a boosted protease inhibitor. After completing PCP treatment, he was started on dapsone and pyrimethamine for secondary prophylaxis.

SUMMARY BOX

Pneumocystis Pneumonia (PCP)

P. jirovecii, a fungus found worldwide, causes *Pneumocystis* pneumonia (PCP) in immunocompromised individuals. Classic symptoms are sub-acute onset of malaise, non-productive cough and progressive exertional dyspnoea; fever may also be present. On examination, desaturation on exertion is the classic sign; this is a useful clinical test in resource-limited settings because it is easy to perform using a simple pulse oximeter.

The chest is often clear on auscultation. Complications include respiratory failure and pneumothorax. Without treatment, PCP is progressive and usually fatal.

Grading of severity at presentation guides management decisions (Table 23.2). Diagnosis is by visualizing *P. jirovecii* on BAL fluid (>90% sensitivity, and sensitivity maintained up to 10 days into treatment). Induced sputum has lower sensitivity (50–90%). PCR of respiratory secretions cannot reliably distinguish infection from colonization. Chest imaging can support the diagnosis, but changes are non-specific and the chest radiograph may be normal. The classic finding is of diffuse perihilar interstitial infiltrates. High-resolution CT scan may show diffuse or patchy "ground-glass" infiltrates. A normal CT scan has a high negative predictive value for PCP.

First-line treatment is with co-trimoxazole, which in severe cases should initially be intravenous. The addition of high-dose corticosteroids in moderate to severe PCP improves outcomes if started within 72 hours of starting specific PCP treatment. In HIV-positive patients co-trimoxazole should be continued for a total of 21 days; in other types of immunosuppression 14 days may be sufficient. Steroids are weaned over 20 days. ART should be started within the first 14 days of PCP treatment in ART-naïve, HIV-positive patients.

In resource-limited settings, the diagnosis of PCP is most commonly made on clinical grounds. Differentiating PCP from pulmonary TB is often challenging, and dual infections with both TB and PCP also need to be considered. In the absence of intensive care options severely ill patients may have to be empirically treated for both infections. Co-trimoxazole is often available as an oral formulation only.

Adverse effects with co-trimoxazole are common and usually occur at 6 to 14 days of treatment, e.g. cytopaenias (40%), rash (25%), fever (20%) and abnormal liver profile (10%). Second-line treatment is with primaquine and clindamycin or IV pentamidine. For mild-to-moderate cases, dapsone-trimethoprim or atovaquone may be given.

In resource-limited settings alternative treatments are mostly unavailable. In case of a mild rash, the only option may be desensitization with cautious re-exposure to co-trimoxazole.

Secondary prophylaxis with co-trimoxazole (480 mg or 960 mg od) should be given until a CD4 count over 200/μL has been maintained for at least 3 months after commencing ART.

In some resource-limited tropical countries, co-trimoxazole is continued life-long.

Further Reading

1. Miller RF, Doffman S. *Pneumocystis jirovecii* infection. In: Farrar J, editor. *Manson's Tropical Disease*. 23rd ed. London: Elsevier; 2013 [chapter 39].
2. Miller RF, Huang L, Walzer PD. *Pneumocystis* pneumonia associated with human immunodeficiency virus. Clin Chest Med 2013;34(2):229–41.
3. Chiliza N, Du Toit M, Wasserman S. Outcomes of HIV-associated pneumocystis pheumonia at a South African referral hospital. PLoS ONE 2018;13(8):e0201733.
4. Stover DE, Greeno RA, Gagliardi AJ. The Use of a simple exercise test for the diagnosis of *Pneumocystis carinii* pneumonia in patients with AIDS. Am Rev Respir Dis 1989;139:1343–6.
5. Church JA, Fitzgerald F, Walker AS, et al. The expanding role of co-trimoxazole in developing countries. Lancet Infect Dis 2015;15:327–39.

24

A 14-Year-Old Boy from Rural Tanzania With Difficulty in Walking

WILLIAM P. HOWLETT

Clinical Presentation

History

A 14-year-old boy presents to his local hospital in rural Tanzania with a history of difficulty in walking. He had been well until just over 2 years earlier when his illness suddenly started. He describes that he was walking home from school when he first noticed that his legs began to feel heavy and started to tremble, which caused him difficulty in walking, with a tendency to fall over. He slowly completed the journey home; and since that day, he has been unable to stand or walk unaided. He now stands on his toes and drags his legs around with the aid of a stick (Fig. 24.1). He denies any history of fever, pain, sensory, bladder or bowel symptoms or disease progression.

His history is otherwise unremarkable. He lives in a village in northern Tanzania in a rural area with limited agricultural suitability, where the main staple food crop is cassava. His diet for the 2 months before the illness was almost exclusively cassava. He has three other siblings, one of whom is similarly affected, whereas their parents remained fine. He mentions that identical cases had occurred in his own and neighbouring villages at around the same time.

Clinical Examination

Clinically, he is well nourished with normal vital signs. General examination is unremarkable. On neurological examination, he is fully orientated and higher mental function appears normal. Cranial nerves are normal but bilateral optic pallor was noted on fundoscopy. Limbs reveal signs of spastic paraparesis with flexion contractures at both ankles and knees. Power in the legs is graded 3 to 4 out of 5 (= just overcoming gravity), with the knee extensors and foot dorsiflexors involved to the greatest extent (Fig. 24.1). There is bilateral hypertonia, hyperreflexia and sustained ankle clonus with extensor plantar responses. The arms are normal apart from generalized hyperreflexia. There is no impairment or loss of sensation. A lumbar lordosis with thoracic kyphoscoliosis is noticeable only on standing.

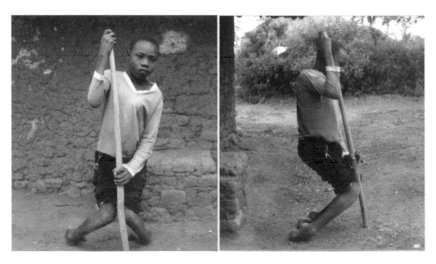

• **Fig. 24.1** A 14-year-old boy from rural Tanzania with spastic paraparesis. His illness started about 2 years earlier and had an acute onset. Several other people are also affected in his own and neighbouring villages.

Investigations

Full blood count, erythrocyte sedimentation rate, blood glucose and creatinine are normal. Urine analysis is normal. Microscopy of urine and stool specimens does not show any ova of *Schistosoma* species. HIV serology and VDRL are negative. Lumbar puncture is normal. Radiographs of the chest and thoracolumbar spine are normal.

Questions

1. What is the clinical diagnosis and the likely cause in this patient?
2. How do you plan to manage this patient?

Discussion

A 14-year-old boy from rural northern Tanzania presents with acute-onset non-progressive spastic paraplegia. There is no history of back pain. On examination, there is no sensory impairment and no bladder dysfunction. The main staple food crop in his village is cassava.

Answer to Question 1

What is the Clinical Diagnosis?

The clinical syndrome is spastic paraparesis. The main differential diagnosis in Africa includes spinal tuberculosis (Pott's disease), transverse myelitis, spinal cord infections such as schistosomiasis and tuberculous myelitis, spinal malignancy (mainly metastases) and tropical nutritional myeloneuropathies.

There are three important features in our case: (1) the isolated involvement of motor neurons without any sensory and bladder involvement; (2) the absence of back pain; and (3) the acute onset with no progression over 2 years. These three clinical points make spinal tuberculosis, spinal cord infection or spinal malignancy very unlikely. Of note, his diet (and probably that of his siblings and other children in the village) for the 2 months before the illness was almost exclusively cassava, and the same disease has affected one of his siblings and more children in the neighborhood. Hence, a nutritional cause must be suspected.

The tropical myeloneuropathies that are nutritional in origin are konzo and lathyrism. Lathyrism in Africa occurs exclusively in Ethiopia. The clinical diagnosis in our patient is konzo. Konzo is a distinct form of tropical spastic paraparesis which occurs exclusively in cassava-growing areas in Africa.

Answer to Question 2

How Do You Plan to Manage this Patient?

There is no cure for patients with konzo because it results in a permanent spastic paraparesis. Management is therefore directed at support, symptomatic improvement and disease prevention. The majority of patients can walk with the aid of a stick or crutches and some will benefit from a wheelchair. Muscle relaxants have a limited role because of relative ineffectiveness as a result of the severity of the spasticity, and these agents' high long-term cost. Surgical treatment involving Achilles tendon lengthening operations have proved useful in improving mobilization in selected patients with konzo. Because of the severity of contractures in this patient, he should be assessed for surgery.

The Case Continued...

At follow-up examination at 6 and 12 months, the findings were unchanged, with a permanent spastic paraparesis. The patient had not been referred for surgery because of the lack of resources and the extent of the epidemic, with many other similar cases in the community. He uses one stick with very restricted mobility and works as a shoe repairer in his village.

SUMMARY BOX

Konzo

Konzo is a distinct form of tropical spastic paraparesis, which occurs exclusively in cassava-growing areas in Africa. The word "konzo" means "tied legs" in the language of the Yaka tribe in the DRC. It is characterized by an abrupt onset of a permanent but non-progressive form of spastic paraparesis related to cassava consumption. It occurs mainly as epidemics, typically during droughts, famines or armed conflict when there is an overreliance on cassava as a staple food for weeks or months. It also occurs in an endemic form but at much lower rates. It affects mainly children and breastfeeding mothers.

The following are the clinical criteria for diagnosing konzo:
- symmetrical spastic paraparesis without sensory or genitourinary involvement
- abrupt onset in less than 1 week with a non-progressive course
- occurring in a cassava-growing area, usually with other cases emerging at the same time
- no other cause found

Its cause is attributed to chronic high dietary exposure of cyanogenic glycosides from insufficiently processed cassava tubers, but the exact pathogenic mechanisms of konzo remain unknown.

Cassava is a staple food for more than 600 million people. It grows well in poor soils and is resistant to drought, plant diseases, insects and animal predators, but it contains cyanogenic glycosides, mainly linamarin. Processing disrupts the tubers releasing cyanide, which makes the food safe for human consumption. Konzo is associated with high intake of insufficiently processed cassava tubers in combination with low or absent levels of the essential amino acids methionine or cysteine. Oxidative stress and glutamate-mediated neuro-excitatory cell death appears likely to be the final pathogenic mechanism. This results in a clinically exclusive pattern of upper motor neurone disease.

Further Reading

1. Aronson J. Plant Poisons and Traditional Medicines. In: Farrar J, editor. Manson's Tropical Diseases. 23rd ed. London: Elsevier; 2014 [chapter 76].
2. Howlett WP, Brubaker GR, Mlingi N, et al. Konzo, an epidemic upper motor neuron disease studied in Tanzania. Brain 1990;113 (Pt 1):223–35.

3. Nzwalo H, Cliff J. Konzo: from poverty, cassava, and cyanogen intake to toxico-nutritional neurological disease. PLoS Negl Trop Dis 2011;5(6):e1051. https://doi.org/10.1371/journal.pntd.0001051.

4. Howlett WP. Paraplegia. In: Howlett WP, editor. Neurology in Africa. Norway: Kilimanjaro Christian Medical Centre, Moshi, Tanzania and University of Bergen; 2012. Available at: https://bora.uib.no.

5. Kashala-Abotnes E, Okitundu D, Mumba D, et al. Konzo: a distinct neurological disease associated with food (cassava) cyanogenic poisoning. Brain Res Bull 2019;145:87–91.

25

A 72-Year-Old Male Farmer from Laos With Extensive Skin Lesions on the Lower Leg

GÜNTHER SLESAK, SAYTHONG INTHALAD AND PAUL N. NEWTON

Clinical Presentation

History

A 72-year-old male farmer is admitted to a provincial hospital in northern Laos with extensive, painful verrucous skin lesions on his left foot and lower leg.

Ten years prior, he had a leech bite on the dorsum of his left foot. One week later a small painless red nodule developed at the site of the bite. Over the following years the lesion slowly increased in size; further lesions developed and spread up to his knee. Three days before admission his ankle became painful and swollen.

Clinical Findings

Vital signs are normal and the patient is afebrile. His left lower leg and foot are grossly swollen (Fig. 25.1); the skin is hyperaemic and feels hot. There are several cauliflower-like masses and oval plaque-like lesions on his left lower leg and foot. The lesions are partly erythematous, partly fungating and purulent, oozing a bad odour.

Investigations

Radiography of the left leg and foot showed no bone involvement.

Questions

1. What are the important differential diagnoses?
2. Which diagnostic tests should be done?

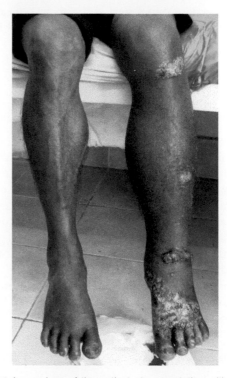

• **Fig. 25.1** Lower legs of the patient at presentation with fungating lesions on his left foot that spread centripetally up to his knee. The left lower leg is also swollen and hyperaemic.

Discussion

A male Lao farmer presents with several verrucous, partially fungating skin lesions on his left leg and foot, which have been growing over the past 10 years after a minor trauma. The affected leg has additionally swollen up and become painful over the previous 3 days.

Answer to Question 1

What Are the Important Differential Diagnoses?

Chronic verrucous skin lesions can typically be seen in fungal infections such as sporotrichosis (*Sporothrix schenckii*) and chromoblastomycosis, which is caused by various pigmented fungi. Mycetoma ("Madura Foot") is a chronic subcutaneous infection caused either by fungi ("eumycetoma") or actinomycetes ("actinomycetoma"). Fistulating lesions discharging granules are the hallmark feature of madura foot but verrucous manifestations may occur. The colour of the granules may indicate the causing pathogen. Despite being common in other parts of Asia, Mycetoma has rarely been described from Laos.

Mycobacterial infections (cutaneous tuberculosis, lepromatous leprosy and infections with atypical mycobacteria) also need to be considered. Cutaneous leishmaniasis can present with verrucous lesions, however it has not been reported in Laos. In HIV-positive patients, Kaposi's Sarcoma may look very similar.

Non-infectious causes such as squamous cell carcinoma, sarcoidosis, chronic eczema and psoriasis should be borne in mind.

Acute localized inflammatory signs are indicative of bacterial superinfection or deep vein thrombosis.

Answer to Question 2

Which Diagnostic Tests Should be Done?

Direct microscopy of skin scrapings taken from the lesions can help detect pigmented fungi in chromoblastomycosis and may be useful to visualize amastigotes in cutaneous leishmaniasis.

Sporotrichosis differs from the other subcutaneous mycoses in that culture is the most reliable mode of diagnosis because there are few organisms present in lesions and these may be difficult to find.

In leprosy, slit skin smears are fairly easy to obtain; however, for other mycobacterial infections biopsy and/or culture may be necessary.

The Case Continued...

Secondary bacterial superinfection was suspected and so iodine-based antiseptics were applied locally and oral antibiotics were started, initially cloxacillin and metronidazole. After bacterial culture of the pus grew *Escherichia coli*, antibiotics were changed to co-trimoxazole, guided by susceptibility testing.

Simple direct microscopic investigations of wet film lesion scrapings revealed characteristic brownish, round, thick-walled, multiseptate sclerotic cells typical of chromoblastomycosis (Fig. 25.2). Use of 10% potassium hydroxide solution made the fungal cells more readily visible. Antifungal treatment was initiated with itraconazole (400 mg/d for 7 days monthly pulse therapy) and surgical debridement of all lesions performed. PCR from skin tissue was positive

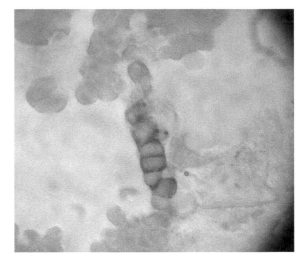

• **Fig. 25.2** Characteristic brownish sclerotic cells in skin scrapings (100×, oil immersion, wet film).

and sequencing revealed 100% similarity with *Fonsecaea pedrosoi*, *F. monophora* and *F. nubica*. When oral terbinafine could be obtained this was added (initially 500 mg/d, later 750 mg/d) for 9 months and local terbinafine ointment was applied for 6 months. Liver function tests and serum glucose were monitored during treatment and remained normal. The lesions healed uneventfully with some residual swelling and hypopigmentation.

SUMMARY BOX

Chromoblastomycosis

Chromoblastomycosis is a chronic fungal infection of the skin and subcutaneous tissue, most commonly of hands, feet and lower legs. It is typically caused by traumatic percutaneous inoculation of the genera *Fonsecaea*, *Phialophora* and *Cladophialophora* which are found in plant debris or forest detritus. Infection occurs worldwide but is most common in rural tropical and subtropical areas. Male agricultural workers are most commonly affected.

Painless lesions develop slowly over years from the site of inoculation as verrucous nodules or plaques, gradually spreading centripetally by lymphatic or cutaneous dissemination. Typical complications are ulcerations, bacterial superinfection and chronic lymphoedema, which may be confused with elephantiasis in regions co-endemic with lymphatic filariasis.

Diagnosis is made by direct microscopic detection of pathognomonic sclerotic cells in skin scrapings ('Medlar bodies', fumagoid or muriform cells). These are brownish, round, thick-walled structures of 4 to 12 µm length, which are already visible on a simple wet film. Hyphae can be more readily seen on a potassium hydroxide preparation. More sophisticated techniques such as culture as well as serology and PCR are rarely available in endemic areas and are often reserved for research purposes; but species identification can also guide treatment schemes.

Treatment is challenging and effectiveness depends on the causative agent, the clinical form and the severity of the lesions. Antifungal therapy commonly comprises oral itraconazole

(200–400 mg/d) alone or in combination with terbinafine or flucytosine (which may be hard to obtain). Antifungals have to be given for at least 6 to 12 months and, in advanced stages, for years to avoid relapse. Cure rates range from 15% to 80%. Multi-drug therapy seems more effective but is expensive. Itraconazole pulse therapy (7 d/month) is cost-saving.

In addition, topical heat therapy, phototherapy, cryosurgery, surgical debridement and/or combination therapy may be helpful.

Further Reading

1. Hay RJ. Fungal infections. In: Farrar J, editor. Manson's Tropical Diseases. 23rd ed. London: Elsevier; 2013 [chapter 38].

2. Queiroz-Telles F, de Hoog S, Santos DW, et al. Chromoblastomycosis. Clin Microbiol Rev 2017;30:233–76.

3. Slesak G, Inthalad S, Strobel M, et al. Chromoblastomycosis after a leech bite complicated by myiasis: a case report. BMC Infect Dis 2011;11:14.

4. Agarwal R, Singh G, Ghosh A, et al. Chromoblastomycosis in India: review of 169 cases. PLoS Negl Trop Dis 2017;11(8): e0005534.

5. Coelho RA, Brito-Santos F, Figueiredo-Carvalho MHG, et al. Molecular identification and antifungal susceptibility profiles of clinical strains of Fonsecaea spp. isolated from patients with chromoblastomycosis in Rio de Janeiro, Brazil. PLoS Negl Trop Dis 2018;12:e0006675.

26

A 14-Year-Old Boy from Malawi Who Has Been Bitten by a Snake

GREGOR POLLACH

Clinical Presentation

History

A 14-year-old Malawian boy presents to a local hospital because of an extensive necrotic wound on his right foot.

Three weeks earlier he was playing with his friends on a path leading through rocky grassland to the maize field of his family when he stepped on a snake. The snake was brown with V-shaped black bands on its back, and it was approximately one metre long. His friends told his mother later that the snake had hissed loudly but did not move away before biting him – which the boy did not even realize, being busy chasing a football. Shortly after the bite, haemorrhagic bullae formed on the right leg. His gums started to bleed and he vomited extensively. He was taken to a local traditional healer for treatment. His bleeding and vomiting settled; however, he developed intense pain and swelling at the site of the bite.

Clinical Findings

14-year old boy, who appears weak and is in respiratory distress. Temperature 39.4°C, pulse 126 bpm, blood pressure 85/60 mmHg, respiratory rate 30 breath cycles per minute. There is an extensive, foul-smelling necrosis affecting his right foot and ankle where the tendons are exposed (Fig. 26.1). The right lower leg is swollen and he is unable to bend the ankle of his right foot. The inguinal lymph nodes are enlarged on the right side.

The urine is clear, rectal exam does not show any signs of bleeding and upon provoked coughing there is no haemoptysis. Fundoscopy is normal.

Investigations

The 20-minute whole blood clotting test (WBCT20) is normal. The results of the other blood tests are shown in Table 26.1.

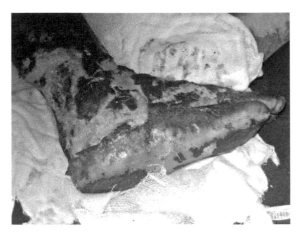

• **Fig. 26.1** The right foot and ankle with extensive tissue necrosis 3 weeks after a snake bite.

TABLE 26.1	Laboratory Results on Admission	
Parameter	Patient	Reference Range
WBC (×10⁹/L)	19	4–10
Haemoglobin (mg/dL)	9.5	12–14
Platelets (×10⁹/L)	60	150–400
K⁺ (mmol/L)	4.2	3.5–5.2

Questions

1. Which snake most probably caused this bite?
2. What first-aid measures should have been taken?

Discussion

A 14-year-old boy from rural Malawi who was bitten by a snake 3 weeks earlier presents to a local hospital. He is septic with an extensive foul-smelling necrotic wound on the right ankle, exposed tendons and oedema of the right leg.

Answer to Question 1

Which Snake Was Most Probably Responsible for the Bite?

The African puff-adder (*Bitis arietans*) is the most likely snake to have caused his bite. Puff-adders are about one metre long and stout. They show a distinctive 'V' or 'U' pattern on their back. When disturbed, they behave aggressively, hissing loudly and inflating their body. The puff-adder is a highly dangerous snake, with large quantities of a potent venom and long fangs. It commonly lives in densely populated areas. Throughout the African savannah, this species is responsible for a large number of serious bites. The main problem is massive local swelling, which may spread to involve the whole limb and cause hypovolaemic shock. Bullae filled with haemorrhagic fluid may develop at the site of the bite. Extensive necrosis may occur. Cardiotoxic effects of the venom may lead to arrhythmias, and the venom may cause systemic haemorrhage.

The puff-adder, along with the saw-scaled or carpet viper (*Echis* species), which produces similar symptoms, are responsible for most fatalities after snake bites in Africa. In contrast, bites by mambas, the most feared snakes in Africa, are relatively uncommon.

Answer to Question 2

What First-Aid Measures Should Have Been Taken?

First-aid should include reassurance of the victim. Paracetamol should be used for pain relief because aspirin might aggravate haemorrhage and morphine can enhance respiratory depression caused by the venom. Any tight jewellery should be removed. The affected limb should be immobilized along with the whole patient, because any muscular contractions will increase the absorption of the venom.

If a neurotoxic venom cannot be excluded, a pressure immobilization technique should be used; e.g. a long elastic bandage can be wrapped around the affected limb incorporating a splint. However, in cytotoxic venoms the local effects may be worsened through such pressure techniques.

The wound itself should be left alone to avoid infection and absorption of the venom.

The patient should gently but quickly be taken to the nearest appropriate health facility. Patients should be placed in a recovery position if vomiting or if their level of consciousness is reduced. All patients bitten by snakes should ideally be observed in hospital for at least 24 hours.

Finally, helpers should not try to kill the snake, risking further bites. However, if the snake has already been killed it should be taken to the healthcare facility for identification. Even a dead snake needs to be handled with great caution as it still may bite by reflex. Smart-phone photography of the culprit snake is another alternative.

Some widely popular first-aid measures have never been proven to be of any help in the management of snake bites; these include local cuts with a knife or razor blade, attempts to suck the venom out of the wound, the often disastrous application of an arterial tourniquet, cauterization, chemicals, ice, electric shocks and the use of 'magic stones'.

The Case Continued...

The snake bite had occurred 3 weeks earlier, therefore application of antivenom was not deemed useful. Because the boy was septic upon admission, he was managed according to the international sepsis treatment guidelines, crucially including early start of broad-spectrum antibiotics, 'ventilatory support' and fluid resuscitation. He also received tetanus prophylaxis.

The wound was managed surgically: After several debridements (Fig. 26.2) it stayed clean and mesh-grafting was successfully performed. Further reconstructive surgery was not necessary and severe local complications (e.g. compartment syndrome, deep tissue infection and ischaemia) did not develop. The boy was discharged several weeks later. Some functional impairment of his right foot remained and he was booked for outpatient physiotherapy.

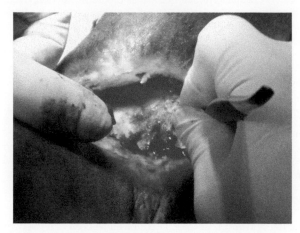

• **Fig. 26.2** After several debridements the wound looks clean.

TABLE 26.2   Principal Effects of African Snake Venoms in Humans

Venom Activity	Clinical Manifestations	African Snake Responsible
Cytotoxic	Massive local swelling, blistering, necrosis; plasma extravasation with consecutive fluid loss, hypotension. Eye: keratoconjunctivitis, corneal ulcer, blindness (spitting cobra)	Puff-adder and other large *Bitis* species, saw-scaled vipers (*Echis*), burrowing asps (*Atractaspis* species); spitting cobra
Auto-pharmacological	Release of vasoactive compounds (e.g. NO, histamine, serotonin, bradykinin); anaphylaxis, acute profound hypotension, urticaria, vomiting, diarrhoea	Burrowing asps (*Atractaspis* spp.), *Bitis* species, boomslang
Haematotoxic	Spontaneous systemic bleeding (gums, brain, gastrointestinal, uterine), bleeding from trauma and recent wounds	Puff-adder and other large *Bitis* spp., saw-scaled vipers, boomslang, vine snake
Cardiotoxic	Hypotension, shock, arrhythmias, conduction abnormalities	Puff-adder and other large *Bitis* species, burrowing asps
Neurotoxic	Cranial nerve palsies, bulbar and respiratory paralysis	Elapids (mamba, cobra, rinkhals) berg adder, Peringuey's adder
Myotoxic	Trismus; rhabdomyolysis with myalgias, myoglobinuria, renal failure, hyperkalaemia, respiratory failure	Sea snake
Nephrotoxic	Acute kidney injury, renal necrosis	Boomslang, vine snake, saw-scaled vipers

Source: After Warrell, 2013[3]

SUMMARY BOX

Snake Bite

Snake bite is a common problem in rural areas of many tropical countries. The true numbers are unknown because many patients may never reach a health facility or seek the help of a traditional practitioner. Snake bites are most common among farm workers, herdsmen, plantation workers and their children. Most bites occur at the beginning of the rainy season. Even though there is a large variety of venomous snakes, the toxic effects of snake bites can be classified into one or more of seven groups (Table 26.2).

The therapeutic approach in hospital has to consider local and systemic effects of the bite and the complications that might arise. Tetanus prophylaxis, antibiotic coverage, wound cleansing and sterile dressing are mandatory.

Antivenom should be given in case of systemic envenoming, indicated by clinical signs and symptoms or deranged laboratory parameters.

Of note, loosening of tourniquets or improvement of circulation may lead to an increased systemic load of venom. In severe local envenoming, antivenom should be given if the swelling involves more than half of the bitten limb and in patients bitten by snakes known to cause local necrosis.

Antivenom is most effective when administered by slow IV injection or infusion. Children need the same dose of antivenom as adults because the same amount of venom has been injected. Antivenom mostly consists of non-human hyperimmunoglobulin; it therefore may lead to severe side effects including fever, anaphylaxis or late serum sickness-like reactions.

Necrotic wounds require careful debridement. Wound infection, compartment syndrome or osteomyelitis must be suspected and treated early. Skin grafts, reconstructive surgery, fasciotomy or amputation may be necessary. Massive local oedema carries the risk of hypovolaemic shock.

In severe haemorrhagic complications with hypotension, patients should be transfused; if blood is unavailable, sufficient IV fluids should be administered.

For neurotoxic complications mechanical ventilation is often required and anticholinesterase drugs should be attempted.

Further Reading

1. Warrell DA. Venomous and poisonous animals. In: Farrar J, editor. Manson's Tropical Diseases. 23rd ed. London: Elsevier; 2013 [chapter 75].
2. Warrell DA. Treatment of bites by adders and exotic venomous snakes. BMJ 2005;331(7527):1244–7.
3. Warrell DA. Venomous and other dangerous animals. In: Mabey D, Gill G, Parry E, et al., editors. Principles of Medicine in Africa. 4th ed. Cambridge: Cambridge University Press; 2013. p. 849–74.
4. Dellinger RP, Levy MM, Rhodes A, et al. Surviving sepsis campaign: international guidelines for management of severe sepsis and septic shock: 2012. Crit Care Med 2013;41(2):580–637.

27

A 16-Year-Old Boy from Sri Lanka With Fever, Jaundice and Renal Failure

RANJAN PREMARATNA

Clinical Presentation

History

A 16-year-old Sri Lankan boy presents to a local hospital with fever, frontal headache and severe body aches for 2 days. He has vomited two to three times during the illness and has not passed any urine for the previous 12 hours. He does not have a cough, coryza or shortness of breath. He has been attending school until his illness. He had been fishing in an urban water stream 5 days before falling ill.

Clinical Examination

The boy appears ill and drowsy. He is jaundiced and has subconjunctival haemorrhages (Fig. 27.1). Temperature is 38.3°C (100.9°F), the pulse rate is 100 bpm (low in volume). The blood pressure is 90/60 mmHg.

There is no neck stiffness, however there is severe muscle tenderness, mainly involving the abdominal wall and the calves such that the patient finds it difficult to walk. There is no lymphadenopathy. The cardiac apex is not shifted and heart sounds are clear. Examination of the lungs is

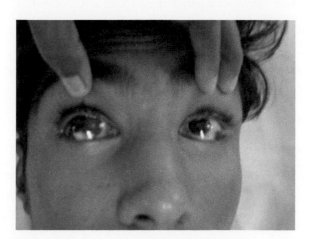

• **Fig. 27.1** Jaundice and subconjunctival haemorrhages

TABLE 27.1	Laboratory Results on Admission	
Parameter	Patient	Reference
WBC (×10⁹/L) (neutrophils: lymphocytes)	5.7 (68%: 31%)	4–10
Haemoglobin (g/dL)	14.8	12–16
Platelets (×10⁹/L)	96	150–350
AST (IU/L)	64	13–33
ALT (IU/L)	58	3–25
ALP (IU/L)	246	40–130
Serum bilirubin total (µmol/L)	77	13.7–30.8
Serum bilirubin direct (µmol/L)	54.7	<5
Blood urea nitrogen (µmol/L)	20.7	2.5–6.4
Serum creatinine (µmol/L)	212.2	71–106
C-reactive protein (mg/L)	48	<5

normal. The liver is palpable at 4 cm below the right costal margin and is tender. The spleen is not palpable. There is mild bilateral renal angle tenderness. Neurological examination is normal.

Further Investigations

The laboratory findings are summarized in Table 27.1. The urine microscopy shows 20 red blood cells per high-power field, proteins '+' and granular casts '+'. A chest radiograph is normal. An ECG shows sinus tachycardia.

Questions

1. What is the most likely diagnosis and what are your differentials?
2. What tests are indicated to confirm the diagnosis?

Discussion

A Sri Lankan teenage boy presents with fever, severe body aches and a reduced urine output. He is jaundiced with subconjunctival haemorrhage and has a tender hepatomegaly. He has had contact with a water stream before his ill health.

His laboratory results show signs of cholestasis with only mildly elevated transaminases. The creatinine is increased twofold and there is thrombocytopenia. The leucocyte count is normal.

Answer to Question 1

What is the Most Likely Diagnosis and What Are Your Differentials?

An acute febrile illness accompanied by jaundice, renal failure and subconjunctival haemorrhage should raise the suspicion of leptospirosis, particularly in case of a history involving exposure to potentially contaminated water.

Scrub typhus is another very common infection in South Asia. It may present with an acute onset of fever, hepatomegaly and renal failure. There usually is lymphadenopathy; and on careful examination, one may spot an eschar. Subconjunctival haemorrhage has been described but is less common than in leptospirosis, and complications such as renal failure tend to occur late in the infection (after about 7 days).

Hantavirus infection may cause a haemorrhagic fever with renal syndrome. It has a similar epidemiology to leptospirosis and is also associated with contact with rodent excreta.

Dengue haemorrhagic fever (DHF) is another differential diagnosis to consider. It also presents with fever, severe myalgias, thrombocytopenia and haemorrhages. Acute kidney injury and jaundice are uncommon for DHF.

Answer to Question 2

What Tests Are Indicated to Confirm the Diagnosis?

The microscopic diagnosis of leptospirosis requires a dark-field or a phase-contrast microscope because the bacteria stain poorly. However, dark-field microscopy is of poor sensitivity and specificity and only yields positive results during the early bacteraemic phase of the disease.

Leptospira may be cultured from blood, CSF or urine. Isolation of the bacteria from blood or CSF is only possible during the first week of illness. Samples have to be incubated for at least 8 weeks and analysed weekly with a dark-field microscope. This technique is laborious and not routine practice in a standard microbiological laboratory.

Polymerase chain reaction (PCR) detection has been used on blood, CSF and urine. PCR performance varies between types of samples taken and depends on the time the sample was taken in relation to duration of illness. Sensitivity and specificity appear to be higher in urine than in blood and are better in blood samples taken early rather than later during the course of illness.

For indirect diagnosis, the historical reference serological test is the microscopic agglutination test (MAT). MAT relies on incubation of patient serum with *Leptospira* antigen suspension and determines agglutination with a dark-field microscope. This method requires a high level of expertise and is limited to expert centres.

The MAT cannot differentiate between current or past infections. Therefore two consecutive serum samples should be examined to look for seroconversion or at least a fourfold rise in titre. The significance of titres in single serum specimens is a matter of debate.

Various ELISA tests detecting anti-*Leptospira* IgM are now commercially available, facilitating the diagnosis outside reference centres. It appears that sensitivity of these tests is highly variable if blood is examined during week one of the illness, it improves (75% and 100%) if blood is taken after day 7. A positive IgM ELISA should be confirmed by MAT.

The Case Continued...

Severe leptospirosis was suspected and the patient was commenced on empirical benzylpenicillin. Despite rehydration he developed acute renal failure warranting haemodialysis (HD). He developed myocarditis and atrial fibrillation, but luckily tolerated further HD. He gradually recovered over 10 days with intensive care management.

SUMMARY BOX

Leptospirosis

Leptospirosis is a zoonotic disease that occurs worldwide. It is caused by pathogenic *Leptospira* species, which belong to the spirochaetes. The most common species causing disease in humans and animals are *L. interrogans* and *L. borgpetersenii*.

Humans become infected through direct contact with urine of infected mammalian hosts, contact with contaminated water or animal abortion products. The major reservoirs are rodents, canines, livestock and wild mammals. Most at risk are slum dwellers and people with an occupational or recreational exposure involving animal contact or immersion in water. Also, natural disasters such as hurricanes and floods may put people at risk.

The bacteria enter the human body through cuts or abrasions of the skin or through intact mucous membranes. The incubation period is 2 to 30 days. The spectrum of disease ranges from asymptomatic to severe infection.

The classical presentation of leptospirosis is that of a biphasic illness. The initial leptospiraemic phase usually starts abruptly. Symptoms are non-specific with fever, headache, sore throat, abdominal pain and a rash. Severe myalgias, most notably of the calves and the lumbar area, and subconjunctival haemorrhage have been mentioned as distinguishing physical findings. This first phase lasts for a week and is followed by a second phase dominated by immune-mediated pathology.

Five to ten per cent of those with clinical infection will develop severe leptospirosis with cholestatic jaundice, acute kidney injury and haemorrhagic diathesis (Weil's syndrome). Further complications include pulmonary involvement, aseptic meningitis and myocarditis.

Leptospirosis is usually treated with antibiotics, although the usefulness of antibiotic treatment in particular during the second phase of illness, which is immune-mediated, has been disputed.

For uncomplicated cases, oral doxycycline is the drug of choice. Alternatives include amoxicillin and azithromycin. In severe infection benzylpenicillin, IV doxycycline, ceftriaxone or cefotaxime seem to have similar efficacy. Doxycycline 200 mg weekly has been suggested as exposure prophylaxis.

Further Reading

1. Chierakul KW. Leptospirosis. In: Farrar J, editor. Manson's Tropical Diseases. 23rd ed. London: Elsevier; 2013 [chapter 37].
2. WHO. Human leptospirosis: guidance for diagnosis, surveillance and control, In: World Health Organization and International Leptospirosis Society. editors. Geneva: WHO; 2003.
3. Bharti AR, Nally JE, Ricaldi JN, et al. Leptospirosis: a zoonotic disease of global importance. Lancet Infect Dis 2003;3(12):757–71.
4. Eldin C, Jaulhac B, Bediannikov O, et al. Values of diagnostic tests for the various species of spirochetes. Med Mal Infect 2019;49 (2):102–11.

28

A 67-Year-Old Female Expatriate Living in Cameroon With Eosinophilia and Pericarditis

SEBASTIAN DIECKMANN AND RALF IGNATIUS

Clinical Presentation

History

A 67-year-old German woman who has lived as an expatriate in Cameroon for the past 4 years presents with palpitations at a tropical medicine clinic in Germany. She also reports transient subcutaneous swellings for the past year. There is no history of fever or constitutional symptoms and the past medical history is otherwise unremarkable.

24-hour ECG recording was done elsewhere, which showed paroxysmal supraventricular extrasystoles. Echocardiography revealed a minimal pericardial effusion.

Clinical Findings

Vital signs are normal and the patient is afebrile. There are no visible subcutaneous swellings. Heart sounds are clear and regular, and there are no murmurs. No pathological findings are noted on physical examination.

Laboratory Results

Full blood count results are shown in Table 28.1.

Further Investigations

The chest radiograph does not show any abnormalities.

Questions

1. What are the key findings?
2. What are your differential diagnoses?

TABLE 28.1 Full Blood Count Results at Presentation

Parameter	Patient	Reference
WBC ($\times 10^9$/L)	6.20	4–10
Haemoglobin (g/dL)	13.8	12–15
Platelets ($\times 10^9$/L)	155	150–450
Neutrophils (%)	45	20–50
Eosinophils (%)	14	0–6
Absolute eosinophil count ($\times 10^9$/L)	0.868	<0.45
Band neutrophils (%)	1	0–5
Lymphocytes (%)	36	20–40
Monocytes (%)	4	0–10
Basophils (%)	0	0–2

Discussion

A 67-year-old expatriate living in Cameroon for 4 years presents with eosinophilia and reports transient subcutaneous swellings. Additionally, the patient suffers from cardiac arrhythmia.

Answer to Question 1

What Are the Key Findings?

The pattern of transient subcutaneous swellings, eosinophilia and the history of living in Cameroon for several years are the key pieces of clinical information suggestive of a filarial infection.

Some filarial infections may affect the heart, and chronic eosinophilia is known to be cardiotoxic and may cause endomyocardial fibrosis. The cardiac findings in this patient, however, may warrant further work-up.

Answer to Question 2

What Are the Differential Diagnoses?

The differentials of skin swellings and eosinophilia include non-specific urticaria, Calabar swellings in loiasis, cysticercosis, larva currens in *Strongyloides stercoralis* infection and infection with *Mansonella perstans.*

Acute schistosomiasis (Katayama syndrome) may present with eosinophilia, fever and an urticarial rash; however, this patient is afebrile and the migratory swellings she describes do not fit the clinical picture of schistosomiasis.

Gnathostomiasis and sparganosis may also cause eosinophilia and migratory swellings; however, these infections are more common in East Asia than in Africa. Sparganosis has been reported from Kenya and Tanzania and gnathostomiasis occurs in the Okavango Delta, Botswana.

The Case Continued...

Serology for filarial infections was positive. Day-blood samples were collected, filtered and stained with Giemsa, which revealed sheathed microfilariae with a tapered tail characteristic for *Loa loa* (Fig. 28.1). In contrast, microfilariae of *M. perstans,* another filarial nematode endemic in West and Central Africa, which may cause similar symptoms, would have been smaller and unsheathed with a blunt tail. The microfilarial count was 1400/mL.

Despite the low microfilarial count the patient was treated with caution, first with albendazole followed by ivermectin. Therapy was tolerated well. The absolute eosinophil count (AEC) returned to normal and the microfilarial count

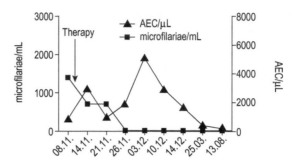

• **Fig. 28.2** Development of microfilaraemia and absolute eosinophil count (AEC) in the patient after treatment.

declined (Fig. 28.2). No sequelae were observed and the palpitations settled.

Follow-up echocardiography 3 months later was normal, the pericardial effusion had resolved and 24-hour ECG was also normal.

Loiasis and other conditions causing high eosinophil counts have been implicated in the development of endomyocardial fibrosis; however, it remains unclear in this case whether there was any association between the infection and the patient's transient cardiac problems.

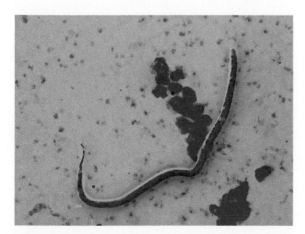

• **Fig. 28.1** Sheathed microfilaria of *Loa loa.* The tail is tapered and nuclei are extending into the tip of the tail. (Giemsa staining; magnification 200×)

TABLE 28.2	Treatment of Loiasis Matched to Levels of Microfilaraemia (After Boussinesq 2012)
Level of Microfilaraemia	**Recommended Drug Regimen**
High (>8000 mf^a/mL)	Albendazole 200 mg bd for 21 days, followed by ivermectin 150 µg/kg stat, then DEC at slowly increasing doses.
Moderate (2000–8000 mf/mL)	Ivermectin 150 µg/kg stat, repeat after 1–3 months until microfilaraemia is <2000 mf/mL, this is followed by treatment with DEC.
Low (<2000 mf/mL)	DEC: start with low doses of 3–6 mg/d if there are parasites in the blood, 50 mg/d if amicrofilaraemic, divided into 2–3 doses. The dose is doubled every day up to 400 mg/d, still divided into 2–3 doses. Start treatment in hospital. Oral antihistamines or corticosteroids may be useful during the first days of treatment to reduce side effects (arthralgias, pruritus, headache, fever). Several 3- to 4-week courses of DEC administered at intervals of 2–3 weeks may be required to achieve a complete cure.

mf^a = microfilariae.

SUMMARY BOX

Loiasis

Loiasis is the symptomatic infection with the filarial nematode *L. loa*. It is common in West and Central Africa. The infective larvae of *L. loa* are transmitted by female *Chrysops* species horseflies.

Inside the human host larvae develop into adult worms, which takes several months. Adult *L. loa* migrate through the subcutaneous and connective tissues of the human body. Migration may cause urticaria and transient painless subcutaneous swellings ('Calabar swellings'), a localized angioedema which may last from several hours to a few days.

Adult worms may be spotted when migrating through the bulbar conjunctiva, which is noticed by the patient as intense itching of the eye, pain and photophobia. Passage of the palpebral conjunctiva is associated with swelling of the eyelid and the periorbital region.

Loiasis may cause renal complications (glomerulonephritis, nephrotic syndrome, etc.) and a wide range of neurological symptoms.

The female worms release sheathed microfilariae that are detectable in the peripheral blood during daytime with a peak around noon, but are usually absent at night. This diurnal periodicity corresponds to the day-biting habits of the *Chrysops* vectors.

Microfilaraemia in *L. loa* infection tends to be higher than in lymphatic filariasis, where microfilariaemia is usually betweeen 1 and 1000 mf/ml. However, there is also a high percentage of amicrofilaraemic individuals ('occult loiasis') in endemic areas, which poses a diagnostic challenge.

Clinical diagnosis in loiasis relies on the typical passage of the adults through the bulbar conjunctiva ('eye worm').

Microfilariae of *L. loa* may be detected in a thick blood film or filtered blood using day-blood samples. PCR (polymerase chain reaction) is currently the best diagnostic method for amicrofilaraemic patients with occult loiasis. Serology has to be interpreted with caution. Serological tests for *L. loa* are usually based on antigens derived from another filarial species, e.g. *Dirofilaria immitis*. Therefore serology is unable to distinguish between the different filarial diseases. Furthermore, cross-reactions with antibodies against other nematodes are common.

For treatment of loiasis, diethylcarbamazine (DEC), ivermectin and albendazole are used. DEC is effective against microfilariae of *L. loa* and also kills a proportion of the adult worms. It has long been considered the drug of choice for the treatment of loiasis; however, it may cause severe side effects in patients with high levels of microfilariae. Furthermore, DEC is difficult to access in non-endemic countries and repeated courses of treatment may be required for final cure.

Ivermectin is only microfilaricidal, and albendazole may have embryostatic activity; however, the precise mechanism of action and the nature and degree of its effect on adult *L. loa* remain to be elucidated.

In contrast to other filarial nematodes (e.g. *O. volvulus, W. bancrofti*), *L. loa* does not harbour any endosymbiotic *Wolbachia* bacteria. Therefore there is no role for doxycycline in the treatment of loiasis.

When patients with high microfilarial counts are treated with DEC or ivermectin, the rapid death of microfilariae can lead to severe side effects, including glomerulonephritis, encephalopathy, coma or death. Sequential treatment has therefore been suggested, depending on the degree of microfilaraemia (Table 28.2).

To safely administer ivermectin in the context of mass drug treatment campaigns for onchocerciasis or lymphatic filariasis in regions co-endemic with *L. loa,* a mobile phone–based videomicroscope has proven useful as a point-of-care device to identify people with high levels of *L. loa* microfilariae under field conditions and postpone their ivermectin treatment.

Further Reading

1. Simonsen P, Fischer PU, Hoerauf A, et al. The filariases. Manson's Tropical Diseases. 23rd ed. London: Elsevier; 2013 [chapter 54].
2. Boussinesq M. Loiasis. Ann Trop Med Parasitol 2006;100:715–31.
3. Boussinesq M. Loiasis: new epidemiologic insights and proposed treatment strategy. J Trav Med 2012;19(3):140–3.
4. D'Ambrosio MV, Bakalar M, Bennuru S, et al. Point-of-care quantification of blood-borne filarial parasites with a mobile phone microscope. Sci Tranl Med 2015;286:1–10.
5. Metzger WG, Mordmueller B. Loa loa – does it deserve to be neglected? Lancet Infect Dis 2014;14:353–7.

29

A 35-Year-Old Woman from Malawi With Fever and Severe Anaemia

CAMILLA ROTHE

Clinical Presentation

History

A 35-year-old Malawian woman presents to a local hospital because of fever and weakness.

The fever started 3 days earlier, but the weakness has progressed over the past several months. There is no cough and no night sweats, but she reports some weight loss. There is no diarrhoea, no dysuria and no history of abnormal bleeds.

Two months earlier she presented to a local health centre because of her weakness. She was found to be clinically pale and was prescribed iron tablets, which she took. Nevertheless, the weakness progressed. Otherwise, the patient does not report any abnormalities.

She is divorced, with three children (17, 15 and 12 years old), who are all well. She works as a small-scale farmer and sells vegetables on the local market. The family can afford three meals a day and occasionally meat or fish.

Clinical Findings

A 35-year-old woman, wasted, body mass index $17 \, kg/m^2$. Blood pressure 90/60 mmHg (difficult to measure because of the low upper arm circumference), pulse 110 bpm, temperature 37.8°C (100°F), respiratory rate 25 breath cycles per minute, oxygen saturation 97% on ambient air, Glasgow Coma Scale 15/15.

Her conjunctivae are very pale, but there is no jaundice. The examination of her mouth is normal, there is no oral thrush, no Kaposi's sarcoma lesions and no oral hairy leukoplakia. The chest is clear. The abdomen is soft, with slight diffuse tenderness, but no guarding. The spleen is palpable 3 cm below the left costal margin. The rectal examination is normal.

Investigations

The malaria rapid diagnostic test is negative. The HIV serology comes back positive.

TABLE 29.1	Laboratory Results on Admission		
Parameter		Patient	Reference
WBC ($\times 10^9$/L)		3.0	4–10
Haemoglobin (mg/dL)		4.8	12–14
MCV (fL)		90	80–99
Platelets ($\times 10^9$/L)		112	150–400

The results of her full blood count are shown in Table 29.1.

Questions

1. What is the suspected diagnosis?
2. How would you manage this patient?

Discussion

A 35-year-old Malawian woman presents in a state of sepsis without any clear focal symptoms. She is wasted and severely anaemic and she newly tests HIV-positive.

This is a very common clinical scenario in a high-prevalence setting for HIV in sub-Saharan Africa.

Answer to Question 1
What is the Suspected Diagnosis?

The patient presents with a septic picture without a clear focus; she is newly diagnosed HIV-positive and her wasting and anaemia suggest advanced immunosuppression and/or possible concomitant tuberculosis (TB).

The most common cause of sepsis in HIV-positive adults in many parts of sub-Saharan Africa is infection with invasive non-typhoidal *Salmonellae* (iNTS). The slight abdominal tenderness and her splenomegaly would also fit with this diagnosis.

Enteric fevers (typhoid or paratyphoid) are clinically indistinguishable from infection with iNTS, they are however far less common than iNTS in HIV-positive patients in sub-Saharan Africa. The reason for this is unclear.

Severe anaemia led to the non-specific feeling of progressive 'weakness' in this patient. It is most likely a consequence of infection of her bone marrow with HIV, *Salmonellae* and possibly also with *Mycobacterium tuberculosis*.

Other causes of severe anaemia, such as iron deficiency, helminth infections and malaria, are less common in an HIV-positive urban adult population but may have to be considered in other patients, in particular children, pregnant women or in the rural poor. Thalassaemia usually leads to a microcytic anaemia.

Severe anaemia is very common in sub-Saharan Africa. Patients commonly present to healthcare facilities late, at times only when they are developing heart failure secondary to severe anaemia.

Visceral leishmaniasis may also cause fever and pancytopenia as seen in this patient. It usually causes gross hepatosplenomegaly which our patient does not have. It also appears not to be endemic in Malawi, but should be considered in other parts of Africa, e.g. South Sudan, Northern Uganda and Northern Kenya, Ethiopia or Somalia.

Answer to Question 2

How Would You Manage This Patient?

Fluids and broad-spectrum antibiotics need to be started immediately. Before starting antibiotic treatment, blood cultures should be taken. Because bacteraemia may be low, it is important to inoculate a decent volume of blood (at least 20–40ml) for culture.

Severe anaemia in an HIV-infected person commonly is a sign of TB. Therefore the patient should be assessed for underlying tuberculosis. A chest radiograph and an abdominal ultrasound scan should be done. If the CD4-count is <100 cells/μl, a lateral flow urine lipoarabinomannan (LAM) may also help confirm TB.

Of note, anaemia may be the only finding in a patient with TB hiding in the bone marrow; and even if all routine investigations are unremarkable, TB should still be high on the list of possible diagnoses if the patient does not make a satisfactory recovery, i.e. remains febrile and/or anaemic or continues to lose weight.

The baseline CD4 count should be checked and the patient should be started on co-trimoxazole preventive treatment as prophylaxis against *Pneumocystis pneumonia,* toxoplasmosis and other opportunistic infections. Antiretroviral therapy (ART) should be started as soon as possible, once the acute infection is under control and concomitant opportunistic infections have been ruled out. The latter is important to prevent unmasking immune reconstitution inflammatory syndrome (IRIS). Her children and her current and past sexual partners should be encouraged to go for an HIV test.

The Case Continued...

Blood cultures were taken and the patient was started on IV ceftriaxone 2 g od, as well as on fluid resuscitation. Blood cultures grew *Salmonella enterica* var Typhimurium. Her

antibiotic treatment was changed to oral ciprofloxacin 500 mg tds which was continued for 14 days. TB screening revealed prominent hilar lymph nodes and the patient was also commenced on antituberculous treatment and on antiretroviral therapy. She also received co-trimoxazole prophylaxis, vitamin B_6 to prevent peripheral neuropathy and therapeutic feeding.

She was discharged after 4 weeks in hospital. On review in ART clinic 3 months later she was feeling much better. She had gained weight and her haemoglobin levels were picking up. Her three children tested negative for HIV. Her ex-husband refused to go for HIV-testing.

SUMMARY BOX

Invasive Non-Typhoidal Salmonellae (iNTS) Infection

S. enterica is a leading cause of community-acquired bloodstream infection in Africa and Asia. Typhoidal *Salmonella* species cause typhoid and paratyphoid, i.e. enteric fever. They are restricted to human hosts. Non-typhoidal *Salmonellae* are host generalists, colonizing and infecting a broad range of vertebrate animals.

Non-typhoidal salmonellae (NTS) usually cause a self-limiting enterocolitis in immunocompetent individuals. In contrast, in sub-Saharan Africa (SSA) NTS commonly cause invasive disease resulting in sepsis and death. Important populations at risk for development of iNTS infection are infants and children living in areas of high transmission intensity for falciparum malaria and/or with severe malnutrition, and adults with advanced HIV-infection.

In Asia, enteric fever still prevails as a cause of invasive salmonellosis, which may be associated with the lower prevalence of iNTS risk factors in the population.

Both the reservoir and source of infection for iNTS remain unclear. S. Typhimurium and S. Enteritidis are the most common serovars, but it is unknown if the same strains cause invasive and diarrhoeal disease and if the modes of transmission are the same.

Infection with iNTS commonly presents as a non-specific febrile illness. Some patients report abdominal pain or a history of diarrhoea, but often the focus remains clinically unclear. Mild splenomegaly occurs in more than one-third of patients, hepatomegaly is less common. About 30% of patients with iNTS have a concomitant lower respiratory tract co-infection, with pathogens such as *M. tuberculosis* or *Streptococcus pneumoniae*. Severe anaemia is common and should prompt the clinician to look carefully for signs of TB co-infection.

Blood culture remains the diagnostic standard; however, it is not widely available in many African settings. Also, sensitivity of blood culture is suboptimal because of the low magnitude of bacteraemia (median <1 CFU/mL). Care should therefore be taken to inoculate large enough volumes of blood for culture.

Antimicrobial resistance among iNTS strains in Africa is increasing. Empirical management is similar to enteric fever and includes either a fluoroquinolone or azithromycin, depending on the local resistance pattern and drug availability. If oral intake is not possible, a third-generation cephalosporin should be administered. Effective antibiotic treatment should be given for 10 to 14 days. Antiretroviral therapy should be started urgently to prevent relapse. The case fatality rate of patients with iNTS is much higher than in enteric fever (22–47% vs 1%).

Further Reading

1. Feasey NA, Gordon MA. Salmonella infections. In: Farrar J, editor. Manson's Tropical Diseases. 23rd ed. London: Elsevier; 2013 [chapter 25].

2. Feasey NA, Dougan G, Kingsley RA, et al. Invasive non-typhoidal salmonella disease: an emerging and neglected tropical disease in Africa. Lancet 2012;379(9835):2489–99.

3. Lewis DK, Whitty CJ, Walsh AL, et al. Treatable factors associated with severe anaemia in adults admitted to medical wards in Blantyre, Malawi, an area of high HIV seroprevalence. Trans R Soc Trop Med Hyg 2005;99(8):561–7.

4. Reddy EA, Shaw AV, Crump JA. Community-acquired bloodstream infections in Africa: a systematic review and meta-analysis. Lancet Infect Dis 2010;10(6):417–32.

5. Crump JA, Heydermann RS. A perspective on Invasive Salmonella Disease in Africa. Clin Infect Dis 2015;61(S4):235–40.

30

A 12-Year-Old Boy from Rural Kenya With Painful Eyes

HILLARY K. RONO, ANDREW BASTAWROUS AND NICHOLAS A.V. BEARE

Clinical Presentation

History

A 12-year-old boy is brought to a health centre in rural north-west Kenya. He reports 2 months of painful, watery, red eyes. The watering of his eyes is worse in the sun and he is struggling to keep his eyes open.

Six months previously he was treated at a dispensary for less severe symptoms. He was given tetracycline eye ointment but his symptoms did not improve. After this, he went to a traditional healer who applied some juice extracts from the ecucuka plant (*Aloe vera* species). After instillation he experienced severe eye pain and discharge, both eyes became very red and he could hardly see.

The boy lives with his parents in Loima, Turkana County, a hot, dusty and dry area of Kenya. They fetch water from a dried riverbed about 6 kilometres from home. They keep herds of cows and sheep, and the boy helps with herding and watering.

Clinical Findings

A 12-year-old boy who appears systemically well. Very poor vision in both eyes: His visual acuity is 6/60 with the left eye, but he can only perceive hand movements with the right eye. The findings on examination are shown in Table 30.1 and Figures 30.1 and 30.2.

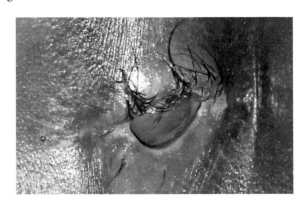

• **Fig. 30.1** The right eye showing lid scarring, trichiasis and extensive corneal opacification.

TABLE 30.1	Findings on Inspection of Both Eyes	
	Right Eye	**Left Eye**
Lid	Fibrotic lids with loss of lid architecture and tightening of palpebral aperture Loss of lashes from lower lid, misdirected and in-turned upper lid lashes (trichiasis)	Lids swollen, mucus deposits, eyelashes misdirected Eversion of lower lid margin
Conjunctiva	Severely inflamed >5 follicles (subepithelial inflammatory foci) identified on eversion of lids Scarring of the upper tarsal conjunctivae	
Cornea	Diffuse corneal opacification (scarring) with central thinning and irregular surface Fibrovascular pannus on the upper cornea	Focal inferocentral corneal scars, one with adherent iris indicating previous perforation Thin central cornea
Anterior chamber	Not visible	Shallow
Pupil	Not visible	Distorted towards the leucoma (corneal scar)

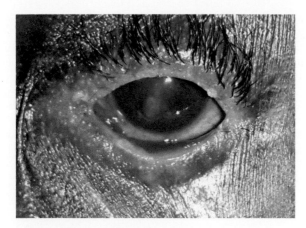

• **Fig. 30.2** The left eye with a focal corneal scarring including a perforated corneal ulcer with adherent iris (leucoma).

Questions

1. What are your differential diagnoses?
2. What features fit the criteria for trachoma?

Discussion

A 12-year-old Kenyan boy from a pastoralist community in an arid area presents with painful, red eyes, discharge and poor vision. He has a history of using traditional eye medicine. On examination he has lid, conjunctival and corneal scarring associated with severe follicular inflammation and trichiasis (in-turning lashes). One eye has a perforated corneal ulcer with scarred iris adhesion (leucoma).

Answer to Question 1

What Are Your Differential Diagnoses?

The most important diagnoses to consider are:

1. Corneal and conjunctival damage from use of traditional eye medicine.
2. Trachomatous trichiasis.
3. Vitamin A deficiency.

Further useful information includes dietary intake, history of measles predisposing to vitamin A deficiency and ideally blood retinol (vitamin A) levels (this only drops once hepatic stores of vitamin A are severely depleted).

Answer to Question 2

What Features Fit the Criteria for Trachoma?

For the diagnosis of trachoma, two out of five clinical criteria need to be fulfilled. This boy has all five criteria:

1. Follicles on the tarsal (inner) conjunctiva. These are 0.5 to 2 mm pale, raised inflammatory foci with hyperaemic surround. Multiple follicles give a rough or dimpled appearance to the surface of the conjunctiva.
2. Conjunctival scarring of the upper tarsal conjunctiva. White bands or strands evident on everting (flipping) the upper eyelid which can also sometimes be seen on the inner lower lid.

3. Limbal follicles or Herbert's pits. Follicles can occur at the edge of the cornea (limbus), and they leave 0.5 to 2 mm dark circular lesions (Herbert's pits).
4. Fibrovascular pannus, mostly affecting the upper cornea. Ingrowth of fibrovascular tissue from the limbus ruining the transparency of the cornea.
5. Trichiasis on the upper lid. In-turning of the lashes so they scuff the cornea.

The Case Continued...

The child was diagnosed with bilateral trachomatous trichiasis (TT), corneal opacity (CO) and a left perforating corneal ulcer. These may have been exacerbated by the application of traditional medicine.

He was admitted and given oral azithromycin and oral vitamin A supplements. He was referred to the ophthalmologist for lid surgery to redress trichiasis, and for a conjunctival flap to seal the corneal defect.

SUMMARY BOX

Trachoma

Trachoma, caused by *Chlamydia trachomatis,* is the leading infectious cause of blindness in the world. It accounts for about 1.4% of the world's blindness, but rates in affected communities in Africa are much higher. In endemic areas, active trachoma prevalence in pre-school children can be as high as 60% to 90%.

Trachoma is common in poor rural communities, where there is scarcity of water, poor sanitation and low socioeconomic status. The spread occurs because of overcrowding within households. Women are affected more than men and younger children are at greater risk of infection, especially children under 5 years old.

After repeated infections in childhood, signs of trachoma progress from conjunctival inflammation to scarring. Scarring of the tarsal conjunctiva leads to inversion of the lid resulting in trichiasis. Repetitive damage and infections lead to corneal scarring and consequent visual impairment or blindness.

A simplified scheme for assessing and classifying trachoma based on clinical signs has been developed. The stages are:
Trachomatous inflammation with follicles (TF)
Intense trachomatous inflammation (TI)
Trachomatous conjunctival scarring (TS)
Trachomatous trichiasis (TT) and
Corneal opacity because of trachoma (CO).

TF and TI are prevalent in young children and are manifestations of moderate and severe active infection, while TT is common in adults.

WHO has a global programme to eliminate trachoma as a disease of public health importance by 2020 (GET 2020). This programme includes mass antibiotic administrations to reduce the prevalence of *Chlamydia* infections, facial cleanliness, environmental improvement and surgery – the SAFE strategy:

S   Surgery for advanced cases.
A   Antibiotic treatment.
F   Facial cleanliness to reduce transmission.
E   Environmental improvement.

Both tetracyclines and macrolides are effective against trachoma in its acute stage (TF and TI). Tetracycline ointment can be applied twice daily for 6 weeks. However, adherence to this treatment is poor. A single oral dose of azithromycin is equally effective and more convenient (20 mg/kg for children, 1 g for adults). The WHO recommends 3 years of annual azithromycin as part of a trachoma control programme in communities where active trachoma is present in >10% of children. However, without additional environmental and economic improvement antibiotic treatment will not have a permanent effect. Communities need to secure suitable water supply, build and use well-designed latrines, safely dispose of rubbish and house animals apart from the family home.

Further Reading

1. Beare NAV, Bastawrous A. Ophthalmology in the tropics and sub-tropics. In: Farrar J, editor. Manson's Tropical Diseases. 23rd ed. London: Elsevier; 2013 [chapter 67].

2. Mabey DC, Solomon AW, Foster A. Trachoma. Lancet 2003;362 (9379):223–9.

3. Negrel AD, Mariotti SP. Trachoma rapid assessment: rationale and basic principles. Community Eye Health/Int Cent Eye Health 1999;12(32):51–3.

4. Emerson PM, Burton M, Solomon AW, et al. The SAFE strategy for trachoma control: using operational research for policy, planning and implementation. Bull WHO 2006;84(8):613–9.

5. WHO. Trachoma. Available from https://www.who.int/news-room/fact-sheets/detail/trachoma (accessed 27.06.2019.).

31

A 6-Year-Old Boy from Malawi With Fever, Cough and Impaired Consciousness

CHARLOTTE ADAMCZICK

Clinical Presentation

History

You review a 6-year-old boy in the paediatric high dependency unit of a Malawian Central Hospital. The boy was admitted the night before because of high fever, dyspnoea and a dry cough which had started 3 days before. On admission, he was started on presumptive antimalarial treatment; the results of the malaria smear are pending.

The boy is known to be HIV-positive but is not yet on antiretroviral therapy (ART).

Clinical Findings

Examination reveals a sick child with a temperature of 39.8°C (103.6°F) and laboured breathing. The Blantyre coma score is 3/5. The boy has coryza and bilateral conjunctivitis. Behind both ears and on the forehead, you notice a fine maculopapular rash that has not been described before. There is bilateral axillary lymphadenopathy.

Questions

1. What is your differential diagnosis?
2. What complications do you expect and how do you manage the child?

Discussion

An HIV-positive Malawian boy presents with high fever, dry cough, coryza, conjunctivitis and impaired level of consciousness together with a fine maculopapular rash on the neck and face.

Answer to Question 1
What is Your Differential Diagnosis?

The symptoms and signs are rather non-specific and the list of differential diagnoses is long, ranging from malaria and typhoid fever to atypical pneumonia and various viral infections. Also a combination of different diagnoses has to be considered, given his state of immunosuppression.

However, the boy shows the three 'Cs' of "cough, coryza and conjunctivitis". Together with his rather conspicuous rash starting behind his ears, measles should be suspected.

Bright red spots with a whitish centre ('Koplik's spots') on the buccal mucosa would be pathognomonic; however, they may be absent, or may appear only for a short period of time.

Other viral infections presenting with a similar rash are rubella, enterovirus infection and infectious mononucleosis. Bacterial infections to consider include scarlet fever, meningococcal disease and rickettsial infections.

Answer to Question 2
What Complications Should You Expect and How Do You Manage the Patient?

Complications in measles are much more common in individuals with cellular immune defects than in the immunocompetent. Severe diarrhoea, septicaemia, giant cell pneumonia, superimposed bacterial pneumonia, encephalitis, otitis media and corneal ulcerations can complicate the course of disease. In this case, with a reduced Blantyre Coma Scale and laboured breathing, encephalitis and pulmonary involvement have to be considered.

Because the rash in this boy has only just appeared, he is still contagious and needs to be isolated and nursed in a separate room.

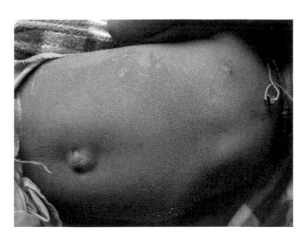

• **Fig. 31.1** Scaling of the erythematous rash.

The Case Continued…

The boy required IV fluids, and vitamin A was given for corneal protection. Malaria treatment was stopped as smears turned out to be negative. Within the next 3 days, the rash covered the trunk and skin scaling started over the chest (Fig. 31.1). The boy developed severe pneumonia and received antibiotic treatment. After recovery, antiretroviral therapy was started in the out-patient-clinic.

SUMMARY BOX

Measles

Measles is a highly contagious viral infection, caused by a para-myxovirus and transmitted through droplets. The course of the disease is strongly influenced by both nutritional and immune status of the affected individual.

Despite the availability of a highly effective vaccine, large measles outbreaks continue to occur worldwide. After an incubation period of 8 to 12 days, the non-specific prodromal stage presents with fever, conjunctivitis, rhinitis and cough, followed after a few days by a maculopapular rash, evolving behind the ears and in the face, spreading over the trunk and limbs. Severe desquamation of the skin may develop during the course of the illness. The patient is highly contagious from about 4 days before until up to 4 days after the appearance of the exanthema.

Immunocompromised individuals may not show the rash ('white measles'), nevertheless they are highly vulnerable to developing complications. Furthermore, a sub-acute 'inclusion-body' encephalitis has been described in the immunocompromised, which occurs a few months after the acute measles infection.

A late complication after several years is subacute severe sclerosing panencephalitis (SSPE), which is invariably fatal. SSPE has an incidence of one in 10 000 to one in a million cases of measles.

The Case Fatality Rate (CFR) in well-resourced settings is around 0.3 per 1000 whereas worldwide CFRs range between 3 and 5% and up to 30% in refugee settings. More than 95% of deaths occur in developing countries, mostly in children below the age of 5 years old.

There is no specific antiviral treatment. In developing countries, all children with measles should receive vitamin A supplementation, which prevents blindness and death. Vaccination or application of human immunoglobulin within 6 days of exposure may help protect non-vaccinated contacts.

Routine measles vaccination of children is recommended by WHO. Recent adaptations in international vaccination schedules are recommending measles vaccination in infants of 9 months of age. Almost 100% of children vaccinated with two doses of the safe live measles vaccine will have protective immunity. However, since measles is highly contagious, around 95% of a population need to be vaccinated to preserve herd immunity.

Asymptomatic and not severely immunocompromised children with HIV should receive measles vaccine because the risk of severe measles complications outweighs possible side effects of the vaccine. In severely immunocompromised persons with HIV, ART should be started and measles vaccination should be delayed until immune reconstitution. However, immune response may be hampered in HIV-positive individuals, particularly if the viral load is high at the time of vaccination.

Further Reading

1. Munoz FM. Viral exanthemas. In: Farrar J, editor. Manson's Tropical Diseases. 23rd ed. London: Elsevier; 2013 [chapter 20].
2. Maldonado A, Shetty A. Rubeola Virus: Measles and Subacute Sclerosing Panencephalitis. In: Long S, editor. Pediatric Infectious Diseases. 5th ed. Philadelphia: Elsevier; 2018 [chapter 227].
3. Mekki M, Ely B, Hardie D, et al. Subacute sclerosing panencephalitis: clinical phenotype, epidemiology, and preventive interventions. Dev Med Child Neurol 2019;61(10):1139–44. https://doi.org/10.1111/dmcn.14166.
4. Haban H, Benchekroun S, Sadeq M, et al. Seroprevalence of measles vaccine antibody response in vertically HIV-infected children in Morocco. BMC Infect Dis 2018;18:680. https://doi.org/10.1186/s12879-018-3590-y.

32

A 44-Year-Old Male Farmer from Laos With Diabetes and a Back Abscess

SAYAPHET RATTANAVONG, VALY KEOLUANGKHOT, SIHO SISOUPHONH, VATTHANAPHONE LATTHAPHASAVANG, DAVID A.B. DANCE AND CAOIMHE NIC FHOGARTAIGH

Clinical Presentation

History

A 44-year-old male rice farmer presents to a provincial hospital in Southern Laos in the rainy season with a 1-month history of fever, headache, generalized myalgia and arthralgia and a painful swelling over the left scapula. The swelling has gradually increased in size, without any history of preceding trauma. He has not noticed any lesions elsewhere. He was diagnosed with type 2 diabetes 4 years previously but was not compliant with oral antidiabetic drugs or follow-up. The lesion on his back was incised and drained at a local health centre the previous week, since when he has been taking cloxacillin 1 g four times daily. However, there has been no improvement and during the 2 days prior to admission he has deteriorated, with high fever, chills and severe malaise.

Clinical Findings

The patient appears septic, with a fever of 40°C (104°F), a heart rate of 136 bpm, blood pressure of 140/80 mmHg and a respiratory rate of 30 breath cycles per minute. He is pale and jaundiced. In the left scapular region, there is an erythematous swelling of 2.5 × 4 cm with pus discharging from a central wound (Fig. 32.1). There is no regional lymphadenopathy. On chest auscultation there are bilateral crepitations and reduced breath sounds at both lung bases. Heart sounds are normal. The abdomen is soft, without any palpable organomegaly.

Laboratory Results

The laboratory results are shown in Table 32.1.

Questions

1. What are your differential diagnoses?
2. What additional investigations would you like to do?

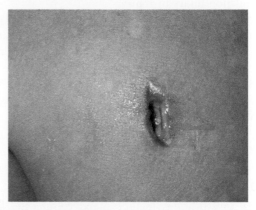

• **Fig. 32.1** Wound on the patient's left shoulder, after incision and drainage of the abscess. (Side finding: hypopigmented macular skin lesions of *Pityriasis versicolor* (*Malassezia* spp.), commonly seen in humid tropical climates.)

TABLE 32.1 Laboratory Results

Parameter	Patient	Reference Range
WBC (×10⁹/L)	16.2	6.0–8.0
Polymorphs (%)	92.1	45–70
Haemoglobin (g/dL)	12.5	12.0–16.0
Platelets (×10⁹/L)	112	150–300
Glucose (mmol/L)	20.6	4.1–6.1
Serum creatinine (μmol/L)	56	62–120
Urea (mmol/L)	6.8	5.4–16.1
AST (U/L)	131	0–37
ALT (U/L)	83	0–40
Serum total bilirubin (μmol/L)	111.2	1.71–20.5
Serum direct bilirubin (μmol/L)	56.4	0–7

Discussion

A male Lao rice famer presents during the rainy season with prolonged fever, jaundice, a back abscess and chest signs. He is a known type 2 diabetic but has been non-adherent to his antidiabetic medication.

Answer to Question 1

What Are Your Differential Diagnoses?

Bacterial abscess with sepsis may be caused by *Staphylococcus aureus*, *Streptococcus pyogenes* or other *Streptococcus* species, *Klebsiella pneumoniae*, *Vibrio vulnificus* or anaerobes. This patient, however, has epidemiological and clinical risk factors for melioidosis, caused by *Burkholderia pseudomallei*. This may cause a spectrum of disease in immunocompromised patients, especially diabetics, ranging from localized abscesses to pneumonia and septicaemia with disseminated abscess formation and high mortality. There is often no history of an inoculation injury or trauma.

Tuberculosis should also be considered with the sub-acute history of abscess with respiratory findings; however, tuberculous abscesses are usually 'cold', without much pain, erythema or warmth.

Disseminated fungal infection seems unlikely but would be possible if there was additional immunocompromise such as HIV.

Answer to Question 2

What Additional Investigations Would You Like to Do?

Essential investigations include blood culture and abscess swab (or deep pus) for microscopy and culture. A throat swab, or sputum sample if there is pulmonary involvement, may also be cultured on selective media, such as Ashdown's agar. A chest radiograph (CXR) should be done looking for evidence of pneumonia or pleural effusion. An ultrasound of the abdomen, or other imaging such as CT or MRI scan, should also be considered, because the findings of liver and splenic abscesses would strongly support a diagnosis of melioidosis while culture results are awaited. Biochemistry assays to check glucose and creatinine are important to optimize glycaemic control and adjust drug dosage respectively. Depending on the CXR findings, sputum, pleural fluid and pus may be sent for staining for acid-fast bacilli (e.g. Ziehl–Neelsen stain) and M. tuberculosis-PCR (e.g. Xpert MTB/RIF).

The Case Continued...

Pus culture yielded *B. pseudomallei* after 48 hours, and later his blood culture also grew the same bacterium. Three throat swabs were cultured on selective media but failed to grow the organism. The CXR revealed bilateral pleural effusions (Fig. 32.2). A shoulder radiograph showed no evidence of bony involvement. Abdominal ultrasound showed hepatosplenomegaly without evidence of liver or splenic abscesses.

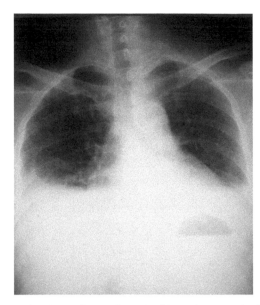

• **Fig. 32.2** Admission chest radiograph of the patient, showing bilateral pleural effusions.

The patient was empirically treated with ceftriaxone and gentamicin while awaiting the culture results. Treatment was switched to ceftazidime after 48 hours when the laboratory alerted the clinicians to the suspicion of melioidosis. The patient improved after 7 days of treatment and was afebrile by day 14, when he was switched to oral co-trimoxazole to complete 20 weeks. Glycaemic control was established. No other foci of infection were detected by locally available investigations. The patient was discharged after 21 days of hospitalization and continued on oral 'eradication' treatment for 5 months. He remains well.

SUMMARY BOX

Melioidosis

Melioidosis is an infectious disease caused by *B. pseudomallei*, an environmental saprophyte endemic to South and South-east Asia and northern Australia. The disease is being described with increasing frequency both in non-endemic and in endemic areas. This may be because of a combination of greater awareness, improving laboratory facilities and research and possibly also as a result of a genuine increase in incidence. A modelling study has estimated 165,000 human melioidosis cases with 89,000 deaths per year worldwide making it a significant neglected tropical disease (NTD), even though it does not feature on the WHO's list of NTDs.

North-eastern Thailand and northern Australia are highly endemic areas, where *B. pseudomallei* is an important cause of community-acquired sepsis and pneumonia. It is probably widely distributed elsewhere outside the endemic region and may be greatly underdiagnosed.

Humans are thought usually to become infected by percutaneous inoculation through cuts and abrasions (e.g. when working in rice fields), inhalation/aspiration during severe weather events and ingestion (e.g. ingestion of contaminated and unchlorinated water supplies), although it is often difficult to determine precisely the mode of acquisition. Host factors are very important; the majority of cases occur in those who are immunocompromised, especially with diabetes mellitus, but also alcoholism, chronic lung disease, chronic renal disease, thalassaemia, steroid use, immunosuppressive therapy and cancer, but surprisingly not HIV infection. The disease is highly seasonal, with 80% of cases presenting during the wet season.

Clinical presentation varies from benign localized infection to rapidly progressive septicaemia. The bacteraemic form accounts for 40% to 60% of cases; and over half present with pneumonia, which carries a case fatality rate of 10% to 40%. The lethality is even higher in resource-poor settings where there is limited access to early diagnosis, appropriate antibiotic treatment and intensive care facilities. The organism may localize in the lungs, liver, spleen, prostate, parotid, skin and soft tissue, bones and joints, or the central nervous system, causing abscesses and granulomas; but approximately 10% to 15% of bacteraemic cases have no evident clinical focus. It is important to use available imaging to identify the extent of infection and monitor the course of treatment. The confirmation of the diagnosis of melioidosis is based on the isolation and identification of *B. pseudomallei* in clinical samples, and in endemic areas it may be possible to reduce the time to diagnosis using immunofluorescence and lateral flow immunoassay on clinical specimens, and *B. pseudomallei* antigen latex agglutination on isolates. Serology has relatively low sensitivity and specificity with high rates of background seropositivity in those living in endemic regions. PCR assays on clinical specimens, aiming to provide a more rapid diagnosis, showed high specificity however the sensitivity on blood specimens depends on adequate bacterial concentration.

Parenteral antibiotics (e.g. ceftazidime, meropenem) are usually given for 2 weeks in the acute phase, followed by oral co-trimoxazole to complete 3 to 6 months eradication therapy to minimize risk of relapse. For patients unable to take co-trimoxazole, co-amoxiclav is an alternative but has higher relapse rates. Supportive treatment of sepsis and surgical drainage of abscesses, as well as control of predisposing factors are also critical in optimizing outcome.

Further Reading

1. Dance DB. Melioidosis. In: Farrar J, editor. Manson's Tropical Diseases. 23rd ed. London: Elsevier; 2014 [chapter 16].
2. Currie BJ. Melioidosis: evolving concepts in epidemiology, pathogenesis, and treatment. Seminars in respiratory and critical care medicine 2015;36(1):111–25.
3. Limmathurotsakul D, Golding N, Dance DA, et al. Predicted global distribution of Burkholderia pseudomallei and burden of melioidosis. Nat Microbiol 2016;1(1):15008.
4. Wiersinga WJ, Virk HS, Torres AG, et al. Melioidosis. Nat Rev Dis Primers 2018;4:17107.
5. Dance D. Treatment and prophylaxis of melioidosis. Int J Antimicrob Agents 2014;43(4):310–8.

33

A 53-Year-Old Man from Malawi With a Chronic Cough

CAMILLA ROTHE

Clinical Presentation

History

A 53-year-old Malawian man presents to a local hospital with a productive cough and whitish sputum for 3 months. He also reports night sweats and some weight loss, which he is unable to quantify.

Two months earlier he presented to a health centre with the same complaints. He was given presumptive antimalarials and amoxicillin for 5 days, but to no avail.

The patient is not aware of any tuberculosis (TB) contacts. He is currently not on any medication and his past medical history is unremarkable. He is a subsistence farmer. He has never worked in a mine or in the construction industry. He is a non-smoker. He is married with five children; all are well.

Clinical Findings

53-year-old man, slightly wasted. Temperature 38.8°C (101.8°F), blood pressure 100/80 mmHg, pulse 88 bpm, oxygen saturation 97% on ambient air. He appears mildly anaemic. On inspection of his mouth there is no oral thrush, no Kaposi's sarcoma and no oral hairy leukoplakia. His chest is clear and there are normal heart sounds without any murmurs. There is no lymphadenopathy; liver and spleen are not enlarged.

Investigations

The HIV-test is reactive. His further laboratory results are shown in Table 33.1.

Chest Radiography

His chest radiograph on admission shows a prominent hilar region bilaterally but is otherwise normal (Fig. 33.1).

TABLE 33.1 Laboratory Results on Admission

Parameter	Patient	Reference
WBC (×10⁹/L)	3.2	4–10
Haemoglobin (g/dL)	9.8	13–15
MCV (fL)	90	80–98
Platelets (×10⁹/L)	305	150–350
CD4 count (cells/µL)	54	500–1200
Sputum for AFB	2 × negative	Negative
Malaria RDT	Negative	Negative
Thick smear for *Plasmodium* spp.	Negative	Negative

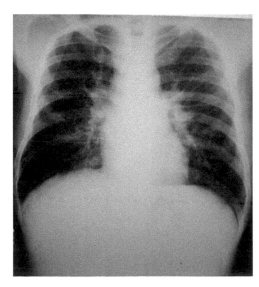

• **Fig. 33.1** Chest radiograph on admission showing a prominent hilar region.

Questions

1. What is your suspected diagnosis?
2. How would you approach this patient?

Discussion

A 53-year-old Malawian man presents with chronic cough and constitutional symptoms. A course of oral antibiotics did not yield any improvement. The patient is not aware of any TB contacts. On admission he is newly diagnosed with HIV-infection and advanced immunosuppression. His sputum microscopy is negative for acid-fast bacilli (AFB). Chest radiography shows a prominent hilar region but is otherwise normal.

Answer to Question 1

What is Your Suspected Diagnosis?

In all HIV-positive patients with cough and weight loss who do not respond to antibiotic therapy, tuberculosis is top of the list of differential diagnoses. In this case the most likely diagnosis is smear-negative pulmonary TB.

TB in patients with advanced immunosuppression often presents with a clinical picture that is very different from immunocompetent individuals: sputum smear-negative TB, which is uncommon in HIV-negative patients, is commonly seen in HIV-infected patients, particularly if immunosuppression is advanced as in this case. The slightly prominent hilar region seen on the patient's chest radiograph is compatible with the intrathoracic lymphadenopathy: typical though not specific for TB. Physical examination of the chest is normal in about half of HIV patients with pulmonary TB.

The fact that the patient does not report any TB contact should not be overvalued. Firstly, TB in immunosuppression is often a consequence of reactivation and the primary infection may have been decades ago. Secondly, in resource-limited countries, practically everyone is exposed to TB – this could occur during a ride on an overcrowded minibus or when congregating with friends and family in someone's small home.

Given the fact that our patient is in an advanced stage of immunosuppression and has not taken any co-trimoxazole prophylaxis, an alternative or possibly co-existing diagnosis to consider is *Pneumocystis jirovecii* pneumonia (PCP). A concomitant bacterial chest infection is possible but unlikely to explain the whole 3 months of illness.

Kaposi's sarcoma (KS) of the lung is another differential diagnosis to consider, but patients with pulmonary KS usually have manifestations of KS elsewhere (skin, oral mucosa). On chest radiography of patients with pulmonary KS, patchy infiltrations are commonly seen in the lower lung zones. Neither was the case in our patient, which makes this diagnosis unlikely.

Pulmonary malignancy or pulmonary sarcoidosis, which would be high on the list of differential diagnoses in industrialized countries, are much less likely than an infectious cause in the given setting.

Apart from chest infections, Gram-negative sepsis secondary to invasive non-typhoidal *Salmonellae* (iNTS) needs to be considered in this febrile and anaemic patient with advanced immunosuppression.

Answer to Question 2

How Would You Approach This Patient?

Induced sputum should be examined for acid-fast bacilli. Real-time PCR-based tests such as XPert MTB/RIF are easy to use, more sensitive than microscopy and also help detect rifampicin resistance. Thanks to an endorsement by WHO and international donor support, XPert MTB/RIF is increasingly available even at remote hospitals in rural areas.

Mycobacterial cultures of the sputum should be done but results will take several weeks, too long to guide the clinician's imminent decision.

Ideally, bronchoscopy with bronchoalveolar lavage should be done and material assessed for *M. tuberculosis* (PCR, culture, microscopy) and *Pneumocystis jirovecii* (PCR, microscopy). Pulmonary Kaposi's sarcoma could also be diagnosed on endoscopy.

Urine lipoarabinomannan (urine-LAM) is a simple lateral-flow assay helpful to look for TB in patients with advanced immunosuppression (CD4 <100/μl). A positive test indicates disseminated TB with renal involvement.

Ultrasound is also very useful and simple to look for signs of extrapulmonary/disseminated TB in patients with advanced immunosuppression. Simple and very useful algorithms have been published to guide clinicians not ultrasound-experienced in the diagnosis of TB.

If none of these investigations is available, it is well justifiable to empirically start the patient on antituberculous treatment, because sputum smear-negative TB is common and fatal if untreated. Adding prednisolone for the first 4 weeks of antituberculous treatment has been shown to reduce the incidence of immune-reconstitution inflammatory syndrome (IRIS).

Additional antibiotic treatment should be considered in this febrile patient with advanced immunosuppression. If available, blood cultures should be taken in any febrile patient before starting antibiotic treatment. Also, adding high-dose co-trimoxazole to antituberculous therapy as presumptive treatment for PCP has to be considered if the patient does not clinically improve. The optimal timing to initiate antiretroviral therapy (ART) is within the first 8 weeks of starting antituberculous treatment and within the first 2 weeks for patients who have CD4 cell counts <50 cells/μl.

The Case Continued…

Induced sputum results came back negative for AFB and there was no sputum PCR available. The patient's exercise test (walking down the hospital corridor three times at a fast pace) showed oxygen saturation of 98% as opposed to 97% at rest, and was therefore negative.

The patient was treated for a possible bacterial chest infection, covering also for Gram-negative bacteria. He received ceftriaxone 2g IV od and erythromycin 500 mg qid for 5 days. It was decided not to treat him for PCP and he received the prophylactic dose of co-trimoxazole (480 mg bid according to local national guidelines). Nonetheless, his fever persisted, even though the cough subjectively improved slightly.

On day 7 in the hospital, the patient was started on empirical treatment for smear-negative TB with four antituberculous drugs (Isoniazid (H), Rifampicin (R), Pyrazinamide (P) and Ethambutol (E). After the first week of treatment, he started to feel better. His fever went down and the cough gradually settled. He was discharged home. Three weeks into the TB treatment he was seen at the HIV clinic. He was doing well and had started antiretroviral therapy.

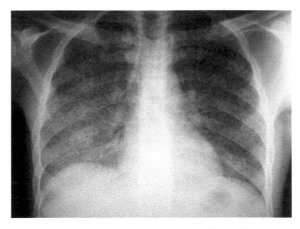

• **Fig. 33.2** Chest radiograph of a patient with miliary TB.

TABLE 33.2	**Clinical Presentation of TB in Patients With and Without Immunosuppression**	
	HIV-negative or high CD4 count (>200/µL)	**Low CD4 count (≤200/µL)**
Cough and sputum production	Severe, productive	Often mild, small amounts of whitish sputum
Haemoptysis	Common	Rare
Chest radiography appearance	Cavities, upper lobe infiltrates and destruction	No cavities Infiltrates Hilar lymphadenopathy Miliary pattern May be completely normal
Sputum smear result	Often positive	Often negative
Extrapulmonary and disseminated TB*	≤20% of TB cases	Common, about 50%

*Disseminated = involving two or more non-contiguous organs concomitantly.
(After Harries, A.D., et al., 2004. and Sharma, S.K., et al., 2005.)

Cavitating smear-positive pulmonary TB, as seen classically in HIV-negative individuals, is uncommon in advanced immunosuppression. Instead, patients more commonly present with sputum smear-negative pulmonary TB. CXR may be completely normal and clinical symptoms are often discrete; patients may produce little sputum and haemoptysis is rare.

HIV-positive individuals are also more likely to present with extrapulmonary TB manifesting as pleural effusion, pericardial disease, lymph node TB, abdominal TB, TB meningitis and miliary disease or a combination of these (Fig. 33.2). Severe anaemia is a common clinical clue to a co-infection with HIV/TB and reflects bone marrow involvement.

When treating HIV/TB co-infected patients, pharmacokinetic interactions between rifampicin and antiretroviral drugs have to be considered. Adding prednisolone during the first 4 weeks of antituberculous treatment may help decrease the risk of immune-reconstitution inflammatory syndrome (IRIS).

Further Reading

1. Thwaites G. Tuberculosis. In: Farrar J, editor. Manson's Tropical Diseases. 23rd ed. London: Elsevier; 2013 [chapter 40].
2. Lawn SD. Advances in diagnostic assays for Tb. Cold Spring Harb Perspect Med 2015;5:a017806.
3. Lawn SD, Brooks SV, Kranzer K, et al. Screening for HIV-Associated Tuberculosis and Rifampicin Resistance before Antiretroviral Therapy Using the Xpert MTB/RIF Assay: A Prospective Study. PLoS Med 2011;8(7). e1001067. https://doi.org/10.1371/journal.pmed.1001067.
4. Heller T, Wallrauch C, Goblirsch S, et al. Focused assessment with sonography for HIV-associated tuberculosis (FASH): a short protocol and a pictorial review. Crit Ultrasound J 2012;4:21.
5. Meintjes G, Stek C, Blumenthal L, et al. Prednisone for the Prevention of Paradoxical Tuberculosis-Associated IRIS. N Engl J Med 2018;379:1915–25. https://doi.org/10.1056/NEJMoa1800762.

SUMMARY BOX

Tuberculosis in HIV-Infected Patients

TB and HIV infection are the most important 'tropical' diseases in adults in many parts of sub-Saharan Africa. Co-infection with HIV and TB is common and poses a particular challenge to the clinician.

Clinical presentation of TB changes with declining peripheral CD4 counts (Table 33.2).

34

A 35-Year-Old Male Farmer from Peru With a Chronic Ulcer and Multiple Nodular Lesions on the Arm

FERNANDO MEJÍA CORDERO, BEATRIZ BUSTAMANTE AND EDUARDO H. GOTUZZO

Clinical Presentation

History

A 35-year-old farmer from the Peruvian highlands presents to a reference hospital in the capital, Lima, with a 2-month history of a slowly growing ulcer and multiple painless nodules on his left arm.

Two months before presentation, the patient suffered a scratch on his left hand from a tree branch while working in the fields. After a few days, he noticed a small painless erythematous papule that later developed into a pustule. He took antibiotics without improvement. Over the following weeks new pustules appeared, and the lesion started to ulcerate and increased in size, despite continued antibiotics and topical traditional medicines. Four weeks after the initial papule the patient noticed painless firm nodules on his left forearm. The patient was seen at a regional hospital and treated empirically for cutaneous leishmaniasis with a 20-day course of pentavalent antimonials, but showed no improvement. He was then referred for further diagnosis and treatment.

The patient was previously healthy. He denied recent contact with animals or travel.

Clinical Findings

The patient appears generally well. His vital signs are normal and he is afebrile.

On his left hand there is a single ulcerative lesion (20 × 30 mm) with irregular elevated borders (Fig. 34.1) and multiple subcutaneous erythematous nodules (10 × 10 mm) along the lymphatic tract of the left arm (Fig. 34.2). The rest of the physical examination is normal.

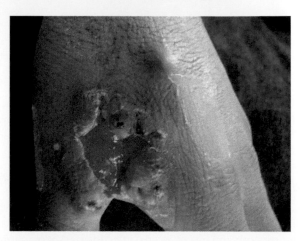

• **Fig. 34.1** Initial ulcerated lesion on the left hand. Note the pustular lesion near the ulcer.

Laboratory Results

The WBC is 4.5×10^9/L (reference range $4–10 \times 10^9$/L) with normal differential count; haemoglobin is 11.3 g/dL (12–16 g/dL). The remainder of the full blood count is normal.

Questions

1. What are your differential diagnoses?
2. How would you approach this patient?

Discussion

A Peruvian farmer presents with a chronic ulcerative lesion on his left hand and contiguous involvement of the lymphatic tract compatible with nodular lymphangitis. The

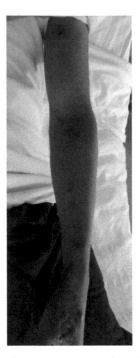

• **Fig. 34.2** Multiple subcutaneous nodules along the lymphatic tract.

lesions started after a minor traumatic injury. The patient denies systemic symptoms. Laboratory examination shows mild anaemia.

Answer to Question 1
What Are Your Differential Diagnoses?

In Peru, the common differential diagnoses of a chronic ulcer with nodular lymphangitis include cutaneous leishmaniasis, sporotrichosis and mycobacterial infection by *Mycobacterium tuberculosis* or *M. marinum*.

Leishmaniasis is endemic in the Andes between 1000 and 3000 m altitude and in the Amazon Basin. The patient's origin and clinical presentation are highly suggestive of cutaneous leishmaniasis. However, the lack of clinical improvement after a complete course of pentavalent antimonials (>80% cure rate) makes this diagnosis unlikely.

Sporotrichosis is the second most important diagnosis to consider. The patient's clinical features are typical and the disease is commonly seen in Peru. Another diagnosis to keep in mind is secondary cutaneous tuberculosis, especially because the patient has likely been exposed to *M. tuberculosis* during his lifetime. The patient has no history of exposure to fresh and saltwater environments to suggest infection with *M. marinum*. Nocardiosis (*Nocardia brasiliensis*) and tularaemia (*Francisella tularensis*) are other causes of nodular lymphangitis but are unlikely in this patient, because nocardiosis is rare and tularaemia has never been reported in the southern hemisphere.

Answer to Question 2
How Would You Approach This Patient?

The first step is the collection of specimens for microscopy (smears for Gram, Giemsa and Ziehl–Neelsen stains), culture and, if available, PCR for *Leishmania and Mycobacterium* species and *Sporothrix schenckii*. Specimens should be collected by scraping of the base of the active ulcer, biopsy of the edge of the lesion, and fine-needle aspiration of one of the lymphatic nodules. If available, a leishmanin skin test would be a useful diagnostic tool. Fungi such as *S. schenckii* grow on special media and the laboratory should be informed of the clinical suspicion of sporotrichosis. The initial evaluation should also include chest radiography and a PPD skin test to rule out tuberculosis.

The Case Continued...

The chest x-ray was normal and PPD skin testing was negative. No leishmania parasites were observed by direct microscopy, and the leishmanin skin test was negative. *Leishmania* culture was not performed. Mycobacterial cultures were negative. However, culture of the ulcer scraping and nodule aspiration were positive for *S. schenckii*.

A diagnosis of lymphocutaneous sporotrichosis was made. The mild anaemia was likely to be unrelated. The patient was started on itraconazole PO 200 mg/day. After 8 months of treatment the ulcer and nodular lesions had resolved and the patient was considered to be cured.

SUMMARY BOX

Sporotrichosis

Sporotrichosis is a sub-acute to chronic fungal infection caused by *S. schenckii*, a dimorphic fungus with a worldwide distribution, existing as a saprophytic mould in soil and plants and as a yeast in tissues. Cutaneous sporotrichosis is the most common form of the disease, which is acquired by inoculation during minor injury by animal bites, plant thorns or other cutting vegetation. Sporotrichosis has in addition emerged as a zoonosis transmitted mainly by infected cats, with epidemic outbreaks in Brazil and some countries in South America, caused by *S. brasiliensis*. The upper limbs are most commonly affected. The infection is usually limited to the cutaneous, subcutaneous and lymphatic tissues surrounding the injury. The initial papule at the inoculation site typically grows slowly into a nodule and then ulcerates. Contiguous lymphatic spread is very common (48–92%) and is referred to as 'nodular lymphangitis' or 'sporotrichoid lymphangitis'. The majority of cases are sporadic. Farmers, veterinarians, rose gardeners and others regularly engaged in outdoor activities are at highest risk. Persons with pre-existing chronic conditions (e.g., alcohol abuse) or immunosuppression (e.g., HIV/AIDS) are at risk of developing pulmonary sporotrichosis after mould inhalation or disseminated sporotrichosis after haematogenous spread from the cutaneous lesion.

The fungi are scarce in tissues and generally not detected on microscopy. Serology is not useful because of low sensitivity and specificity. Diagnosis is based on isolation of the organism by culture of the skin biopsy, lesion aspirate, or sputum. *S. schenckii* grows on Saboraud agar at 25 to 27°C. Also, molecular methods may be used.

Spontaneous resolution of the lesions is rare. Itraconazole PO 200 mg/day is considered the drug of choice for cutaneous sporotrichosis. The treatment should be continued for 2 to 4 weeks after resolution of all lesions, typically 3 to 6 months but sometimes even requiring years. Saturated solution of potassium iodide, a cheap and effective drug, has also been widely used but its low tolerability and many unpleasant side effects (e.g., salivary gland swelling, metallic taste, rash and fever) limit its use. Terbinafine is also an alternative treatment. Itraconazole (200 mg PO bd for 1–2 years) is also the preferred drug for pulmonary or osteoarticular sporotrichosis. In severely ill patients or patients with disseminated disease, initial therapy with amphotericin B is recommended, with conversion to oral itraconazole after a favourable response and stabilization. Relapses are infrequent with all forms and therapy, although long-term secondary prophylaxis might be required in patients with HIV/AIDS.

Further Reading

1. Hay RJ. Fungal infections In: Farrar J, editor. Manson's Tropical Diseases. 23rd ed. London: Elsevier; 2013 [chapter 38].
2. Sanchotene KO, Madrid IM, Klafke GB, Bergamashi M, Terra PPD, Rodrigues AM, Xavier MO. Sporothrix brasiliensis outbreaks and the rapid emergence of feline sporotrichosis. Mycoses 2015;58:652–8.
3. Barros MB, de Almeida Paes R, Schubach AO. *Sporothrix schenckii* and sporotrichosis. Clin Microbiol Rev 2011;24(4):633–54.
4. Kauffman CA, Bustamante B, Chapman SW, et al. Clinical practice guidelines for the management of sporotrichosis: 2007 update by the Infectious Diseases Society of America. Clin Infect Dis 2007;45 (10):1255–65.
5. Hay R, Denning DW, Bonifaz A, Queiroz-Telles F, Beer K, Bustamante B. The Diagnosis of Fungal Neglected Tropical Diseases (Fungal NTDs) and the Role of Investigation and Laboratory Tests: An Expert Consensus Report. Trop Med Infect Dis 2019;4(4):E122.

35

A 32-Year-Old Woman from Malawi With Headache and Blurred Vision

CAMILLA ROTHE

Clinical Presentation

History

A 32-year-old Malawian woman presents to a local hospital with a 3-week history of headache and blurred vision. The headache has been gradual in onset and does not respond to over-the-counter painkillers. There is no fever and no history of convulsions or of head trauma.

The patient presented to a local health centre where she received presumptive antimalarial treatment (artemether/lumefantrine) and a course of antibiotics (amoxicillin 500 mg tds for 5 days), which was of no benefit.

Clinical Findings

The patient appears wasted and slightly anaemic. All vital signs are normal and she is afebrile. The GCS is 15/15. There is no neck stiffness. The visual acuity is normal on both sides. On left lateral gaze there is an abduction deficit of the left eye with 'blurring of vision' reported by the patient (Fig. 35.1). The rest of the examination is normal.

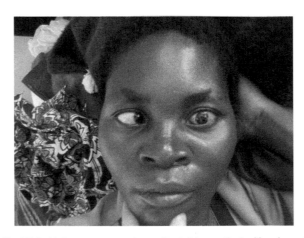

• Fig. 35.1 Abducens nerve palsy on the left in a patient with sub-acute headache.

TABLE 35.1 Laboratory Results on Admission

Parameter	Patient	Reference
WBC ($\times 10^9$/L)	3.7	4–10
Haemoglobin (g/dL)	10.2	12–16
MCV (fL)	92	80–98
Platelets ($\times 10^9$/L)	91	150–350
Fasting blood glucose (mmol/L)	5.43	5.0–6.7
Malaria RDT	Negative	Negative

Laboratory Results

See Table 35.1.

Questions

1. What are your differential diagnoses?
2. What investigations would you like to do?

Discussion

A Malawian woman presents with a chronic headache and 'blurred vision'. She is wasted and has a unilateral abducens nerve palsy. She is afebrile and has no neck stiffness. The full blood count shows normocytic anaemia and thrombocytopenia.

Answer to Question 1

What Are Your Differential Diagnoses?

The patient's clinical presentation suggests chronic meningitis. The two most important differential diagnoses are cryptococcal meningitis and tuberculous meningitis. Also, partially treated bacterial meningitis is a possibility because she received amoxicillin at the health centre, but the gradual onset of symptoms makes this less likely.

Chronic meningitis is commonly associated with immunosuppression. The patient lives in a part of the world with a high HIV prevalence. Her laboratory findings (anaemia and thrombocytopenia) are also common in untreated HIV infection.

Even though malaria may present with non-specific symptoms and both thrombocytopenia and anaemia are commonly seen in malaria patients, the absence of fever, the negative rapid diagnostic test (RDT) and the history of taking artemisinin combination therapy make it an unlikely differential diagnosis. Also, malaria usually does not cause cranial nerve palsies.

Answer to Question 2

What Investigations Would You Like to Do?

An HIV test is crucial and a lumbar puncture should be done without delay. Cerebrospinal fluid (CSF) opening pressure should be measured and documented. Routine CSF examination should include India Ink stain and bacterial and fungal cultures. Cryptococcal antigen (CrAg) should be tested in blood and CSF.

The Case Continued...

A lumbar puncture was done on admission. The CSF looked clear, but the opening pressure was increased at $50\,cmH_2O$ (normal: $10–18\,cmH_2O$). The CSF results are shown in Table 35.2.

A diagnosis of cryptococcal meningitis was made based upon a positive fungal culture result. India Ink was negative, but sensitivity is only at around 50–70%. CrAg, which is >95% sensitive, was not available.

The HIV serology came back positive. The CD4 count was very low at $22/\mu L$. The patient was started on oral fluconazole 1200 mg (see Summary Box), because the preferred fungicidal drugs Amphotericin B and flucytosine were not available.

She was also started on co-trimoxazole prophylaxis. She received repeated therapeutic lumbar punctures until the headache settled.

Antiretroviral therapy was commenced 4 weeks into her antifungal treatment. The patient returned to her village yet died 6 weeks later of an unknown cause.

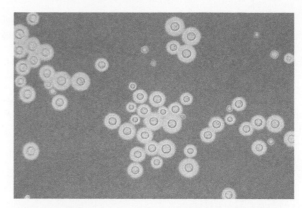

• **Fig. 35.2** Photomicrograph of *Cryptococcus neoformans* (India Ink stain). (**Source:** www.cdc.gov; www.cdc.gov/fungal/cryptococcosis-neoformans/)

SUMMARY BOX

Cryptococcal Meningitis

Cryptococcal meningitis (CM) occurs worldwide. Ninety-five per cent of CM cases in developing countries are HIV-associated. CM is the most common cause of adult meningitis in sub-Saharan Africa and parts of Asia where HIV prevalence is high.

Cryptococcal meningitis is caused by the encapsulated environmental yeast, *Cryptococcus neoformans*. It is an opportunistic infection, which occurs at advanced stages of immunosuppression, in HIV mostly at CD4 counts below $100/\mu L$. Patients usually present with a sub-acute headache of several days to weeks duration. Other common clinical findings are cranial nerve palsies (N VI), confusion and impaired consciousness. Altered mental state is associated with increased lethality. CM is clinically indistinguishable from tuberculous meningitis (TBM), although fever and neck stiffness are more common in TBM.

CSF opening pressure is often markedly elevated. Further CSF findings are commonly non-specific, and the CSF may even be normal. Diagnosis of CM is made by demonstrating the fungus in the CSF. This is traditionally done by light microscopy after India-Ink staining (Fig. 35.2), but this method is user-dependent and the sensitivity is therefore variable. Detection of CrAg e.g. by latex-agglutination test or lateral flow assay (LFA) is better. Fungal culture of CSF is required to isolate the organism for antimicrobial susceptibility testing. CM treatment consists of three phases: induction, consolidation, and maintenance. The gold standard is an induction therapy with two fungicidal drugs that rapidly decrease the fungal burden in the CSF i.e. combined (liposomal) amphotericin B plus flucytosine (IV or oral) for the initial 2 weeks, followed by oral fluconazole 400 mg daily for at least 8 weeks and fluconazole maintenance therapy 200 mg daily until immune reconstitution.

The reality in many resource-limited settings is however hampered by poor drug availability and therefore commonly differs from the gold standard. Oral fluconazole is often the only available drug, thanks to a drug donation programme by the manufacturing company. Fluconazole is only fungistatic, which may be effective as a secondary prophylaxis, but is less useful as induction therapy when potent fungicidal drugs are needed to rapidly bring down the fungal burden. Studies in low-income settings have demonstrated that even short courses of Amphotericin B (5–7 days) are preferable to treatment with fluconazole alone. Flucytosine, the other fungicidal drug, is expensive; and despite its great value in the treatment of CM, remains unlicensed in many African and Asian countries. Steroids are of no benefit in the treatment of HIV-associated cryptococcal meningitis.

TABLE 35.2	CSF Results on Admission	
Parameter	Patient	Reference
Leukocytes (cells/μL)	18	0–5
Protein (g/L)	0.8	0.15–0.40
Glucose (mmol/L)	1.97	2.22–3.88
India Ink	Negative	Negative
Culture	*C. neoformans*	Negative

Many patients with CM suffer from severe headaches, which do not respond to analgesics. The headache is caused by raised intracranial pressure (ICP) and therapeutic lumbar punctures (LPs) bring immediate pain relief. LPs may have to be repeated on a daily basis until the ICP has come down and sustained pain control has been achieved.

HIV-positive patients with CM should start antiretroviral therapy, but the optimum timing is not yet clear. Introduction of ART 4 to 10 weeks after starting antifungal treatment is currently considered the safest approach.

Prognosis of CM in resource-limited settings is poor and 10-week lethality on fluconazole monotherapy may exceed 60%.

Further Reading

1. Wood R. Clinical features and management of HIV/AIDS. In: Farrar J, editor. Manson's Tropical Diseases. 23rd ed. London: Elsevier; 2013 [chapter 10].

2. Perfect JR, Dismukes WE, Dromer F, et al. Clinical practice guidelines for the management of cryptococcal disease: 2010 update by the Infectious Diseases Society of America. Clin Infect Dis 2010;50(3):291–322.

3. Sloan DJ, Dedicoat MJ, Lalloo DG. Treatment of cryptococcal meningitis in resource limited settings. Curr Opin Infect Dis 2009;22(5):455–63.

4. Sloan DJ, Parris V. Cryptococcal meningitis: epidemiology and therapeutic options. Clin Epidemiol 2014;6:169–82.

5. Molloy SF, Kanyama C, Heyderman RS, et al. Antifungal Combinations for Treatment of Cryptococcal Meningitis in Africa. N Engl J Med 2018;378:1004–17.

36

A 23-Year-Old Farmer from Myanmar With Unilateral Scrotal Swelling

KENTARO ISHIDA AND CAMILLA ROTHE

Clinical Presentation

History

A 23-year-old farmer presents to a district hospital in Myanmar with a 3-year history of left-sided scrotal swelling. The swelling is non-tender and has gradually increased in size. There is no history of fever. He has attempted to treat the swelling with traditional herbal medicine to no avail.

The patient comes from the central part of Myanmar. He reports that scrotal swelling is not an uncommon problem in his home region.

Clinical Findings

The patient is a 23-year-old man in fair general condition. His vital signs are normal and he is afebrile. There is unilateral scrotal swelling, which cannot be reduced (Fig. 36.1). There are no palpable inguinal lymph nodes.

Questions

1. What is the differential diagnosis?
2. What investigations would you like to do?

Discussion

A young Burmese farmer presents with progressive unilateral scrotal swelling. On examination, the swelling is non-tender and non-reducible. He does not have any other symptoms or signs.

Answer Question 1

What is Differential Diagnosis?

The most common differentials to consider in a chronic, non-tender, unilateral scrotal swelling are inguinal hernia and hydrocoele. A testicular tumour also needs to be taken into consideration. Unlike hydrocoeles, hernias can often be manually reduced. Hydrocoeles may be verified by trans-illumination with a penlight.

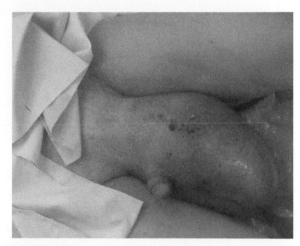

• **Fig. 36.1** Massive unilateral scrotal swelling. The swelling is non-tender and non-reducible.

The patient reports that scrotal swelling is common in the region where he comes from. This may suggest a possible infectious aetiology. The most important infectious disease to consider in this patient is lymphatic filariasis (LF) caused by *Wuchereria bancrofti*. Hydrocoele is the most common clinical abnormality in men with bancroftian filariasis.

Also, urogenital schistosomiasis *(Schistosoma haematobium)* may lead to unilateral scrotal swelling, but it is not endemic in South-east Asia. Testicular tuberculosis is another infectious disease that may manifest with scrotal swelling. However, the long duration of the swelling in the absence of other signs and symptoms make this unlikely, and it would not explain the large number of cases seen in his home region.

Answer Question 2

What Investigations Would You Like to Do?

Ultrasound can help distinguish a testicular tumour from a hydrocoele or hernia. Also, in case of lymphatic filariasis, adult worms may be seen on scrotal ultrasonography ("filarial dance sign").

99

The traditional diagnostic gold standard for lymphatic filariasis is the proof of microfilariae in the blood. Samples should be collected when microfilaraemia is highest. For the majority of filarial species, this is between 9 PM and 3 AM because of the nocturnal biting activities of most vectors. Microfilarial PCR assays have a sensitivity and specificity comparable to microscopy with an experienced microscopist, but are usually not available in a district hospital setting.

Circulating filarial antigen (CFA) tests detect antigens released by adult *W. bancrofti*. They are available as immunochromatographic card tests and can use finger-prick blood. Because there is no periodicity of adult-worm antigens, CFA tests can be taken at any time. Their sensitivity and specificity are high. CFA tests are also the preferred method for diagnosis and treatment monitoring of bancroftian filariasis within national control programmes. Antifilarial antibody testing lacks specificity and is of limited value.

The Case Continued...

Hydrocoele was confirmed on ultrasound. The patient underwent hydrocoelectomy, and 3 litres of clear fluid could be drained during the operation. He also received antifilarial treatment. He lived in a remote area and was lost to follow-up afterwards.

TABLE 36.1	Direct Effect of Most Commonly Used Drugs on Different Stages of *W. bancrofti* and *Brugia* species

	Microfilariae	Adults
Diethylcarbamazine (DEC)	++	+
Ivermectin	++	−
Albendazole	−	+
Doxycycline	−	++

++ = most eliminated; + = few/some eliminated; − = no effect.

The most advanced stage of chronic lymphoedema (stage III) is also referred to as 'elephantiasis'. Chronic ulceration with bacterial and fungal superinfection is a common problem.

Moreover, in areas of high HIV prevalence, lymphatic filariasis was found to increase susceptibility to HIV infection by inducing systemic CD4 T-cell activation.

Drugs used for treatment and control of lymphatic filariasis include diethylcarbamazine (DEC), ivermectin, albendazole and doxycycline.

Albendazole 400 mg STAT with either DEC (6 mg/kg) or ivermectin (200 µg/kg) reduces microfilaraemia to very low levels (Table 36.1). A triple therapy combining all three drugs appears even more efficacious.

However, DEC should not be given in areas co-endemic for onchocerciasis or loiasis because of potentially severe side effects, and care must be taken to administer ivermectin in areas with *Loa loa* co-endemicity.

Treatment in mass drug administration (MDA) programmes is recommended annually; whereas individual patients should get treatment every 6 months until microfilariae and CFA tests are negative, or life-long, if transmission goes on.

Doxycycline kills endosymbiotic *Wolbachia* bacteria, which adult worms require for viability and reproduction. Several weeks of treatment are required, and doxycycline is contraindicated in pregnancy and in children under the age of 8 years, which make it an unsuitable option for mass treatment. Its role may be in individual treatment of LF patients who lack any of the contraindications.

For management of lymphoedema, meticulous hygiene is crucial, such as daily washing with water and soap and careful drying of the affected limb. Bacterial and fungal infections should be treated early. Specialized shoes should be worn to prevent injury if the lower limbs are affected. Integration of lymphoedema care and leprosy or diabetic foot care programmes are being promoted.

Small hydrocoeles sometimes regress after anthelmintic treatment. Large hydrocoeles require surgery.

SUMMARY BOX

Lymphatic Filariasis

LF is caused by filarial nematodes (*W. bancrofti, Brugia malayi* and *B. timori*). LF is transmitted by a variety of mosquito species. It is endemic in South and South-east Asia, sub-Saharan Africa and parts of South America and the Caribbean. Around 68 million people worldwide are estimated to be infected with filarial parasites; an additional 20 million are suffering from chronic morbidity.

Lymphatic filariasis is a result of chronic, repeat exposure to filarial nematodes. It is therefore not a problem relevant for short-term travellers to endemic regions.

Adult worms reside in the lymphatic vessels of the human host. They shed microfilariae which are ingested by female mosquitoes during blood-meals.

The most common features of bancroftian filariasis are hydrocoele, acute adenolymphangitis (ADLA) and lymphoedema.

Hydrocoele results from the accumulation of fluid in the tunica vaginalis surrounding the testes. Most cases are unilateral. In endemic areas, hydrocoeles start to develop in early adulthood. Prevalence rates rise steadily with age. Rupture of dilated abdominal lymphatic vessels into the urinary tract may lead to chyluria. Brugian filariasis is milder than infection with *W. bancrofti*, and urogenital complications do not occur.

Acute ADLA occurs in episodic events that start with fever, chills and severe malaise. Regional lymph nodes are tender and enlarged, the affected limb may become swollen and hot and the skin may peel off. Repeated episodes of ADLA can lead to lymphoedema.

Chronic lymphoedema most commonly affects the lower leg, but may also involve the arms, breasts and genitals, as shown in this case.

Further Reading

1. Simonsen P, Fischer PU, Hoerauf A, et al. *The Filariases.* In: Farrar J, editor. Manson's Tropical Diseases. 23rd ed. London: Elsevier; 2013 [chapter 54].

2. Taylor MJ, Hoerauf A, Bockarie M. Lymphatic filariasis and onchocerciasis. Lancet 2010;376(9747):1175–85.

3. WHO. Lymphoedema and the chronic wound. The role of compression and other interventions. In: Macdonald JM, Geyer MJ,

editors. Wound and Lymphoedema Management. Geneva: World Health Organization; 2010. p. 1–136.

4. Thomsen EK, Sanuku N, Baea M, et al. Efficacy, safety and pharmacokinetics of co-administered diethylcarbamazine, albendazole and ivermectin for treatment of Bancroftian filariasis. Clin Inf Dis 2016;62(3):334–41.

5. Kroidl I, Saathoff E, Maganga L, et al. Effect of Wuchereria bancrofti infection on HIV-incidence in southwest Tanzania: a prospective cohort study. Lancet 2016;388:1912–20.

37

A 29-Year-Old Woman from Malawi With Confusion, Diarrhoea and a Skin Rash

CAMILLA ROTHE

Clinical Presentation

History

A 29-year-old woman is brought to a hospital in Malawi by her relatives. She has been confused, restless and irritable for the past month. She also has watery diarrhoea, which started 1 week ago. She does not have a fever. It is January, which is the rainy season in Malawi.

Her past medical history has been uneventful. There have been no psychiatric disorders in the past. Her HIV status is unknown. She is not taking any medication. There are no known intoxications, no use of alcohol or recreational drugs.

The patient is married with four children. She is a housewife. Her husband works as a farmhand on a local chicken farm. They live in a grass-thatched mud-hut and collect their water from a borehole. There is no electricity at home. They eat two meals a day, mainly maize porridge with a few vegetables. Only rarely can the family afford fish or meat.

Clinical Findings

The patient is slim but not wasted. Glasgow Coma Scale 14/15 (confusion), the remaining vital signs are normal and she is afebrile. There is no neck stiffness. The conjunctivae are pale. There is a noticeable skin rash around the patient's neck (Fig. 37.1), on her forearms, hands and feet (Fig. 37.2), where the skin appears hyperpigmented and dry. The skin changes are clearly demarcated. The rest of the physical examination is unremarkable. When asked, her relatives report that the rash had been present for the past 2 months.

Questions

1. What is the suspected diagnosis and what are your differential diagnoses?
2. How would you manage this patient?

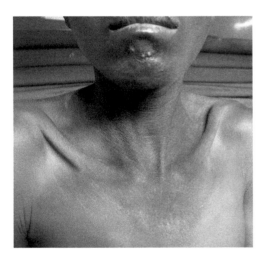

• **Fig. 37.1** Hyperpigmented skin rash on sun-exposed skin.

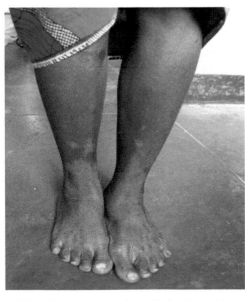

• **Fig. 37.2** The skin changes involve both hands and feet. The skin appears dry and scaly.

Discussion

A young Malawian woman presents during the rainy season with a 1-month history of confusion, acute watery diarrhoea and a rash that mainly seems to affect the sun-exposed areas of the skin. The family appear to be poor villagers; they live on an imbalanced diet.

Answer to Question 1

What is the Suspected Diagnosis and What Are Your Differential Diagnoses?

The patient presents with a triad of neuropsychiatric changes, watery diarrhoea and a photosensitive dermatitis. This clinical triad – diarrhoea, dermatitis, dementia – is typical of pellagra (vitamin B_3 deficiency). The rainy season, during which the patient presents, is not only the peak of malaria transmission but is also the 'hungry season'. Stocks have been consumed, the new crop is not ready for harvesting yet and in poor, rural areas large parts of the population go hungry.

A combination of confusion, diarrhoea and skin changes in a sub-Saharan African setting should also prompt any clinician to rule out HIV infection. Persistent confusion in the context of HIV is commonly seen in tuberculous meningitis, cryptococcal meningitis and progressive multifocal leukoencephalopathy (PML), or may be caused by the human immunodeficiency virus (HIV-associated neurocognitive disorder). Both diarrhoea and skin changes of various aetiologies commonly occur in HIV infection.

A further differential diagnosis to consider in a patient with photosensitive dermatitis, anaemia and neuropsychiatric changes is systemic lupus erythematosus.

Answer to Question 2

How Would You Manage This Patient?

Even though the clinical presentation is very typical of pellagra, other differential diagnoses should actively be ruled out: A diagnostic HIV test should be carried out. The fact that the patient is currently unable to receive counselling and give her consent should not lead to a delay of testing because its result determines immediate further management. Once confusion has settled, the HIV test should be repeated to include a pre- and post-counselling session. In case of a reactive HIV serology, a lumbar puncture should be done to rule out tuberculous or cryptococcal meningitis.

A full blood count would help assess the cause of the patient's clinical anaemia. If normocytic anaemia is found, creatinine should be checked, because chronic kidney disease is very commonly seen in the tropics. Patients often present late, and both confusion and dermatitis can be signs of uraemia.

In case of a microcytic, hypochromic anaemia patients should be treated with iron and possibly also receive folic acid substitution, because a poor diet usually is not limited to just one nutritional component. β-thalassaemia, commonly seen in tropical countries, also presents with microcytic anaemia and should be considered if there is no response to iron supplementation. In β-thalassaemia the so-called Mentzer index (MCV [fL] : Erythrocyte count [$\times 10^{12}$/L]) is typically below 13; in iron deficiency it is above 13.

Intestinal helminth infection can contribute to anaemia. Because reliable stool microscopy may not be feasible in a resource-constrained setting, pragmatic anthelmintic treatment appears justifiable. Vitamin B_3 (niacin) should be supplemented and it should be evaluated how the family's diet could be improved despite their poor socioeconomic circumstances. A simple affordable trick is to advise the patient to eat some of the maize directly from the cob, because it is the husks that harbour tryptophan and that go lost during preparation of white maize flour.

It is a slight irony in this case that the husband is working on a local chicken farm and still cannot afford a balanced diet that includes eggs and poultry for his family.

The Case Continued...

The HIV test came back negative. The full blood count showed a microcytic anaemia with a haemoglobin of 6.7 g/dL and a Mentzer index >13. The patient received an appropriate dose of vitamin B-complex, iron and folic acid supplementation and a single dose of albendazole. Her confusion settled within a week and the diarrhoea stopped. The patient and her family received dietary counselling. She was prescribed soothing applications for her skin lesions and was told to avoid sun exposure. She was discharged and asked to come back at 3 months for an outpatient follow-up visit including a repeat full blood count.

SUMMARY BOX

Pellagra

Pellagra is a nutritional disorder caused by the deficiency of vitamin B_3 or its precursor, the essential amino-acid tryptophan. 'Pellagra' is derived from the Italian *pelle agra,* meaning 'rough skin'. It continues to be a problem in central and southern Africa where maize is the main staple food. Maize is poor in tryptophan, which is required for niacin synthesis. In some parts of Africa white maize is mainly consumed, which is nutritionally poorer than the yellow maize used in this region as animal feed. Milling maize and removing its husks further deprives it of nutritious components. In many poor African countries with little crop diversity, diet may literally consist of just maize, whereas niacin-containing food items such as fresh fruits, vegetables, peanuts, fish, meat, milk and eggs are not affordable. Most nutritional disorders peak during the rainy season, including kwashiorkor and marasmus in children. Apart from a poor diet, pellagra may be caused by malabsorption, alcoholism, antituberculous treatment and other aetiologies. The roll-out of INH-preventive therapy (IPT) for HIV patients has led to an increase in pellagra cases in some areas in Africa. Single cases of pellagra continue to be described from all over the world.

Patients present with the three 'Ds' of dermatitis, diarrhoea and dementia. The dermatitis often presents in a typical shape around the neck, which is referred to as 'Casal's necklace' after the Spanish physician who first described it in poor peasants in the 18th century. The skin tends to be dry, tender to touch and exposure to sunlight may be very painful.

'Dementia' stands for a large spectrum of possible neuro-psychiatric symptoms including anxiety, depression, hallucinations, ataxia and spastic paraparesis. A fourth 'D', death, occurs if pellagra is left untreated. The diagnosis is made clinically.

Treatment is with niacin or nicotinamide. Recommended doses in adults range from 50 to 400 mg daily in the acute phase. In severe cases, doses of up to 1000 mg IV per day have been recommended. Once acute symptoms have settled, continuation treatment is with 50 to 150 mg niacin daily for 2 weeks. Therapy should also include other B vitamins, zinc, magnesium and a diet rich in calories. Skin lesions should be covered with soothing applications and the patient should avoid sun exposure until the lesions have resolved. Patients and their families require intense dietary counselling on how to improve their diet despite socio-economic challenges.

Further Reading

1. Abrams S, Brabin BJ, Coulter JBS. Nutrition-associated disease. In: Farrar J, editor. Manson's Tropical Diseases. 23rd ed. London: Elsevier; 2013 [chapter 77].

2. Hegyi J, Schwartz RA, Hegyi V. Pellagra: dermatitis, dementia, and diarrhea. Int J Dermatol 2004;43(1):1–5.

3. Matapandeu G, Dunn SH, Pagels P. An outbreak of Pellagra in the Kasese Catchment Area, Dowa. Malawi Am J Trop Med 2017;96 (5):1244–7.

4. Kipsang JK, Chogea JK, Marindac PA, et al. Pellagra in isoniazid preventive and antiretroviral therapy. ID Cases 2019;17:e00550.

5. Narasimha VL, Ganesh S, Reddy S, Shukla L, Mukherjee D, Kandasamy A, Chand PK, Benegal V, Murthy P. Pellagra and alcohol dependence syndrome: findings from a tertiary care addiction treatment centre in India. Alcohol Alcohol 2019;54(2):148–51.

38

A 24-Year-Old Female Globetrotter With Strange Sensations in the Right Side of Her Body

JURI KATCHANOV AND EBERHARD SIEBERT

Clinical Presentation

History

A 24-year-old Dutch yoga instructor presents to an emergency room in Berlin, Germany, with one episode of strange sensations in the right side of her body. This started in the right side of her face, marched to her right arm and then continued to involve her right leg. She describes the feeling as 'pins and needles' lasting for about 2 minutes. She had a similar episode several months ago. At that time, she did not consult a doctor.

Four years before this presentation, after finishing school, she had left her home town in The Netherlands to go backpacking for 2 years. She travelled extensively through South America (Ecuador, Peru, Argentina) and South-east Asia (Thailand, Laos, Cambodia), staying in hostels or private accommodations. She describes herself as an 'eco-traveller', visiting the countryside and staying with local people. She has been a strict vegan for the past 8 years. She would eat food from local vendors but never any animal products. Her main diet during her travelling consisted of fruits, vegetables, nuts and rice.

Clinical Findings

On examination she looks well and is afebrile. Her neurological examination is completely unremarkable. The rest of her physical examination is also normal.

Laboratory Results

Her routine blood investigations, including differential blood count and C-reactive protein are completely normal. Her CSF examination is unremarkable.

Imaging

The MRI of her brain with gadolinium enhancement shows multiple cortical and subcortical cystic lesions in both hemispheres (Fig. 38.1).

Questions

1. What is the clinical syndrome the patient presents with and what is the most likely diagnosis in light of the imaging findings and the patient's travel history?
2. How would you treat this patient?

Discussion

A young Dutch woman presents with paraesthesias that spread over the right side of her body, lasting for about 2 minutes. Four years previously she went on an extensive backpacking trip around the world, visiting various places in South America and Asia. She lives on a vegan diet. Her physical examination including her neurological status are completely normal. The basic blood and CSF results are normal and do not reveal any signs of inflammation. The MRI of the brain shows multiple cystic lesions in both hemispheres.

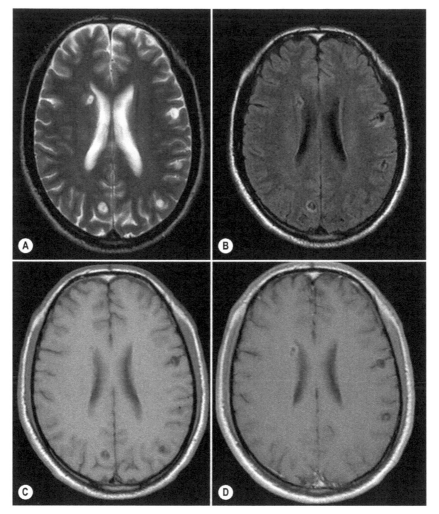

• **Fig. 38-1** Cerebral MRI of the patient. T2-weighted (A), Fluid attenuation inversion recovery (B), T1-weighted (C) and contrast-enhanced T1-weighted (D) images show multiple CSF isointense (cystic) lesions containing a scolex (central dot) in cortical and subcortical distribution. Some lesions show perifocal oedema and ring-enhancement after contrast administration (D).

Answer to Question 1

What is the Clinical Syndrome?

The patient presents with a focal epileptic seizure. Her paraesthesias represent a so-called Jacksonian 'sensory march'. Neuroimaging reveals multiple cortical and subcortical lesions. The cortical lesions in the left hemisphere are likely to be responsible for the patient's epileptic disorder on the contralateral side of her body.

The lesions are cystic, some of them show gadolinium enhancement of the wall and surrounding oedema. Given the presentation (healthy-looking patient, no immunosuppression, no fever, one similar episode a while ago with no progression of symptoms) and her travel history to South America and South-east Asia the most likely diagnosis is neurocysticercosis with multiple cysts in the vesicular and colloidal stage. An enzyme-linked immunoelectrotransfer blot (EITB) for the detection of anticysticercal antibodies in serum and CSF should be done to confirm the diagnosis.

Answer to Question 2

How Would You Treat This Patient?

The patient should receive antiparasitic treatment, corticosteroids and antiepileptic drugs (see Summary Box and Table 38.1).

The Case Continued...

The EITB came back positive for serum and CSF and a diagnosis of neurocysticercosis was made.

The patient was treated with albendazole 400 mg bd pig faeces which contain for 10 days and started on antiepileptic drugs. She declined treatment with steroids. She did not attend her 3-month follow-up but returned as an outpatient 1 year later. She had remained seizure-free for 1 year. MRI of the brain showed regression of all cysts. A CT scan on 2-year follow-up showed two calcifications. Her antiepileptic treatment was stopped after a seizure-free period of 3 years.

TABLE 38.1 Stages of Cysticercal Cyst and Treatment Recommendations[4]

Neuroimaging	Stage	Biology		Anticysticercal Treatment
Isointense/isodense to CSF, no contrast enhancement	Vesicular	Viable, non-immunogenic, can persist asymptomatically for years	1–2 cysts	Albendazole* + steroids for 10–14 days
Enhanced wall ('ring enhancement') on contrast imaging, surrounding oedema	Colloidal	Viable but degenerating, immunogenic	>2 cysts	Albendazole* + Praziquantel* + steroids for 10–14 days
Thickened retracted cyst without oedema	Granulo-nodular	Degenerated		No anthelmintic treatment
Calcification	Calcified	Final involuted stage		

*diffuse cerebral oedema is a contraindication for antihelminthic treatment

SUMMARY BOX

Neurocysticercosis

Neurocysticercosis is a CNS infestation with the larval form of *Taenia solium* (the pork tapeworm). It is widely prevalent in Africa, Asia and Latin America and is considered by the WHO to be the most common preventable cause of epilepsy in the developing world.

Humans acquire neurocysticercosis by eating food, e.g. salad or vegetables, contaminated with *T. solium* eggs. This explains why even individuals who do not eat pork meat for religious or ideological reasons can get neurocysticercosis, as seen in this case. (Consuming infested pork meat leads to intestinal infection with adult pork tapeworm).

Consumed ova release oncospheres that penetrate the intestinal wall to spread haematogenously throughout the host's body. In the CNS they become encysted affecting either the CNS parenchyma or, less commonly, the subarachnoid space.

Symptoms and signs depend on the location of cysts. The most common clinical presentation is focal epileptic seizures. Cysts in the subarachnoid space can cause hydrocephalus, producing headache and altered mental state. Diagnosis is based on neuroimaging, serology and epidemiological evidence.

Only vesicular and colloidal cysts are amenable to anthelmintic treatment (Table 38.1). Albendazole or the combination of albendazole and praziquantel can decrease the number of active lesions and reduce long-term seizure frequency. Adjunctive corticosteroid therapy before antiparasitic drugs is recommended for all patients treated with anthelmintic drugs.

In patients with untreated hydrocephalus or diffuse cerebral oedema, management of elevated intracranial pressure alone without antiparasitic treatment is recommended. The management of patients with diffuse cerebral oedema should be antiinflammatory therapy with corticosteroids; hydrocephalus usually requires a surgical approach.

The duration of antiepileptic therapy depends on the course of the disease. Radiological follow-ups at 6-month intervals are recommended. If the patient has remained seizure-free for 24 consecutive months with cysts resolved on neuroimaging, antiepileptic drugs may be tapered off and then stopped.

Further Reading

1. Heckmann JE, Bhigjee AI. Tropical neurology. In: Farrar J, editor. Manson's Tropical Diseases. 23rd ed. London: Elsevier; 2013 [chapter 71].
2. Baily G, Garcia HH. Other cestode infections: intestinal cestodes, cysticercosis, other larval cestode infections. In: Farrar J, editor. Manson's Tropical Diseases. 23rd ed. London: Elsevier; 2013 [chapter 57].
3. Garcia HH: Neurocysticercosis. Neurol Clin 2018;36(4):851–4.
4. Coyle CM. Neurocysticerosis: an individualized approach. Infect Dis Clin North Am 2019;33(1):153–68. https://doi.org/10.1016/j.idc.2018.10.007.
5. White Jr. AC, Coyle CM, Rajshekhar V, et al. Diagnosis and treatment of neurocysticercosis: 2017 Clinical Practice Guidelines by the Infectious Diseases Society of America (IDSA) and the American Society of Tropical Medicine and Hygiene (ASTMH). Clin Infect Dis 2018;66(8):1159–63.

39

A 30-Year-Old Male Chinese Trader With Fever in Laos

PAUL N. NEWTON, VALY KEOLUANGKHOT, MAYFONG MAYXAY, MICHAEL D. GREEN AND FACUNDO M. FERNÁNDEZ

Clinical Presentation

History

A 30-year-old male Chinese itinerant trader is referred to a hospital in Vientiane, Laos, with 7 days of fever, chills, headache and a dry cough. He developed slide-positive falciparum malaria whilst living in southern Laos and was treated with intravenous infusions and intramuscular artemether 80 mg for 5 days, which he had brought from China as standby therapy, but did not improve. The fever persisted, jaundice developed and he was therefore transferred to the capital Vientiane.

Clinical Findings

On admission he was febrile (39.5°C, 103.1°F) with normal blood pressure and Glasgow Coma Score, but had nausea, dry cough, moderate dehydration, chest pain and abdominal tenderness. His chest was clear and no hepatosplenomegaly was detected.

Investigations

Giemsa smear was negative for malaria parasites but a rapid diagnostic test (HRP-2) was positive for *Plasmodium falciparum,* consistent with recent falciparum malaria. Serum creatinine and glucose were normal. His further laboratory results are shown in Table 39.1.

Questions

1. What are your most important differential diagnoses?
2. How would you approach this patient?

Discussion

A 30-year-old Chinese itinerant trader presents to a hospital in Laos with persistent fever after receiving a 5-day course of antimalarial treatment with artemether for falciparum

TABLE 39.1 Laboratory Results on Admission

Parameter (unit)	Patient	Reference range
ALT (U/L)	301	<40
AST (U/L)	230	<37
ALP (U/L)	470	<120
Total bilirubin (µmol/L)	14	<14.5
Direct bilirubin (µmol/L)	6.4	<4.3

malaria. His blood smear is negative, but his rapid diagnostic test is positive for *P. falciparum.*

Answer to Question 1

What are your most important differential diagnoses?

With falciparum malaria the patient is at risk of bacterial co-infection, especially with *Salmonella* species. He could have another common infectious disease contracted in Laos such as scrub typhus *(Orientia tsutsugamushi),* murine typhus *(Rickettsia typhi),* leptospirosis, tuberculosis or dengue fever.

Artemisinin-resistant falciparum malaria has been described from southern Laos, Cambodia border, the Burma (Myanmar)/Thai border, Myanmar and southern Vietnam, manifested as prolonged parasite clearance times. Other possibilities are that the artemether was given at the incorrect dose, was of poor quality or that there were issues with intestinal absorption of the medicine.

Answer to Question 2

How would you approach this patient?

Repeat history, physical examination and investigations (such as blood culture and chest radiography) looking for other causes of infection, review of the antimalarial dosage

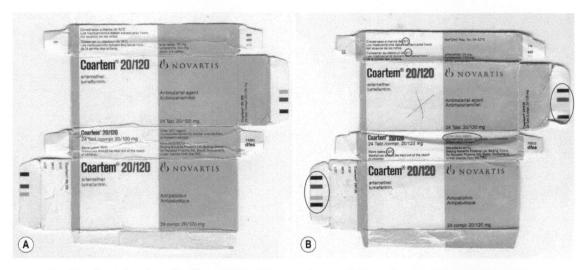

• **Fig. 39.1** Examples of genuine (A) and falsified (B) artemether-lumefantrine discovered in Africa. The red circles indicate errors made by the criminals. The falsifiers confused 'm' with 'rn' in 'lagern' (German for "storing") and printed the packets with the word 'lagem' in error. The falsified samples contained no detectable artemether or lumefantrine but did contain subtherapeutic pyrimethamine. (Reproduced from Newton, P.N., Green, M.D., Mildenhall, D.C., et al., 2011. Poor quality vital anti-malarials in Africa - an urgent neglected public health priority. Malar J. 10, 352.)

received and likely efficacy and consider retreatment with a known, quality-assured antimalarial.

The Case continued...

The patient was treated with oral quinine sulphate 10 mg/kg every 8 hours and doxycycline 100 mg every 12 hours for 7 days. His fever cleared 35 hours after starting this therapy and he was discharged well. No evidence was found for any other infections.

Intramuscular artemether has been widely used for the treatment of severe *P. falciparum* malaria, and clinical trial evidence suggests that it has similar efficacy to parenteral quinine, but is probably inferior to parenteral artesunate. There is a common error of package inserts advising 5 days, rather than the international guidelines of 7 days of monotherapy.

In our case, examination of the vial and packaging of the suspect sample did not reveal any overt differences from genuine samples suggesting that it was not falsified. However, high performance liquid chromatography (HPLC) and mass spectrometry (MS) analysis of the suspect sample demonstrated that it only contained 59 mg artemether (74% of that stated on the vial). Electrospray mass spectra demonstrated that suspect and genuine samples were identical in terms of their qualitative chemical composition, i.e. their "fingerprints", but differed in active ingredient content. The artemether was therefore substandard, containing inadequate amounts of artemether because of factory error or negligence or a good quality genuine product that deteriorated during storage and transport.

The conventional dose of intramuscular artemether is 3.2 mg/kg STAT followed by 1.6 mg/kg once daily for 7 days. The patient probably received an actual dose of only approximately 1.0 mg/kg per day as monotherapy of inadequate duration. The combination of underdosing and poor-quality drug most likely resulted in his poor clinical response. He would presumably have recovered rapidly if oral artemether-lumefantrine had been given, as specified in the Lao national treatment guidelines.

This case emphasizes the importance of appropriate therapy and dosage, of following national guidelines and of checking the quality of a medicine taken if expected improvement does not occur.

SUMMARY BOX

Poor-Quality Medicines

Poor-quality medicines are of two main types – substandard and falsified drugs.

Substandard drugs are produced by authorized manufacturers; but because of unintentional errors in production or negligence, they fail to meet pharmaceutical standards. They often contain reduced amounts of active ingredients or their bioavailability is poor. Medicines may also leave the factory of good quality but deteriorate because of poor storage in the distribution chain. In contrast, falsified drugs are deliberately produced by criminals by fraud and often, but not always, contain none of the stated active ingredients.

In the 1990s and early 2000s, there was a large epidemic of falsified oral artesunate throughout mainland South-east Asia and, most alarmingly, there are increasing reports of falsified and substandard artemisinin-based combination therapies (ACTs) in Africa. Some contain wrong active ingredients that may be toxic or engender resistance.

There have been false reports of antimalarial drug resistance in both Africa and Asia, which upon further investigation were shown to be because of poor medicine quality. The use of artemisinin derivative combinations with subtherapeutic drug content (whether falsified or substandard) and prescriptions for inadequate doses or duration raise concern that these factors may facilitate the spread of resistance to this vital class of antimalarials.

Inspection of packaging, although difficult, is key in detecting falsified medicines (Fig. 39.1).

Unexpectedly low-cost medications, unexpectedly poor patient outcomes, unexpected adverse events and differences in packaging from those that patients and pharmacists are used to should signal alerts that should be reported to national regulatory authorities and the WHO (at rapidalert@who.int). There are very few quality-assured laboratories in malaria-endemic countries for the packaging and chemical analysis of antimalarial quality, making the timely and affordable checking of medicine quality very difficult.

Further Reading

1. Shrestha P, Roberts T, Homsana A, et al. Febrile illness in Asia: gaps in epidemiology, diagnosis and management for informing health policy. Clin Microbiol Inf 2018;24(8):815–26.

2. Ashley EA, Dhorda M, Fairhurst RM, et al. Tracking Resistance to Artemisinin Collaboration (TRAC). Spread of artemisinin resistance in *Plasmodium falciparum* malaria. N Engl J Med 2014;371(5):411–23.

3. Jackson Y, Chappuis F, Loutan L, et al. Malaria treatment failures after artemisinin-based therapy in three expatriates: could improved manufacturer information help decrease the risk of treatment failure? Malar J 2006;5(81):1–5.

4. World Health Organization. WHO Global Surveillance and Monitoring System for substandard and falsified medical products, Geneva: World Health Organization; 2017; http://apps.who.int/medicinedocs/en/m/abstract/Js23373en/.

5. Newton PN, Green MD, Mildenhall DC, et al. Poor quality vital anti-malarials in Africa - an urgent neglected public health priority. Malar J 2011;10:352.

40

A 62-Year-Old Woman from Ethiopia With Difficulty Eating

CHRISTOPHER J.M. WHITTY

Clinical Presentation

History

A 62-year-old woman from rural Ethiopia had flown to Europe to visit her daughter and meet her new grandchild. She was normally fit and well and very physically active, because she worked on her smallholding in Ethiopia. Three days after arrival she began to find it difficult to chew, with what she described through her daughter as 'stiffness of the mouth'. This had never happened before.

Clinical Findings

No abnormal findings are discovered on examination. Her pulse, blood pressure and respiratory rate are within normal limits.

Questions

1. What are the important differential diagnoses and what would help establish the diagnosis?
2. What is the immediate management?

Discussion

A 62-year-old woman from Ethiopia presents with difficulties chewing. She has been fit and well in the past. Her physical examination is unremarkable.

Answer to Question 1

What Are the Important Differential Diagnoses and What Would Help Establish the Diagnosis?

Although there is a range of possible causes of stiffness on mastication, the main cause from less developed countries is early tetanus. The risk factors are agricultural work and being from a country and age group in which vaccination is unlikely to have occurred. An important differential for trismus in older people is giant cell arteritis (GCA), and

an ESR should be performed on this woman to exclude GCA as a matter of urgency, although she is towards the lower end of the age range for this.

The diagnosis of tetanus is purely clinical. Generalized tetanus with spasms is easy to diagnose once it is established, but it is usually preceded by trismus because the muscles of mastication have the shortest motor neurons.

Answer to Question 2

What is the Immediate Management?

The initial treatment for any possible tetanus is to give an antibiotic (metronidazole is the antibiotic of choice) to kill the infection and prevent more toxin production, and an antitoxin injection to neutralize circulating tetanospasmin. The earlier this is undertaken the better the outlook; therefore it is better to over-suspect tetanus than to wait until spasms make the diagnosis obvious.

The time between the high-risk injury and the first symptoms is a guide to prognosis but often it is not known, especially in agricultural populations who may sustain high-risk injuries (which may be minor) regularly.

The Case Continued...

The woman received metronidazole and antitoxin on day 1. On day 2 she presented again, having had two generalized spasms. Over the next 2 days she was nursed in a dark, quiet environment, but her spasms increased in frequency, severity and duration over the next 5 days and she developed dysphagia. She was treated with diazepam and antitoxin was administered intrathecally. A prophylactic tracheotomy was performed because of the risk of laryngeal spasms, the commonest cause of sudden death in tetanus. Her symptoms got no worse after 7 days; she did not have to be paralysed and ventilated, and her respiration was not severely compromised at any point. She made a slow recovery over 3 weeks, and was still experiencing stiffness when seen in clinic 3 months later.

SUMMARY BOX

Tetanus

Severe tetanus is a terrible disease both to have and to witness. Some tetanus stops at trismus, but most will go on to generalized spasms. As these become more severe, respiratory function is compromised; and in the most severe cases, there is autonomic dysregulation with rapid swings in blood pressure, heart rate and pulse. There is a wide variation in the mortality from established generalized tetanus between different units, demonstrating that proper medical and nursing care have a significant influence on outcome. Wounds require meticulous cleaning and debridement. After the initial antibiotics, antitoxin and diazepam (for spasms), it is essential to assess the stage of the patient regularly. Tetanus toxin already in the motor nerves will not be affected by antitoxin and will continue to track to the spinal cord, therefore patients generally continue to deteriorate for several days after initial presentation and treatment. Intrathecal antitoxin should be considered in severe cases. In survivors, the disease then plateaus before a slow recovery. Most deaths are either from laryngeal spasm (rapid), respiratory arrest in prolonged spasms, cardiac dysrhythmia or chest infection. Increased respiratory rate (over 40 breath cycles per minute) or difficulty swallowing should make the treating physician consider the risk of laryngeal spasm and prepare the patient for either elective tracheotomy or paralysis and ventilation in the intensive care unit (ICU). Because of the protracted course of tetanus, weaning from ventilators once started is slow and difficult, with all the complications that a prolonged stay in an ICU brings.

Further Reading

1. Thwaites C, Yen LM. Tetanus. In: Farrar J, editor. Manson's Tropical Diseases. London: Elsevier; 2013.
2. Rodrigo C, Fernando D, Rajapakse S. Pharmacological management of tetanus: an evidence-based review. Crit Care 2014;18:217.
3. Thwaites CL, Beeching NJ, Newton CR. Maternal and neonatal tetanus. Lancet 2015;385:362–70.
4. Yen LM, Thwaites CL. Tetanus. Lancet 2019;393:1657–68.
5. Pollach G, Goddia C, Namboya F, Luiz T, Rothe C. Severe tetanus in Malawi: where are the female patients? J Public Health 2016; 24(5):401–8.

41

A 7-Year-Old Girl from West Africa With Two Skin Ulcers and a Contracture of Her Right Wrist

MORITZ VOGEL

Clinical Presentation

History

A 7-year-old girl is presented to a district hospital in the tropical region of a West African country. After an insect bite, she developed an itchy papule on the back of her right hand, which enlarged over a period of 3 months. A traditional healer had prescribed herbal remedies. When the lesion ulcerated a few weeks later, diclofenac and dexamethasone were administered at the local health post. When a second lesion appeared, treatment with oxacillin was initiated with no effect. The girl became increasingly unable to use her right hand. There is no history of relevant trauma or systemic symptoms.

Clinical Findings

A 7-year-old, anxious girl in good general condition holding her right wrist in a 45° flexion and 20° abduction position. Pulse 108 bpm (normal 70–110), blood pressure 100/70 mmHg, temperature 37.9°C (100.2°F).

Two skin ulcers are present on the back of her right hand (3 × 3 cm) and on the medial side of her right wrist (0.5 × 1 cm). The larger ulcer is filled with necrotic tissue (Fig. 41.1) and surrounded by hypo- and hyperpigmentation, lichenification and desquamation. An ill-defined induration surrounds the ulcers (12 × 8 cm) with oedema extending from the lower arm to the fingers. A 0.5 × 0.5 cm nodule is noticed above the medial right elbow.

Questions

1. What is the most likely diagnosis and what is the differential diagnosis?
2. What is the appropriate clinical approach in the given context?

Discussion

A 7-year-old West African girl presents with two progressive cutaneous ulcers linked by an area of altered skin. The movement in the associated joint is restricted. General symptoms are limited to a mildly elevated temperature.

Answer to Question 1

What is the Most Likely Diagnosis and What is the Differential Diagnosis?

The geographical region of West Africa, the young age of the patient, the location of the lesion on the extremities, the absence of major trauma and the clinical picture lead to a suspected diagnosis diagnosis of Buruli ulcer (BU). The history of an insect bite is an incidental finding, the mode of transmission of the causative organism, *Mycobacterium ulcerans*, remains unknown.

Pain and low-grade fever as seen in this case may also be explained by bacterial superinfection. A careful history and physical examination will provide guidance in differentiating numerous other infectious (bacterial, viral, fungal, parasitic) and non-infectious (trauma, envenoming, autoimmune, haematological, neoplastic) causes of ulcers in tropical countries. In areas endemic for BU, the accuracy of clinical diagnosis in experienced hands is remarkably high.

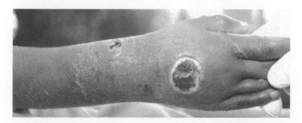

• **Fig. 41.1** Large skin ulcer on the back of the right hand filled with necrotic tissue; second smaller ulcer on the medial side of the wrist.

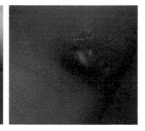

At the end of specific treatment

• **Fig. 41.2** At the end of specific treatment, the ulcer on the back of the hand had healed almost completely. However, the second, smaller ulcer had increased in size.

Answer to Question 2

What is the Appropriate Clinical Approach in the Given Context?

Adequate wound care, including pain relief, according to WHO guidelines should be instituted immediately. The desired sterile, moist atmosphere of the wound can be achieved with saline-soaked gauze changed daily. Colonization with other bacteria may be controlled by povidone-iodine. Antitetanus coverage must be secured. Written documentation of pain control and picture documentation of wound progress is helpful in achieving or maintaining a high-quality wound management standard.

Laboratory confirmation of BU by *M. ulcerans* using PCR is desirable but limited by the availability of reliable laboratory capacity and by its cost, which must be balanced with important supportive measures, such as improved nutrition.

The indication for surgical debridement depends on the clinical picture, but also on the availability of adequate anaesthetic and surgical care.

BU-specific antimycobacterial therapy should be commenced as soon as possible. In the absence of systemic symptoms, the toxicity of the recommended antibiotic treatment may justify a few days of delay until diagnostic results have been obtained.

The Case Continued...

PCR from a wound swab confirmed the presence of *M. ulcerans*. During the 8 weeks of specific treatment and wound care the ulcer on the back of the hand healed almost completely, but the second smaller ulcer increased to 8 × 10 cm in size (Fig. 41.2).

Debridement and skin grafting were performed, and the patient made an uneventful recovery. The restriction of movement was corrected by physiotherapy.

SUMMARY BOX

Mycobacterium ulcerans Disease (Buruli Ulcer)

M. ulcerans disease is a necrotizing infection mainly of the subcutaneous tissue. It is most prevalent among children and adolescents living in rural communities of West Africa; but other continents and temperate regions of Australia, China and Japan are also affected. Endemic areas are associated with water

bodies such as rivers and lakes. However, the exact mode of transmission remains poorly understood.

M. ulcerans is characterized by its particular sensitivity to heat, its propensity to develop local and distant satellite lesions and its production of a necrotizing, locally immunosuppressive and analgesic macrolide exotoxin called mycolactone.

Clinically, *M. ulcerans* disease presents with skin lesions ranging from papules, nodules and plaques to the eponymous ulcers. The latter may involve most of a limb surface or trunk and can simultaneously occur at different body sites. All lesions share skin alterations including induration, hypo- and hyperpigmentation, lichenification, desquamation and possibly local oedema. Ulcers are characterized by undermined edges surrounding a 'cotton wool' like necrosis. Lesions are classically described as painless, but evidence has emerged questioning this doctrine. The diagnosis can be confirmed most reliably by PCR from a wound swab; however, a test for the presence of mycolactone suitable for district-level laboratories is under investigation.

Culture is difficult because of the slow growth rate of the mycobacteria.

The WHO recommends combination therapy with rifampicin (10 mg/kg per day PO) plus either streptomycin (15 mg/kg per day IM) or clarithromycin (7.5 mg/kg twice daily PO) for 8 weeks, which achieve high specific cure rates. Local heat application at temperatures >40°C for several weeks has also been shown to be curative. Special attention must be paid to patients co-infected with HIV, who are at increased risk for complications.

Careful wound management, pain relief, surgical excision and skin grafting as well as physiotherapy for restricted movements remain indispensable cornerstones of BU treatment. Extensive necrosis of subcutaneous tissue at diagnosis may cause a significant increase in ulcer size under treatment. Once secondary bacterial infection has been ruled out, this must not be mistaken for treatment failure. Local or distant new lesions may become evident during or after treatment. This so called 'paradoxical reaction' is thought to be caused by a local host immune reconstitution syndrome because of a fall in mycolactone levels. The distinction between bacterial secondary infection, recurrence and paradoxical reactions remains challenging and should involve expert advice.

Further Reading

1. Junghanss T, Johnson C, Pluschke G. *Mycobacterium ulcerans* disease. In: Farrar J, editor. Manson's Tropical Diseases. 23rd ed. London: Elsevier; 2013 [chapter 42].
2. Laboratory diagnosis of buruli ulcer. A manual for health care providers. World Health Organization; 2014; WHO/HTM/NTD/IDM/2014.1, Available from: https://apps.who.int/iris/bitstream/handle/10665/111738/9789241505703_eng.pdf?sequence=1 (accessed 01.05.19).

3. Treatment of *Mycobaterium ulcerans* disease (Buruli ulcer): guidance for health workers. World Health Organization; 2012; WHO/HTM/NTD/IDM/2012.1, Available from: https://apps.who.int/iris/bitstream/handle/10665/77771/9789241503402_eng.pdf?sequence=1 (accessed 01.05.19).

4. Macdonald JM, Geyer MJ, editors. Wound and Lymphoedema Management. WHO/HTM/NTD/GBUI/2010.1. World Health Organization; 2010. http://whqlibdoc.who.int/publications/2010/9789241599139_eng.pdf (accessed 01.05.19).

5. Yotsu RR, Suzuki K, Simmonds RE, et al. Buruli ulcer: a review of the current knowledge. Curr Trop Med Rep 2018;5(4): 247–56.

42

A 41-Year-Old Male Traveller Returning from Australia With Itchy Eruptions on His Thighs

CAMILLA ROTHE

Clinical Presentation

History

A 41-year-old male yoga teacher presents to a travel clinic in Europe because of itchy skin eruptions on both upper thighs for the past week.

He has just returned from a 10-day trip to northern Australia where he attended a yoga seminar. On his way to Australia he had stopped over on a Thai island for a 3-day beach holiday. Just after his arrival in Australia he developed three intensely itchy skin eruptions on both upper thighs. The itch is so intense that at times it keeps him awake at night.

There has been no fever, no cough or wheeze and he is otherwise completely well.

Clinical Findings

On both upper thighs there are a total of three reddish, serpiginous tracks, about 2 mm in width (Fig. 42.1). The inguinal lymph nodes are not enlarged. The chest is clear. The rest of the examination is unremarkable.

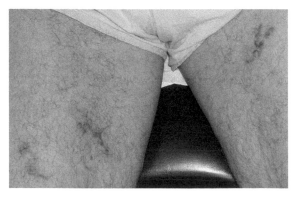

• **Fig. 42.1** Three track-like skin eruptions on both upper thighs causing intense itching.

Questions

1. What is the clinical syndrome and what is the differential diagnosis?
2. What management would you recommend?

Discussion

A 41-year-old European man presents to a travel clinic with itchy serpiginous skin lesions. He has recently returned from a trip to Asia and Australia.

Answer to Question 1

What is the Clinical Syndrome and What is the Differential Diagnosis?

The clinical syndrome is a creeping eruption. A creeping eruption is defined as a linear or serpiginous, slightly elevated, erythematous track that moves forward in an irregular pattern. The most common cause of creeping eruptions seen in returned travellers is cutaneous larva migrans (CLM) caused by larvae of animal hookworms.

Creeping eruptions can also result from infection with larvae of *Strongyloides stercoralis* (larva currens, i.e. running larva), but this can easily be distinguished from CLM. *S. stercoralis* larvae move several centimetres an hour, that is considerably faster than larvae in cutaneous larva migrans. The eruptions in larva currens persist only for a few hours, whereby in CLM the track may stay for weeks.

Creeping eruptions can also be caused by adult nematodes such as *Gnathostoma* species and trematodes (*Fasciola* species). The larvae of parasitic flies have also been shown to cause creeping eruptions (migratory myiasis).

However, cutaneous larva migrans caused by zoonotic hookworms is by far the commonest cause of creeping eruption seen in travel clinics worldwide. The patient was probably infected while lying on the beach or performing yoga exercises in the sand.

Answer to Question 2

What Management Would You Recommend?

The diagnosis of cutaneous larva migrans can be established clinically, supported by the patient's travel history. There are no other investigations required. Antiparasitic treatment can be administered topically or systemically (see Summary Box).

The Case Continued...

The patient was prescribed a single-dose treatment of ivermectin (200 µg/kg). The itchy eruptions settled within a few days of taking the drug.

SUMMARY BOX

Hookworm-Related Cutaneous Larva Migrans

CLM is a creeping eruption resulting from accidental infestation of the human skin by larvae of dog and cat hookworms (*Ancylostoma caninum, A. braziliense* and *Uncinaria stenocephala*). It is one of the most common dermatoses in returning travellers from tropical destinations. Apart from its relevance in travel medicine, it is endemic in resource-poor communities in the developing world, particularly in Central and South America, the Caribbean and South and South-east Asia.

CLM occurs in most warm and humid climates and where stray dogs and cats are common, or pets are not treated regularly with anthelmintics. The animals pass hookworm ova with their stools, and the larval stages develop in sand or soil. CLM is usually acquired when walking barefoot, or sitting or lying on faecally contaminated ground.

Animal hookworm larvae enter the epidermis but are unable to cross the basement membrane and enter the human body. Confined to the skin, they are unable to complete their lifecycle as they would do in their animal host.

There usually is a pruritic papule at the site of larval entry. A raised erythematous track starts progressing in an irregular fashion. The onset of symptoms and the speed by which the creeping eruption progresses vary between different hookworm species, but usually itching starts shortly after larval entry, and the elevated track appears 1 to 5 days later.

The skin eruptions are most commonly found on the feet but may occur in any part of the body that came into contact with infested sand or soil. The itching is intense and may prevent affected people from sleeping. Very rarely, animal hookworms may invade the human body leading to pulmonary eosinophilia.

Diagnosis is made clinically, supported by exposure history. Skin biopsy is not helpful because the larva is invariably in advance of its track. There are no reliable serological tests available, and blood eosinophilia is present in a minority of cases.

The treatment of choice is ivermectin (200µg/kg for 1-2 days.). Albendazole is a good alternative when ivermectin is contraindicated or not available. Albendazole 400 mg should be given twice daily (bd) for 3 days. Topical thiabendazole 10–15% tds for 5 to 10 days is also effective but requires more compliance and can be difficult in multiple lesions.

Without treatment the lesion can persist for several months, and scratching may lead to bacterial superinfection, particularly if hygiene is poor.

For prevention at the community level, cats and dogs should be dewormed and banned from beaches and playgrounds. In resource-limited settings this is usually not feasible. Individual protection can be achieved by wearing appropriate footwear when walking on sand or soil in the tropics and using a sunchair on the beach because towels may be covered with sand and therefore do not protect sufficiently.

Further Reading

1. Brooker S, Bundy DAP. Soil-transmitted helminths (geohelminths). In: Farrar J, editor. Manson's Tropcial Diseases. 23rd ed. London: Elsevier; 2013 [chapter 55].
2. Vega-Lopez F, Ritchie S. Dermatological problems. In: Farrar J, editor. Manson's Tropical Diseases. 23rd ed. London: Elsevier; 2013 [chapter 68].
3. Heukelbach J, Feldmeier H. Epidemiological and clinical characteristics of hookworm-related cutaneous larva migrans. Lancet Infect Dis 2008;8(5):302–9.

43

A 35-Year-Old Malawian Woman With a Painful Ocular Tumour

MARKUS SCHULZE SCHWERING

Clinical Presentation

History

A 35-year-old woman from Malawi presents to the outpatient department of a local tertiary hospital. She was referred by an ophthalmic clinical officer from a district hospital for exenteration of the left eye because of an ocular tumour.

The first symptoms started 8 months prior when she noticed a whitish lesion growing on the conjunctiva of her left eye. She presented at a health centre and was prescribed non-specified eye drops. Yet, over the following months the lesion grew bigger and turned reddish. She went to a traditional healer who prescribed herbal eye drops, which did not help either. The lesion grew constantly bigger and she finally lost her eyesight in the affected eye. Pain also increased which made her present at her local district hospital.

The patient is known to be HIV-positive. She has been on antiretroviral treatment for the past 3 years. The CD4 count is unknown.

Clinical Findings

Localized swelling of the left eyeball and orbit, lid closure incomplete (Fig. 43.1). The visual acuity on the right side is 6/6, whereas the left eye has no light perception. Her left preauricular lymph nodes are swollen. She is afebrile and the rest of her physical examination is unremarkable.

Questions

1. What is the suspected diagnosis?
2. How would you manage the patient?

Discussion

An HIV-positive Malawian woman presents with a painful tumour of her left eye. It started as a whitish lesion on her conjunctiva several months ago. The lesion continued to grow and the affected eye eventually turned blind.

Answer to Question 1

What is the Suspected Diagnosis?

The lesion most likely is an advanced ocular surface squamous neoplasia (OSSN). OSSN are commonly seen in HIV-positive individuals in sub-Saharan Africa. They start as discrete whitish conjunctival lesions (Fig. 43.2) and may develop into large tumours if left untreated. Early stages may be confused with pterygium, with an amelanotic naevus, or a lipoma. Malignant lesions such as amelanotic melanomas, lymphomas or adenocarcinomas may look similar as well.

Answer to Question 2

How Would You Manage this Patient?

The patient should be started on analgesic treatment with nonsteroidal antiinflammatory drugs. She should be counselled and booked for surgery. An extended exenteration of

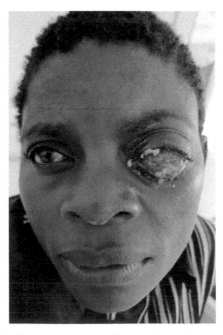

• **Fig. 43.1** Left eye with marked axial proptosis, nasal upper lid covered with tetracycline eye ointment.

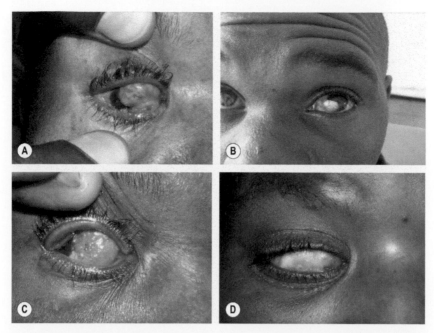

• **Fig. 43.2** Squamous cell carcinoma of the conjunctiva (SCCC). The lesion is commonly seen in HIV patients in the tropics and should not be missed during routine clinical examination. (Courtesy Nicholas A.V. Beare).

the left eyeball and orbit should be done. Control of the patient's HIV infection is crucial, and her HIV viral load should be checked.

Because the patient has lost her eyesight on the left side, the right eye should be carefully examined for possible growth of another OSSN that could be removed at an early stage. A fundoscopy should be performed in order to detect any abnormalities, especially an upcoming cytomegalovirus infection.

The Case Continued...

The patient was admitted to the hospital and counselled several times about the need for surgery. Yet she refused surgical intervention and was only willing to accept conservative treatment.

The patient's left orbit was covered with antibiotics and bandaged. When pain was sufficiently controlled, the patient was discharged with the offer to come back at any time.

She was asked to report to her antiretroviral therapy (ART) clinic for control of the viral load and possible switch of her antiretroviral therapy.

SUMMARY BOX

Ocular Surface Squamous Neoplasia

OSSN are commonly seen in HIV-positive individuals in tropical countries. Early diagnosis is crucial for successful treatment, and any clinician working in a tropical region with high HIV prevalence should be able to recognize an OSSN.

The term OSSN is used to describe dysplastic lesions of conjunctiva and cornea ranging from conjunctival intraepithelial neoplasia (CIN) to invasive squamous cell carcinoma of the conjunctiva (SCCC). The use of ultrasound biomicroscopy (UBM) in OSSN may help detect intraocular invasion. Prominent nodular tumours >5 mm thick can also be taken as risk factors for

intraocular involvement. HIV infection, ultraviolet radiation (UV) and human papilloma virus (HPV) are strongly associated with OSSN. These factors, together with vitamin A deficiency, weaken the tumour surveillance system and allow DNA-damaged cells to proliferate into tumours. A five- to tenfold increase in incidence has been observed in parallel with the HIV epidemic. The current incidence of OSSN in sub-Saharan Africa is estimated to be 2.2 per 100 000, and it continues to rise (USA: 0.3 per 100 000). By which mechanism HIV infection favours development of OSSN is as yet unknown. Co-infection with human papilloma virus (HPV) has been implicated in the aetiology of OSSN, but the virus could only be detected in less than half of cases.

OSSN typically presents as a greyish, elevated, gelatinous mass surrounded by engorged conjunctival vessels. There is no explanation why the disease is mostly unilateral. It often starts to develop at the nasal side of the eye and spreads to involve the whole conjunctiva, lids, local tissue and lymph nodes. In the developing world, patients often present late with sometimes disfiguring lesions. There is a trend towards treating conjunctival lesions suspected to be OSSN based on clinical impression. However, clinical diagnosis by slit lamp – with or without gonioscopy – is difficult because of the overlap in clinical features of OSSN and non–OSSN lesions. Toluidine blue 0.05% vital staining is a good screening tool. Negative staining results indicate that OSSN is relatively unlikely. It does, however, not replace surgical biopsy with histopathological examination.

Early, non-invasive stages of OSSN can be treated with topical chemotherapeutic agents such as topical 5-flurouracil and mitomycin or subconjunctival interferon-α2b. Primary treatment is surgical excision. Inexpensive use of fluorouracil 1% eyedrops for 4 weeks substantially reduces the risk of recurrence. It is a low-cost option listed on the WHO's Essential Drug List. In more advanced disease, surgery may have to involve enucleation of the eye or exenteration of the orbit. Adjuvant treatment can decrease recurrence rate, which after simple excision is high (30%–40%). Possibilities for adjunctive treatment include topical chemotherapy, cryotherapy and intraoperative β-irradiation. Diagnosis of OSSN in an HIV-unknown individual should prompt the clinician to perform an HIV test. Because HIV seems to play a role in tumour development, HIV-reactive patients with OSSN should receive effective ART to achieve virological control.

Further Reading

1. Beare NV, Bestawrous A. Ophthalmology in the tropics and sup-tropics. In: Farrar J, editor. Manson's Tropical Diseases. 23rd ed London: Elsevier; 2013.
2. Tiong T, Borooah S, Msosa J, et al. Clinicopathological review of ocular surface squamous neoplasia in Malawi. Br J Ophthalmol 2013;97(8):961–4.
3. Meel R, Dhiman R, Sen S, et al. Ocular surface squamous neoplasia with intraocular extension: Clinical and Ultrasound Biomicroscopic Findings. Ocul Oncol Pathol 2019;5(2):122–7.
4. Gichuhi S, Sagoo MS, Weiss HA, Burton MJ. Epidemiology of ocular surface squamous neoplasia in Africa. Trop Med Int Health 2013;18(12):1424–43.
5. Gichuhi S, Macharia E, Kabiru J, et al. Topical fluorouracil after surgery for ocular surface squamous neoplasia in Kenya: a randomised, double-blind, placebo-controlled trial. Lancet Glob Health 2016;4(6):e378–85.

44

A 7-Year-Old Girl from South Sudan With Undulating Fever

KAREN ROODNAT AND KOERT RITMEIJER

Clinical Presentation

History

A 7-year-old girl is presented at a clinic in South Sudan with a 4-week history of undulating fever. The fever occurs mainly in the afternoon hours accompanied by chills and sometimes convulsions. Between the febrile episodes she was initially fine and played normally. However, over time she has developed progressive anorexia, dry cough, chest pain, joint and back pain.

She has never been admitted to a hospital, but she has presented at another clinic recently where she received some unspecified tablets that did not bring any improvement.

Clinical Findings

The girl is alert and pale, but not jaundiced. She is severely malnourished (Z-score <3). Her vital signs are: temperature 39.6°C (103.3°F), pulse 96 bpm, blood pressure 100/60 mmHg. Her chest sounds clear; normal heart sounds; soft abdomen with a splenomegaly of 4 cm below the left costal margin. There are multiple enlarged lymph nodes of about 1 cm in diameter in the cervical, axillary, inguinal and epitrochlear region. There are no skin lesions and no peripheral oedema.

Laboratory Results

The patient's blood test results are shown in Table 44.1.

Plasmodium falciparum rapid diagnostic test (RDT) and a blood film for malaria parasites are negative. *Brucella* species serology (IgG and IgM) is negative. Visceral leishmaniasis: rK39-antibody RDT is negative.

Questions

1. What are your most important differential diagnoses?
2. How would you approach this patient?

TABLE 44.1	Laboratory Results on Admission		
Parameter		Patient	Reference
WBC (×10^9/L)		1.35	4–10
Haemoglobin (g/dL)		6.8	12–16
Platelets (×10^9/L)		98	150–300

Discussion

In South Sudan, a young girl presents with a 4-week history of fever, progressive anorexia, general body pains and a dry cough. On examination she is pale and severely malnourished. She has splenomegaly and generalized lymphadenopathy. The full blood count (FBC) shows pancytopenia. Serological rapid diagnostic tests for malaria, brucellosis and visceral leishmaniasis are negative.

Answer to Question 1

What Are Your Most Important Differential Diagnoses?

Chronic fever, splenomegaly and wasting in a child from South Sudan should raise the suspicion of visceral leishmaniasis or brucellosis. Tuberculosis and HIV infection both need to be ruled out, because they can cause chronic fever, anorexia, weight loss, splenomegaly and generalized lymphadenopathy.

Malaria can cause fever, anaemia and splenomegaly, but two different negative tests make this unlikely. In addition, the chronic fever is unusual; in a child one might expect a more acute course. Furthermore, malaria does not cause any lymphadenopathy. Hyperreactive malarial splenomegaly syndrome (HMS) has been described in children. It can cause gross splenomegaly and anaemia in regions hyperendemic for malaria, but HMS does not present with a fever, neither is lymphadenopathy part of the picture.

Typhoid fever can present with persistent fever and splenomegaly; a dry cough is also common. The duration of fever in this case may be slightly too long though, and generalized lymphadenopathy is not a common feature of typhoid.

A splenic abscess could cause chronic fever and splenomegaly, but would not explain the generalized lymphadenopathy and the haematological changes, unless the patient was acutely septic.

Chronic schistosomiasis caused by *Schistosoma mansoni* infection can cause splenomegaly in the context of portal hypertension, but patients would not be febrile and lymphadenopathy is not part of the picture either.

Malignancies like leukaemia and lymphoma should be ruled out.

Answer to Question 2

How Would You Approach this Patient?

The little girl appears very sick and should be admitted to the hospital. The list of differential diagnoses is long and there are many tests that would be requested if the same patient presented in an affluent setting.

In a resource-constrained place like South Sudan, a pragmatic clinical approach is necessary. The history should be taken as accurately as possible to narrow down the differential diagnosis. One should try to find out if the patient comes from an area where visceral leishmaniasis (VL) is endemic. For possible HIV infection, it would be of great importance to find out if the parents and siblings are alive and well; and enquiries should be made if there are any close contacts who are suspected to have TB or who have a history of recent TB treatment.

The clinician has to cope with the investigations available, which may commonly not be in line with the internationally recommended standards. Gold standard for diagnosis of VL is the proof of the parasite in tissue specimens. However, this is often not feasible under field conditions and serological tests are used instead. The rapid antigen test for VL (rK39) used in this case was negative (sensitivity of this test in South Sudan is 85–90%).

Because VL is high on the list of differential diagnoses, a second serological test such as the Direct Agglutination Test (DAT) should be done, and direct proof of the parasite should be attempted.

Sensitivity is highest for splenic aspirates (93–99%), followed by bone marrow (53–86%) and lymph node aspiration (53–65%), which can be further increased by culture and PCR. Splenic aspiration is complicated with life-threatening haemorrhages in about 0.1% of procedures and therefore requires strict precautions, technical expertise and postinterventional monitoring.

Blood cultures, if available, would be helpful for diagnosis of typhoid fever, brucellosis and septicaemia.

The Case Continued…

The mother of the patient reported that the family came from an area where visceral leishmaniasis was known. It turned out that the uncle of the child had been treated for VL before. The girl's sister had recently been treated for TB.

The child's health continued to deteriorate. She had persistently high fever and became increasingly pale.

The DAT came back positive with a high titre (≥1:6.400), which supported the suspected diagnosis of visceral leishmaniasis.

Considering her critical condition, with severe malnutrition and progressive anaemia, the patient was started on liposomal amphotericin B and a broad-spectrum antibiotic (ceftriaxone). The girl also received nutritional support with high-energy/high-protein ready-to-use therapeutic food (RUTF) and vitamin/mineral supplementation.

After 5 days, the fever settled and the patient started to recover. Two weeks later the girl had gained some weight and was again able to walk and play.

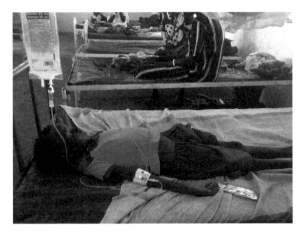

• **Fig. 44.1** A child is receiving liposomal amphotericin B on a paediatric ward in South Sudan.

SUMMARY BOX

Visceral Leishmaniasis (Kala-Azar)

VL is a vector-borne systemic parasitic infection caused by *Leishmania* protozoans, most commonly *L. donovani* and *L. infantum*. Large epidemics have been described in East Africa and the Indian subcontinent. As a result of efforts to eliminate the disease on the Indian subcontinent, the incidence of VL has decreased substantially in the past decade. Ninety per cent of all cases occur in only five countries: India, Sudan, South Sudan, Ethiopia and Brazil.

Transmission can be anthroponotic or zoonotic, differing by region and parasite strain. Humans most commonly acquire VL through the bite of an infected female sandfly, but other modes of transmission have been described.

Leishmania promastigotes invade cells of the human reticuloendothelial system where they metamorphose into amastigotes and multiply. The incubation period varies greatly, from 10 days to several years, but usually takes between 2 and 8 months.

The clinical presentation depends on the infecting species, as well as on the host's genetic background and immune status. Most infections remain asymptomatic.

Clinical VL presents with symptoms and signs of a chronic systemic infection (fever, fatigue, anorexia, weight loss) and of parasite invasion of the mononuclear phagocyte system (enlarged lymph nodes, splenomegaly, hepatomegaly) resulting in severe immunosuppression. In India, hyperpigmentation has led to the name 'kala-azar' (Hindi for 'black sickness'). VL is typically fatal if not treated, and potentially fatal complications include bacterial superinfections and congestive heart failure because of severe anaemia and haemorrhage.

In low-resource settings, diagnostic options for VL are often limited. On FBC all three cell lines can be depleted. Demonstration of *Leishmania* amastigotes in samples from bone marrow, spleen and lymph node is the classic confirmatory test for VL. Under field conditions, direct proof of the parasite is often not feasible, and several serological tests have been developed instead. Sensitivity and specificity of these tests generally vary and they should always be used in combination with a standardized case definition as suggested by the WHO.

The rK39 immuno-chromatographic test (ICT) and the direct agglutination test (DAT) were found to have the highest sensitivity and specificity. The rK39 ICTs are easy to perform, rapid (10–20 minutes), cheap and give easily reproducible results. The semiquantitative DAT has a longer turnaround time of about 24 hours, and requires a laboratory with well-trained technicians.

Treatment of VL is complex: efficacy of the individual drugs varies geographically and depends on parasite susceptibility and the immune status of the patient. Parenteral drugs currently used are pentavalent antimonials, paromomycin and (liposomal) amphotericin B (Fig. 44.1). The oral drug in use is miltefosine. Combinations of antileishmanial drugs seem to help shorten therapy courses, reduce side effects, improve treatment outcomes, delay resistance development and reduce treatment costs.

In HIV patients, VL is even more difficult to treat because it does not respond well to the classic antileishmanial drugs and has a higher tendency to relapse.

Further Reading

1. Boelaert M, Sundar S. Leishmaniasis. In: Farrar J, editor. Manson's Tropical Diseases. 23rd ed. London: Elsevier; 2013 [chapter 47].
2. WHO. Control of the Leishmaniases. WHO Technical Report Series 949. Geneva: World Health Organization; 2010.
3. Burza S, Croft SL, Boelaert M. Leishmaniasis. Lancet 2018;392 (10151):951–70.
4. Chappuis F, Sundar S, Hailu A, et al. Visceral Leishmaniasis: what are the needs for diagnosis, treatment and control? Nat Rev Microbiol 2007;5(11):873–82.
5. Alves F, Bilbe G, Blesson S, et al. Recent development of visceral leishmaniasis treatments: successes, pitfalls, and perspectives. Clin Microbiol Rev 2018;31(4):e00048–18.

45

A 2-Month-Old Girl from Laos With Dyspnoea, Cyanosis and Irritability

MAYFONG MAYXAY, DOUANGDAO SOUKALOUN AND PAUL N. NEWTON

Clinical Presentation

History

You are working in the paediatric intensive care unit (PICU) of a tertiary hospital in Vientiane, Laos. A 2-month-old baby girl is presented with 3 days of irritability, dyspnoea and grunting. Her mother is a 24-year-old rice farmer who describes that the baby suddenly became unwell but was neither feverish nor coughing. The infant was born at term and had been very well until 3 days previously.

Clinical Findings

Irritable infant, crying and grunting, with a temperature of 37.0°C (98.6°F), pulse 140 bpm (normal range 100–160), respiratory rate 40 breath cycles per minute (normal range 30–60). The blood pressure is not taken. The child is dyspnoeic and has central cyanosis, hepatomegaly and oedematous extremities. The rest of the physical examination appears normal, with a clear chest and no heart murmurs.

Questions

1. What are your most important differential diagnoses?
2. What additional information do you need to obtain from the mother and what would be your immediate management?

Discussion

A young Lao mother presents with her 2-month-old baby girl, who has been acutely unwell for the past 3 days. The child has been breastfeeding poorly and was noted to have been grunting, which is a non-specific sign of severe systemic illness in infants. On examination, the child is irritable, cyanosed and shows signs of heart failure.

Answer to Question 1

What Are Your Most Important Differential Diagnoses?

The most important differential diagnoses to consider are congenital heart disease, respiratory diseases (e.g. bronchopneumonia, bronchiolitis and laryngitis), meningitis and infantile beriberi (thiamine or vitamin B_1 deficiency).

However, the absence of cough, wheeze and fever, along with a normal chest examination, suggest that respiratory diseases are unlikely. The fact that the cyanosis has started well after birth along with the sudden onset of symptoms and the absence of a heart murmur suggests that congenital heart disease is unlikely. Absence of fever or bulging fontanels makes meningitis unlikely. The combination of dyspnoea, poor breastfeeding, abnormal cry, grunting and swollen extremities in a suitable endemic setting (South-east Asia) suggest infantile beriberi as the most likely diagnosis.

Answer to Question 2

What Additional Information Do You Need to Obtain from the Mother and What Would be Your Immediate Management?

The most important information to be obtained from the mother is whether the child has been exclusively breastfed, whether the mother had practiced food avoidance during pregnancy and/or post-partum, and whether the mother herself has had any symptoms and signs suggestive of beriberi, such as paresthesias and difficulty rising from a squatting position.

Prolonged food avoidance post-partum is common in lowland Lao culture. It is based upon the traditional belief that certain food items may harm the newborn. Most lowland mothers eat milled glutinous rice but avoid eating fruits and vegetables, which results in low diet diversity for some months before and after delivery.

Thiamine deficiency may be one result of such dietary restriction, and affected mothers secrete insufficient levels of thiamine in their breastmilk. The cardiac form of thiamine deficiency usually manifests during the second or third month of life. Infants present with dyspnoea, cyanosis, vomiting and irritability.

Children with infantile beriberi respond rapidly (i.e. within 30–60 min) to intravenous or intramuscular thiamine (50 mg), which should urgently be administered. The child should be closely monitored.

The Case Continued...

The mother reported that her child had been exclusively breastfed and that she had practiced food avoidance since delivery: She had avoided eating beef, pork, vegetables and fruits. The mother said that she herself had anorexia, weakness, a husky voice, and paresthesias affecting her limbs – symptoms of thiamine deficiency.

Intravenous thiamine (50 mg) was given immediately to the child after admission and she quickly and dramatically responded. Six hours later the baby was able to breastfeed normally and was discharged the following day. Blood samples were taken from the child and the mother. Analysis showed that both were thiamine-deficient.

The mother was given oral thiamine supplementation and advised to return to a well-balanced diet including thiamine-rich foods.

SUMMARY BOX

Infantile Beriberi

Infantile beriberi, or clinical thiamine (vitamin B1) deficiency in infants, is a largely forgotten, fatal but inexpensively treated disease. It mainly occurs in South and South-east Asia, where 50 to 100 years ago it was recognized as a major public health problem. It remains relatively common in Laos, probably because of prolonged maternal food avoidance during pregnancy and postpartum. There is also evidence that it is still of importance in Cambodia, India and Myanmar, and cases have been reported from refugee populations in Thailand.

Infantile beriberi occurs in exclusively breastfed babies of approximately 2 to 3 months of age, whose mothers have thiamine deficiency resulting from inadequate thiamine intake.

It commonly manifests mainly as the "wet" form of beriberi, characterized by heart failure with hepatomegaly and marked peripheral oedema. The disease typically presents as shock, often preceded by a hoarse cry, grunting, poor breastfeeding, irritability, dyspnoea and cyanosis. Clinically unapparent thiamine deficiency was also found to be common among sick infants admitted to the hospitals in Laos.

A thiamine-deficient diet is largely made up of milled, sticky rice that has had most of its thiamine removed as a result of the milling process. In the late nineteenth century, the advent of mechanical rice milling, which removes the main dietary source of thiamine in the rice husk, is thought to be the precipitant for beriberi becoming a major public health problem in Asia, responsible for considerable mortality. However, there has been very little recent epidemiological research, despite evidence that it remains focally important.

The pathophysiology of infantile beriberi remains unclear, but the cardinal problem is usually myocardial dysfunction. Thiamine deficiency may also present with a variety of other clinical syndromes, including encephalopathy, hypoglycemia and lactic acidosis.

Infantile beriberi is usually diagnosed clinically because of the need to act before biochemical results are available and the lack of laboratories in endemic areas that can perform thiamine biochemical assays. Treatment of infantile beriberi with thiamine is simple, inexpensive and highly effective. It should be administered parenterally to rapidly increase tissue thiamine levels. Thiamine supplementation should also be given to the mothers of infants with beriberi. Education about thiamine-rich foods (e.g. pulses, groundnuts, whole wheat, fruits and vegetables) and on the danger of food avoidance should be provided before discharge. Prevention is crucial: better understanding of post-partum diets, and on how to change the practice of food avoidance is very important and thiamine supplementation for mothers is urgently needed.

Further Reading

1. Abrams S, Brabin BJ, Coulter JBS. Nutrition-associated disease. In: Farrar J, editor. Manson's Tropical Diseases. 23rd ed. London: Elsevier; 2013 [chapter 77].
2. Barennes H, Simmala C, Odermatt P, et al. Postpartum traditions and nutrition practices among urban Lao women and their infants in Vientiane. Lao PDR Eur J Clin Nutr 2009;63(3):323–31.
3. Barennes H, Sengkhamyong K, Rene JP, et al. Beriberi (Thiamine deficiency) and high infant mortality in Northern Laos. PLoS Negl Trop Dis 2015;9(3):e0003581.
4. Bhat JI, Ahmed QI, Ahangar AA, et al. Wernicke's encephalopathy in exclusive breastfed infants. World J Pediatr 2017;13(5):485–8.
5. Whitfield KC, Bourassa MW, Adamolekun B, et al. Thiamine deficiency disorders: diagnosis, prevalence, and a roadmap for global control programs. Ann N Y Acad Sci 2018;1430(2018):3–43.

46

A 45-Year-Old Man from Sri Lanka With Fever and Right Hypochondrial Pain

RANJAN PREMARATNA

Clinical Presentation

History

A 45-year-old Sri Lankan man presents to a local hospital with fever, chills, headache, body aches and severe right hypochondrial pain for the past week. He has also developed a dry cough during the past few days. He has vomited twice during his illness and has lost his appetite.

His abdominal pain is constant and dull. It radiates to the right shoulder and is made worse when coughing and resting on the right side.

The patient had been well before the current illness. He admits to consuming locally brewed alcohol ('*toddy*', made of coconut flowers) daily for the past 10 to 15 years.

Examination

The patient looks generally ill, mildly dehydrated and is in pain. Temperature is 38.3°C (100.8°F), blood pressure 100/80 mmHg, pulse 102 bpm, respiratory rate 24 breath cycles per minute. There is no jaundice, no pallor and no lymphadenopathy. The abdominal examination reveals a tender hepatomegaly; however, the tenderness is most prominent over the 6th to 9th intercostal spaces in the right mid-axillary line. The spleen is not enlarged. On auscultation, there are few inspiratory crackles over the right lung base. The cardiovascular system and the nervous system are clinically normal.

Investigations

His laboratory results are shown in Table 46.1. A chest radiograph showed elevated right hemidiaphragm and patchy shadows in the right lower zone.

Questions

1. What is the likely diagnosis?
2. How would you manage this patient?

TABLE 46.1 Laboratory Results at Presentation		
Parameter	Patient	Reference
WBC (×10⁹/L)	14.7	4–10
Haemoglobin (g/dL)	12.3	12–16
Platelets (×10⁹/L)	224	150–350
AST (U/L)	54	13–33
ALT (U/L)	38	3–25
ALP (U/L)	446	40–130
Serum bilirubin total (µmol/L)	10.3	25.7–30.8
Serum bilirubin direct (µmol/L)	1.5	1.7–5.1
Blood urea nitrogen (mmol/L)	7	2.5–6.4
Serum creatinine (µmol/L)	124	71–106
C-reactive protein (mg/L)	48	<6

Discussion

A 45-year-old Sri Lankan man presents with fever, headache, body aches and constant right-sided abdominal pain for a week. He also has a dry cough. His past medical history is unremarkable, but he consumes local alcohol. He is febrile with tender hepatomegaly and intercostal tenderness on the right. There is no jaundice.

His blood results show very mildly elevated transaminases, an elevated alkaline phosphatase (AP) and raised inflammatory markers.

Answer to Question 1

What is the Likely Diagnosis?

Tender hepatomegaly, intercostal tenderness and an elevated right hemidiaphragm in the context of fever point towards an infectious focus in the liver.

His transaminases are only slightly elevated; AST is higher than ALT, which could be explained merely by his regular alcohol consumption. In infectious hepatitis one would expect higher transaminase levels and clinical jaundice.

The most likely diagnosis in this man is a liver abscess, which could be amoebic or pyogenic. Given the Asian setting, hyermucoviscous serotypes of *Klebisella pneumoniae* have to be considered which have been increasingly detected in South and South East Asia since around 1990 and also seem to be spreading to countries outside Asia. Given the epidemiological setting, the relatively young age of the patient and the absence of comorbidities such as diabetes or biliary disease, an amoebic liver abscess is more likely. Also, the alcoholic drink the patient consumes is locally known to be linked with amoebiasis. The precise mechanisms are still under discussion; it is assumed that the parasites contaminate the clay containers used to collect *toddy,* but additional factors may play a role as well.

Another tropical infectious disease to consider in a febrile patient from Asia with any kind of organ abscess is melioidosis. Melioidosis, caused by the environmental bacterium *Burkholderia pseudomallei,* can also present with pulmonary infiltrates and cavities similar to TB, as septic arthritis, with skin manifestations and with cerebral involvement. Cases of melioidosis have been increasingly reported from Sri Lanka. The majority of cases occur in the immunocompromised, especially with type 2 diabetes mellitus, but also alcoholism, chronic lung disease, chronic renal disease, steroid use, immunosuppressive therapy and cancer.

Melioidosis is also endemic in other parts of Asia, such as India, Thailand, Lao PR, Vietnam and in northern Australia, sporadic cases are seen all over the tropics.

Answer to Question 2

How Would You Manage This Patient?

An ultrasound of the liver should be done. *Entamoeba histolytica* serology is highly sensitive and useful as a screening test; however, it may lack specificity in individuals from highly endemic tropical regions like the Indian subcontinent. Recently, multiplex PCR testing on aspirated fluid has been identified as a rapid and robust diagnosis of amoebic liver abscess in patients with cystic focal liver lesions. Stool microscopy for *E. histolytica* trophozoites may be attempted but is less than 50% sensitive.

The Case Continued...

The ultrasound scan of his abdomen revealed a solitary hypoechoic lesion with an irregular wall measuring 7×6 cm in the right liver lobe. There was a small pleural effusion on the right.

Because of its large size, the lesion was aspirated under ultrasound guidance, yielding brownish pus highly suspicious of an amoebic liver abscess.

TABLE 46.2 Treatment of Amoebic Liver Abscesses. (After Anesi, J.A., 2015)

Agent	Medication	Dose	Duration
Tissue Agents	Metronidazole	500–750 mg IV/PO TDS	7–10 days
	Tinidazole	2 g PO OD	3–5 days
	Ornidazole	0.5 g IV BD	3–6 days
	Nitazoxanide	500 mg PO BD	3 days
Luminal Agents	Paromomycin	8–10 mg/kg PO TDS	7 days
	Diloxanide Furoate	500 mg TDS	10 days
	Iodoquinole (Diiodohydroxyquin)	650 mg PO TDS after meals	20 days

PO = orally, IV = intravenously, BD = twice daily, TDS = three times a day.

The patient was treated with metronidazole for ten days and made a rapid and uneventful recovery.

SUMMARY BOX

Amoebic Liver Abscess

Amoebic liver abscess (ALA) is the most common extraintestinal form of invasive amoebiasis caused by *Entamoeba histolytica*. The infection occurs worldwide but is most common in tropical areas with overcrowding and poor sanitation. Rates of ALA are 3 to 20 times higher in men between 18 and 50 years of age than in other populations; the reasons for this are poorly understood but hormonal factors are being discussed, as well as alcohol consumption. Humans acquire the infection by ingestion of faecally contaminated food or water. Trophozoites of *E. histolytica* may penetrate the intestinal wall and haematogenously spread to the liver. Clinical manifestations include fever with chills, right hypochondrial pain, anorexia and weight loss, but most patients with ALA do not have a history of recent dysentery. A dry cough and fine crepitations over the right lung bases are common. Jaundice is unusual. Localized intercostal tenderness helps in the clinical diagnosis. ALA may rupture into the peritoneal cavity or through the skin or diaphragm. Haematogenous spread may cause metastatic abscesses in distant organs such as the brain.

Leukocytosis, raised inflammatory parameters and an elevated alkaline phosphatase are the most common non-specific laboratory findings. Diagnosis is usually made by a combination of imaging studies and serology. Abdominal ultrasound scan is the most suitable imaging technique in resource-limited settings, but CT and MRI scans are also highly sensitive. None of the imaging techniques is specific for ALA. Plain radiography of the thorax may reveal elevation of the right hemidiaphragm.

Serology is highly sensitive but may lack specificity in individuals from endemic countries. Although aspiration of a suspected ALA is not a routine investigation, aspirated fluid can be tested with multiplex PCR testing for the rapid and robust diagnosis of amoebiasis in patients with cystic focal liver lesions. The aspirated fluid is thick, odourless and brownish in colour; it is bacteriologically sterile and amoebic trophozoites are not usually detectable in the aspirate. The term 'abscess' is a misnomer, as the 'pus' is in fact necrotic liver.

Most patients rapidly respond to antibiotic treatment with metronidazole or tinidazole.

Metronidazole 500 to 750 mg tds PO or IV should be given for 7 to 10 days, tinidazole 2 g per day PO for 3 to 5 days. This should be followed by a luminal amoebicide, such as paromomycin, diloxanide furoate, or iodoquinol (Table 46.2).

The role of therapeutic percutaneous aspiration or drainage is still controversial. It may be useful in large abscesses, especially when located in the left liver lobe with high risk for rupturing into the pericardium, and in ALA that do not respond to nitroimidazole therapy within 72 hours when pyogenic infection is a concern. Lesions may take a long time to decrease in size, therefore short-term, follow-up imaging has to be interpreted with caution.

Further Reading

1. Kelly P. Intestinal protozoa. In: Farrar J, editor. Manson's Tropical Diseases. 23rd ed. London: Elsevier; 2013 [chapter 49].
2. Anesi JA, Gluckman G. Amebic Liver Abscess. Clin Liver Dis 2015;6(2):41–3.
3. Siu LK, Yeh KM, Lin JC, Fung CP, Chang FY. *Klebsiella pneumoniae* liver abscess: a new invasive syndrome. Lancet Infect Dis 2012;12:881–7.
4. Weitzel T, Cabrera J, Rosas R, et al. Enteric multiplex PCR panels: a new diagnostic tool for amoebic liver abscess? New Microbes New Infect 2017;18:50–3. https://doi.org/10.1016/j.nmni.2017.05.002.
5. Kumanan T, Sujanitha V, Balakumar S, et al. Amoebic liver abscess and indigenous alcoholic beverages in the tropics. J Trop Med 2018;2018:6901751. https://doi.org/10.1155/2018/6901751.

47

A 32-Year-Old Man from Malawi With a Painfully Swollen Neck

JOEP J. VAN OOSTERHOUT

Clinical Presentation

History

A 32-year-old Malawian man presents to the outpatient department of a local tertiary hospital with a 6-week history of productive cough and chest pain associated with weight loss, fevers and night sweats. He has also noticed that his neck has swollen and is painful. There are no other symptoms. He has never been admitted to a hospital but has been tested HIV positive and was started on antiretroviral therapy (ART) and co-trimoxazole prophylaxis 2 months earlier at a nearby health centre. His health passport (Fig. 47.1) reveals that a recent CD4 count was 95 cells/μL and that the patient had been treated for acid-fast bacilli (AFB) sputum smear-negative pulmonary tuberculosis 12 years ago.

Clinical Findings

He looks moderately ill, is pale, is sweating and has a temperature of 39.2°C (102.56°F), pulse 112 bpm, respiratory rate 28 breath cycles per minute and normal blood pressure. There are large, matted lymph glands palpable in his neck. The rest of the examination is unremarkable.

Investigations

Full blood count: WBC 14.3×10^9/L (reference range: 4–10), haemoglobin 6.3 g/dL (13–15), MCV 66 fL (80–98), platelets 246×10^9/L (150–350).

Three sputum samples are negative for AFB. Fine-needle aspiration (FNA) of a neck gland yields purulent material. Microscopy for AFB is 2+ positive. There is no growth on blood culture.

Initial treatment

The patient is admitted to the hospital and started on TB repeat treatment for tuberculous lymphadenitis with streptomycin, isoniazid, rifampicin, pyrazinamide and ethambutol, while continuing the same ART. Against expectation, he does not improve after 3 weeks. He still has fevers, night sweats, lack of appetite and the glands in the neck have further swollen and are now clearly fluctuant (Fig. 47.2).

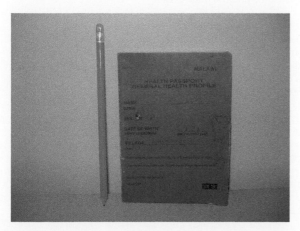

• **Fig. 47.1** The patient's "health passport". The health passport is a booklet all patients in Malawi hold which documents their medical history.

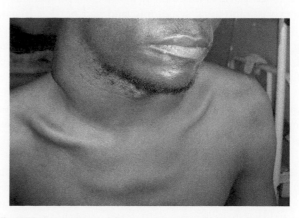

• **Fig. 47.2** Increasing and fluctuant lymphadenitis in the neck.

Questions

1. What could be the reasons for the lack of clinical improvement?
2. Which investigations are indicated?

Discussion

A 32-year-old Malawian man who is known to be HIV positive is admitted with a diagnosis of tuberculous lymphadenitis and immune reconstitution inflammatory syndrome (IRIS) of the unmasking type (see Summary Box). The TB diagnosis is based on microscopic findings. He unexpectedly deteriorates on antituberculous treatment.

Answer to Question 1

What Could Be the Reasons for the Lack of Clinical Improvement?

Although the diagnosis of TB lymphadenitis is very likely when AFB are identified in a lymph gland sample, atypical mycobacteria should also be considered now that the initial response to TB treatment is unsatisfactory, especially given the deep immune suppression the patient had at the start of ART. Other reasons for a poor response to TB treatment are non-adherence, malabsorption and drug resistance. Given the frank fluctuation that is present, a bacterial lymphadenitis is probable, whereas a lymphoma seems much less likely.

Answer to Question 2

Which Investigations Are Indicated?

HIV viral load and a CD4 count should be done to determine the response to ART. A repeat FNA should be performed to check for AFB. A Gram stain and bacterial culture should help rule out bacterial superinfection. Ideally, the aspirate should be examined by PCR (XPert MTB/RIF) and also be cultured to rule out infection with resistant *Mycobacterium tuberculosis* or atypical mycobacteria (culture).

The Case Continued...

The patient denied missing any tablets, had no diarrhoea or other gastrointestinal symptoms, and had not left Malawi, where multi-drug resistance for TB is uncommon. IRIS of the paradoxical type was also considered to explain the lack of improvement (see Box), therefore corticosteroids were initiated.

Further investigations were done, with the following results: CD4 109 cells/µL; HIV-1 RNA < 400 copies/mL. Repeat FBC results were: WBC 7.8×10^9/L, haemoglobin 6.7 g/dL, MCV 84 fL, platelets 428×10^9/L.

Because of the increasingly fluctuant swelling in the neck, a second FNA was done, now showing frank yellowish pus. On microscopic examination, numerous coccoid bacteria and polymorphonuclear lymphocytes were observed. Unfortunately results from a bacterial culture were never received.

The diagnosis at this point was superimposed bacterial lymphadenitis, possibly iatrogenic because of the earlier aspiration, with *Staphylococcus aureus* being the most likely microorganism. The patient recovered well after incision and drainage, antibiotic treatment and a short course of corticosteroids while he continued on TB treatment and ART.

In the first full blood count, severe microcytic anaemia was present. Anaemia is extremely common in patients with advanced HIV immunosuppression and TB co-infection; however, the marked microcytosis is unusual. There was no good explanation for this finding because there was no source of blood loss in the history, and the MCV had normalized in the second full blood count, which was against β-thalassaemia as a cause of microcytic anaemia. The first full blood count also showed a leukocytosis when TB lymphadenitis was diagnosed. This finding is paradoxical because later, when the florid purulent bacterial infection was present, it had resolved. Multiple dynamic factors were apparently influencing the white blood cell count in this patient, including HIV, TB, bacterial infection, immune reconstitution, corticosteroids, antiretroviral and antituberculous drugs and co-trimoxazole.

SUMMARY BOX

Immune Reconstitution Inflammatory Syndrome

HIV-associated immune reconstitution inflammatory syndrome (IRIS) is a deterioration of the clinical situation caused by increased inflammation because of improving immune competence resulting from successful ART.

The clinical manifestations are wide-ranging and depend on the underlying condition, which is mostly an opportunistic infection, but can also be a tumour, an autoimmune disease or another condition. In sub-Saharan Africa, tuberculosis and cryptococcal meningitis are the two most important IRIS presentations. IRIS is very common, occurring in between 10 and 25% of patients who start ART. There are no validated tests for IRIS. The diagnosis is therefore clinical.

A widely accepted definition does not exist, although standardization has been attempted. Definitions include measures of successful ART, exclusion of other causes of the clinical deterioration, such as toxicity, and a relationship in time between the symptoms and the start of ART.

IRIS is classified into two types: In "unmasking IRIS", a condition is present but remains subclinical and undiagnosed because of severe immunosuppression before the start of ART, and becomes clinically apparent within 6 months after ART initiation. In "paradoxical IRIS", a condition has been diagnosed and is being treated successfully, but clinical worsening occurs because of the increased inflammation after immune recovery, e.g. after starting ART. Risk factors for HIV-associated paradoxical IRIS include a low pre-ART CD4 count and haemoglobin level, a high pre-ART viral load, large pre-ART weight loss, large and rapid increase of the CD4 count, rapid reduction of the viral load on ART and a short period between the start of treatment for an opportunistic infection and initiation of ART. Prednisone initiated alongside ART in selected patients with CD4 counts <100 cells/µL seems to reduce the risk of paradoxical IRIS and is not associated with significant adverse effects.

Paradoxical IRIS may also occur in other conditions, e.g. in TB alone without HIV co-infection when TB treatment itself induces immune reconstitution. Patients have to be prepared for the IRIS phenomenon when starting treatment.

Further Reading

1. Thwaites G. Tuberculosis. In: Farrar J, editor. Manson's Tropical Diseases. 23rd ed. London: Elsevier; 2013 [chapter 40].

2. Haddow LJ, Moosa MY, Easterbrook PJ. Validation of a published case definition for tuberculosis-associated immune reconstitution inflammatory syndrome. AIDS 2010;24(1):103–8.

3. Yu G, Zhong F, Ye B, et al. Diagnostic Accuracy of the Xpert MTB/RIF assay for lymph node Tuberculosis: as systematic review and meta analysis. Bio Med Res Int 2019;2019:4878240.

4. Walker NF, Stek C, Wasserman S, et al. The tuberculosis-associated immune reconstitution inflammatory syndrome: recent advances in clinical and pathogenesis research. Curr Opin HIV AIDS 2018;13(6):512–21.

5. Meintjes G, Stek C, Blumenthal L, et al. Prednisone for the Prevention of Paradoxical Tuberculosis-Associated IRIS. N Engl J Med 2018;379(20):1915–25.

48

A 31-Year-Old Woman from Tanzania With Acute Flaccid Paraplegia

WILLIAM P. HOWLETT

Clinical Presentation

History

A 31-year-old woman is referred to a hospital in northern Tanzania with a loss of power and feeling in her legs. She describes being perfectly well up until 2 days earlier when she felt acute back pain which radiated band-like to the level of her umbilicus. The pain was severe, continuous, burning and unrelieved by analgesics or position. Within 12 hours the pain had lessened but she developed numbness in her feet and legs ascending to the level of her waist, loss of power in her legs and loss of control of her bladder. There is a history of a febrile illness 3 weeks previously, treated as malaria. There is no past or family history of similar illness and no history of trauma. She is married with 3 children, the last born is 12 months old. She does not smoke or take alcohol, and her HIV status during her last pregnancy was negative.

Clinical Findings

Clinically, she is well nourished with normal vital signs. General examination is unremarkable; there is no spinal tenderness, deformity or gibbus. On neurological examination she is fully orientated and higher mental functions appear normal. Cranial nerves including fundoscopy and upper limbs are normal. She is unable to move her legs and examination of the lower limbs reveals a flaccid paraparesis with a sensory level at T10. On inspection feet are in a slightly plantar-flexed position (Fig. 48.1). Tone is reduced bilaterally, power is reduced (MRC grade 1/5) in all muscle groups. Reflexes are absent bilaterally, and plantar reflexes are extensor. Sensation is reduced to light touch to the level of the umbilicus. Joint position sense is impaired in the feet and ankles, and vibration sense is absent to the anterior iliac crest bilaterally.

Questions

1. What is the clinical syndrome and where is the lesion?
2. What investigations will you plan to do?

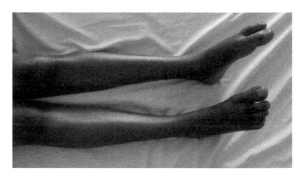

• **Fig. 48.1** A patient with an acute-onset flaccid paraplegia. Note the plantar flexion of her feet.

Discussion

A 31-year-old woman from northern Tanzania presents with an acute-onset inability to walk. She had a febrile illness 3 weeks prior, but has otherwise been well.

Answer to Question 1

What is the Clinical Syndrome and Where is the Lesion?

The clinical syndromic diagnosis is acute flaccid paraparesis. The main neuroanatomical differential diagnoses of flaccid paraparesis are lesions of peripheral nerves, including their roots (polyneuropathies or polyradiculoneuropathies), and acute lesions of the spinal cord (myelopathies). The sensory impairment up to the umbilicus (T10 level) and extensor plantar reflexes localise the site of the lesion to the spinal cord. The flaccidity and loss of reflexes can be explained by the early flaccid phase of acute spinal cord injury when spasticity appears days or weeks later (Table 48.1).

Answer to Question 2

What Investigations Will You Plan to Do?

If available, the following investigations should be performed:

Full blood count, ESR, blood glucose, renal and liver function tests, HIV serology, VDRL test and schistosomiasis

TABLE 48.1 Flaccid versus Spastic Paraparesis

Clinical Presentation		Neuroanatomical Diagnosis	Examples of Common Aetiologies in Tropical Countries
Flaccid paraparesis	with bladder involvement and/or sensory level	Acute spinal cord lesion	inflammation of the spinal cord (= myelitis), ischaemia of the spinal cord (= spinal infarction)
		Acute cauda equina lesion	metastatic malignancy, schistosomiasis
	without bladder dysfunction, without sensory level	Polyradiculoneuropathy	Guillain-Barré-syndrome, tuberculous arachnoiditis, CMV in HIV
		Polyneuropathy	Diabetes, HIV-related, nutritional
Spastic paraparesis		Chronic spinal cord lesion	Compression of spinal cord because of Pott's disease, chronic viral infections such as HTLV-1 and HIV

serology. The latter has to be interpreted with caution because it stays positive after past infection. Urine and stool analysis for ova of *Schistosoma* species should be done.

Lumbar puncture should be performed with measurement of opening pressure and testing cell differentiation, CSF protein, glucose, Gram and Ziehl-Neelsen stain, Xpert MTB/RIF for *M. tuberculosis* and VDRL. Imaging should include x-rays of the chest and spine. Neuroimaging (e.g. spinal CT/MRI) is recommended mainly to exclude a compressive spinal cord lesion but is usually not readily available in sub-Saharan Africa.

The Case Continued...

The patient's full blood count, renal and liver function tests were normal. Results of further blood tests are shown in the Table 48.2.

A spinal tap was done. The CSF opening pressure was normal and looked clear. Further CSF results are shown in the Table 48.3.

TABLE 48.2 Laboratory Results on Admission

Parameter (Unit)	Patient	Normal range
ESR (mm/h)	19	≤10
Random blood glucose (mmol/l)	5.6	3.9–11.1
HIV-Serology and p24 Antigen	negative	negative
VDRL	negative	negative
Schistosomiasis-serology	negative	negative
Urine for ova of S. haematobium	negative	negative
Stool for ova of S. mansoni	negative	negative

TABLE 48.3 CSF Results

Parameter (Unit)	Patient	Normal range
CSF white cell count (cells/μl)	11 (90% lymphocytes)	0–5
CSF protein (g/L)	1.11	<0.45
CSF glucose (mmol/l)	3.9	2.8–3.8*
Gram stain	negative	negative
Ziehl-Neelsen stain	negative	negative
Xpert MTB/RIF	negative	negative
VDRL in the CSF	negative	negative

*{1/2} to {2/3} of paired serum glucose sample

The x-rays of her chest and thoracolumbar spine were normal.

The main differential diagnosis of acute non-compressive flaccid paraparesis that localizes in the spinal cord is acute spinal cord inflammation (acute transverse myelitis), and vascular spinal cord ischaemia ("spinal stroke"). The CSF findings of increased lymphocytes and elevated protein level are suggestive of inflammation in the spinal cord. Hence, the clinicolaboratory diagnosis is that of acute transverse myelitis.

The management is based on principles of establishing and treating the cause and preventing complications. Treatment in this patient includes steroids and acyclovir directed against the main causes of acute transverse myelitis, e.g. autoimmune inflammation and viral infections (see Summary Box). Counselling of patient and family is very important, and family members/guardians should from the beginning on be actively involved in physiotherapy and mobilization of the patient. General measures include strict 2 hourly turning, frequent passive movements, urinary catheterization if non-functioning bladder, and adequate analgesia according to the WHO analgesic ladder.

The patient was treated with corticosteroids and acyclovir. She partially improved and was discharged after 3 weeks. The power in her legs had slightly improved (MRC 2-3/5) and she had a urinary catheter in situ. She will be reviewed in the outpatient department.

TABLE 48.4	Pathophysiology of Acute Transverse Myelitis	
	Pathophysiology	**Treatment**
Idiopathic, (majority of the cases)	Presumably an autoimmune phenomenon. Might be a manifestation of a chronic autoimmune demyelinating CNS disease (such as NMO and multiple sclerosis)	Corticosteroids against inflammation
Associated with infection	Direct invasion of the spinal cord by microorganisms	Causative treatment e.g. acyclovir for VZV myelitis
	Autoimmune phenomenon as a result of infection elsewhere ("parainfectious"). Might be associated with vaccination against the microorganism	Corticosteroids against inflammation
Associated with a systemic autoimmune disorder	Autoimmune phenomenon. Often the autoimmune disorder (e.g. lupus or secondary vasculitis) in the patient is already known	Corticosteroids against inflammation

SUMMARY BOX

Acute Transverse Myelitis

Acute transverse myelitis (ATM) is an inflammation of the spinal cord characterized by an acute (hours) or sub-acute (days) onset, presenting typically with back pain, flaccid paraplegia, a sensory level on the trunk and urinary incontinence. The incidence of ATM in tropical countries is reported to be <1/100 000 but is likely to be much higher particularly in Africa. Women are more frequently affected, typically in their second and fourth decades. Evidence of inflammation within the spinal cord is shown by increased lymphocytes and elevated protein in the CSF. It can be associated with infections and autoimmune disorders. Symptoms that suggest infection include fever, rash, adenopathy, concurrent systemic infection and symptoms of herpes zoster radiculopathy. If the aetiology remains unknown as is frequently the case, the ATM is termed idiopathic (Table 48.4). Idiopathic ATM is considered to be an autoimmune phenomenon. "Idiopathic" ATM can be the first attack of an autoimmune demyelinating disease such as neuromyelitis optica (NMO) and rarely multiple sclerosis. However, multiple sclerosis is very rare in tropical latitudes.

Treatment of idiopathic ATM in adults is largely empirical with high doses of IV corticosteroids followed by oral prednisolone for 2 to 3 weeks. Empirical acyclovir is also recommended if VZV or HSV myelitis cannot be excluded. The majority (70% to 80%) of patients with ATM remain disabled with flaccid paraparesis/paraplegia and incontinence.

Further Reading

1. Heckmann JE, Bhigjee AI. Tropical neurology. In: Farrar J, editor. Manson's Tropical Diseases. 23rd ed. London: Elsevier; 2013 [chapter 71].
2. Borchers AT, Gershwin ME. Transverse myelitis. Autoimmun Rev 2012;11(3):231–48.
3. Howlett WP. Paraplegia, In: Neurology in Africa. Kilimanjaro Christian Medical Centre and University of Bergen; 2012. Available from:www.uib.no/cih/en/resources/neurology-in-africa.
4. Musubire AK, Meya DB, Bohjanen PR, et al. A systematic review of non-traumatic spinal cord injuries in sub-Saharan Africa and a proposed diagnostic algorithm for resource-limited settings. Front Neurol 2017;8:618. https://doi.org/10.3389/fneur.2017.00618.

49

A 33-Year-Old Male Traveller to India With Diarrhoea and Flatulence for Two Weeks

GAGANDEEP KANG AND SUDHIR BABJI

Clinical Presentation

History

A 33-year-old man from Finland who had been backpacking in India for the previous month presents to a private doctor in Chinglepet, Tamil Nadu, with complaints of passage of loose stools (four or five episodes per day) for the past 2 weeks. He reports weight loss, anorexia, malaise, flatulence and abdominal cramping when passing stool. For the past 3 days he has had bloating and distension after intake of milk products with an urge to pass stool. He has mild nausea, but no fever. Stools were watery earlier but he went to a local pharmacy and was given ciprofloxacin, which he took for 5 days ending 2 days previously, and stools are now three or four per day, mushy, greasy and foul-smelling.

Clinical Findings

A 33-year-old man, 180 cm, 72 kg (reports a 4 kg weight loss), mild non-specific abdominal tenderness. No signs of dehydration. The rest of the examination is normal.

Laboratory Results

Stool for reducing substances: positive. Stool examination for enteric parasites: *Giardia* trophozoites are seen in the fresh specimen. *Giardia* cysts are detected on formol-ether concentrated specimens (Fig. 49.1).

Questions

1. What clinical features can be used to establish an aetiological diagnosis of infectious diarrhoea in the tropics?
2. What complications can result from an acute enteric infection?

Discussion

A 33-year-old Finnish traveller to India presents with passage of loose stools, four or five episodes a day for the past 2 weeks. The stools have become greasy and foul-smelling, and he has bloating and distension after consumption of milk or milk products.

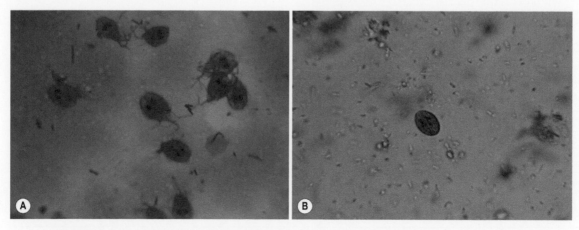

• **Fig. 49.1** Fresh preparation showing trophozoites (A) and formol-ether concentration showing cysts (B) of *Giardia* species.

The presence of *Giardia* trophozoites and cysts in the stool sample is confirmatory of giardiasis. The presence of reducing substances in the stool indicates a carbohydrate malabsorption, most likely of post-infectious origin.

Answer to Question 1

What Clinical Features Can be Used to Establish an Aetiological Diagnosis of Infectious Diarrhoea in the Tropics?

In the absence of a laboratory, clinical features sometimes provide a clue to the cause of infectious diarrhoea (Table 49.1). Diarrhoea caused by small intestinal infection is typically high volume, watery and often associated with malabsorption and dehydration. Colonic involvement is more often associated with frequent small-volume stools, the presence of blood and a sensation of urgency.

Chronic diarrhoea or recurrent episodes of acute diarrhoea should prompt HIV testing.

Answer to Question 2

What Complications Can Result from an Acute Enteric Infection?

Common complications of acute enteric infections are shown in Table 49.2.

TABLE 49.1 Clinical Clues to Pathology and Possible Aetiological Agents of Diarrhoeal Disease

Clinical Observation	Pathophysiology	Possible Aetiology
Few, bulky or large watery stools	Small bowel, secretory	Enterotoxigenic *Escherichia coli* (ETEC), enteropathogenic *E. coli* (EPEC), *Salmonella*, *Vibrio parahaemolyticus*, *Giardia*, possibly *Shigella*
Large volume, watery diarrhoea	Small bowel, enterotoxin mediated	*Vibrio cholerae*, ETEC, *Cryptosporidium*
Many, small volume stools	Large bowel	*Shigella*, *Salmonella*, *Campylobacter*, *Yersinia enterocolitica*, *Clostridium perfringens*, *Entamoeba histolytica*
Tenesmus, faecal urgency, dysentery	Colitis	*E. histolytica*, enteroinvasive *E. coli* (EIEC), enterohaemorrhagic *E. coli* (EHEC), *Shigella*, *Campylobacter*, *Y. enterocolitica*, *Clostridioides difficile*
Associated with vomiting	Gastroenteritis or toxin mediated	Noroviruses, rotavirus in children, *Bacillus cereus*, *Staphylococcus aureus* (food poisoning)
Associated with fever	Mucosal invasion or in children	*E. histolytica*, EIEC, EHEC, *Shigella*, *Salmonella*, *C. difficile*, *Campylobacter*, viral agents
Persistent diarrhoea (>2 weeks)	Secondary malabsorption, invasion	*Giardia*, *Cryptosporidium*, *E. histolytica*, *Aeromonas*. In immunosuppression: *Cystoisospora belli*, *Cryptosporidium*, *Microsporidium*

TABLE 49.2 Common Complications of Acute Enteric Infections

Complication	Pathogen
Carbohydrate intolerance or malabsorption	*Giardia lamblia/intestinalis*, rotavirus and other forms of viral gastroenteritis,
Fat malabsorption	*Giardia lamblia/intestinalis*
Haemolytic uraemic syndrome	Enterohaemorrhagic *Escherichia coli* (EHEC), *Shigella dysenteriae*
Guillain–Barré syndrome	*Campylobacter jejuni*
Reactive arthritis	*Campylobacter*, *Salmonella*, *Shigella*, *Yersinia* spp.
Erythema nodosum	*Campylobacter*, *Salmonella*, *Shigella*, *Yersinia* spp
Enteritis necroticans	*Clostridium perfringens* type C
Liver abscess and other forms of extraintestinal amoebiasis	*Entamoeba histolytica*
Chronic fatigue syndrome	*Giardia lamblia/intestinalis*, particularly described from Scandinavia

The Case Continued...

The patient was given tinidazole 2 g as a single oral dose. He was advised to restrict milk and high sugar products for a period of 2 weeks. He was counselled on food and water safety when travelling and was asked to return after 3 days. On review, he stated that his stool consistency had returned to normal and the frequency had decreased, he had no nausea and his anorexia had decreased. He had eaten a local dessert the previous day without realizing that it was made of reduced milk and had experienced some bloating and discomfort, but was otherwise feeling much better.

SUMMARY BOX

Giardiasis

Giardiasis is caused by *Giardia intestinalis* (also called *G. lamblia*), a flagellate protozoan. The parasite is present throughout the world, with several species found in animals. Not all infections result in symptoms, particularly in tropical countries where local populations with constant exposure rarely develop disease.

Symptomatic giardiasis is common in travellers to regions of South and South-east Asia, Africa, the Middle East and Latin America, particularly where clean water supplies and standards of food hygiene are low.

Giardia trophozoites are found in the small intestine of humans, and these non-invasive parasites appear to cause diarrhoea by blocking the absorptive surfaces of the gut and possibly by inducing fluid secretion. The trophozoites produce an environmentally resistant form, the cyst, which is passed in stool and enters the soil, water, food, or other surfaces after bowel movements. The most common method of infection is by drinking contaminated water. However, people may also become infected through hand-to-mouth transmission. This involves eating contaminated food or touching contaminated surfaces and unknowingly swallowing the parasite. The signs and symptoms of giardiasis usually occur within 7 to 14 days of exposure. Symptoms include diarrhoea, pale greasy stools, stomach cramps, gas, nausea, vomiting, bloating, weight loss and weakness. The symptoms usually last for 1 to 2 weeks, but may last longer. Giardiasis can cause malabsorption of vitamin A, vitamin B_{12}, iron, fat and carbohydrates in up to 20–40% of patients. Malabsorption can sometimes be prolonged and take several weeks to disappear. Chronic and multiple infections in young children have been shown to cause long-term effects on growth leading to stunting. The most common treatment is administration of drugs of the nitroimidazole group, with tinidazole being the drug of choice followed by metronidazole. Tinidazole is effective as a single dose of 2g, and metronidazole 500mg is given tds for 5 to 7 days. Non-responsiveness to nitroimidazole treatment is increasingly seen, in particular in travellers to South Asia where rates can reach up to 50%. Other drugs used are e.g. quinacrine, nitazoxanide and furazolidone.

Further Reading

1. Kelly P. Intestinal protozoa. In: Farrar J, editor. Manson's Tropical Diseases. 23rd ed. London: Elsevier; 2013 [chapter 49].
2. Ross AG, Olds GR, Cripps AW, et al. Enteropathogens and chronic illness in returning travelers. N Engl J Med 2013;368(19):1817–25.
3. Kaiser L, Surawicz CM. Infectious causes of chronic diarrhoea. Best Pract Res Clin Gastroenterol 2012;26(5):563–71.
4. Wright SG. Protozoan infections of the gastrointestinal tract. Infect Dis Clin North Am 2012;26(2):323–39.
5. Watkins RR, Eckmann L. Treatment of giardiasis: current status and future directions. Curr Infect Dis Rep 2014;16(2):396.

50

A 24-Year-Old Man of Turkish Origin With Jaundice and Cystic Liver Lesions

MARIJA STOJKOVIC

Clinical Presentation

History

A 24-year-old man of Turkish origin presents at a hospital in Germany because of right upper quadrant pain, nausea and vomiting.

The patient is a German resident but visits his family in rural eastern Turkey (Anatolia) every year for about 6 weeks.

Three years earlier the patient had presented with right upper quadrant pain. Then, an ultrasound and a CT scan of the liver had revealed two calcified cystic lesions, one in the right liver lobe, another smaller cyst in the left liver lobe (Figs. 50.1A and B and 50.2). Serology was positive for *Echinococcus granulosus* and a diagnosis of cystic echinococcosis (CE) was made.

Since both cyst walls were already calcified, anthelmintic treatment was not considered an option as the bioavailability

of albendazole in cysts with calcified cyst walls is rather poor. Being free of symptoms, the patient refused surgical treatment. The cysts were monitored regularly by ultrasound for signs of spontaneous involution.

Clinical Findings

A 24-year-old man in fair general condition with scleral jaundice. Blood pressure 110/70 mmHg, pulse 64 bpm, temperature 36°C (96.8°F). There is right upper quadrant and epigastric tenderness, but no guarding.

Laboratory Findings

The full blood count is normal. Additional results are shown in Table 50.1.

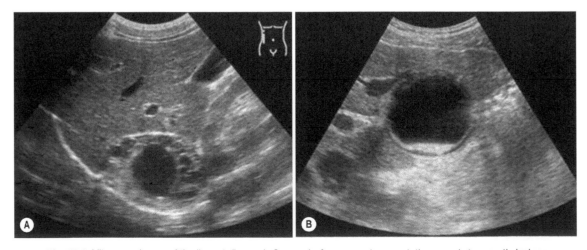

• **Fig. 50.1** Ultrasound scan of the liver at diagnosis 3 years before current presentation reveals two cystic lesions. One lesion is located in the right liver lobe (7 × 6 cm). Cyst content shows a solid cyst matrix containing multiple smaller cysts (A). The cyst wall is partially calcified (WHO classification CE3b). (B) Second cystic lesion in the left liver lobe (5 × 4 cm). The cyst wall is up to 4 mm thick with partial calcification. Cyst content is liquid; there is a double line sign, a feature of WHO CE1, and hydatid sand. (Copyright W. Hosch, Department of Radiology, Heidelberg University Hospital.)

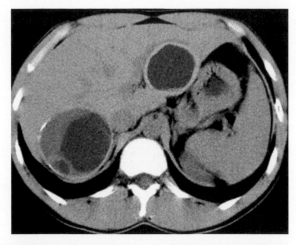

• **Fig. 50.2** Computed tomography of the same patient. Both cyst walls show calcification. (Copyright W. Hosch, Department of Radiology, Heidelberg University Hospital.)

TABLE 50.1	Laboratory Results on Presentation	
Parameter	Patient	Reference
AST (U/L)	145	<35
ALT (U/L)	454	<35
GGT (U/L)	394	<55
ALP (U/L)	402	38–126
Total bilirubin (µmol/L)	120	<19.0
ESR (mm/h)	17/40	≤10/20
CRP (mg/L)	49	<5

Questions

1. What is the suspected diagnosis and how would you approach this patient?
2. Which differential diagnoses should be considered in a patient with cystic liver lesions?

Discussion

A young man of Turkish origin presents with right upper quadrant pain and jaundice. He was diagnosed with CE 3 years earlier and has not been on any specific treatment.

Answer to Question 1

What is the Suspected Diagnosis and How Would You Approach This Patient?

His presentation should raise suspicion of a cystobiliary fistula with biliary obstruction, which is the most common acute complication in cystic echinococcosis and may be complicated by bacterial cholangitis.

In case of biliary obstruction, the first step is to restore the biliary flow by endoscopic retrograde cholangiography (ERC). ERC is both a diagnostic and therapeutic tool in cases of biliary obstruction; cyst content can be extracted from the hepatic or common bile duct. In case of bacterial cholangitis, the patient should receive antibiotic treatment to cover for Gram-negative bacteria and anaerobes.

Once biliary flow is restored and cholangitis has settled, the cyst can be surgically removed in a second step.

Answer to Question 2

Which Differential Diagnoses Should be Considered in a Patient With Cystic Liver Lesions?

The main differential diagnoses in this patient with cystic liver lesions and liquid cyst content are a congenital simple hepatic cyst and pseudocysts (necrotic cavity) in alveolar echinococcosis (*E. multilocularis*).

Depending on the presence of systemic symptoms and signs and liquid versus solid cyst content, infectious causes like abscesses (bacterial, amoebic) or tuberculoma must be considered.

In addition, benign and malignant liver tumours or metastases are relevant differentials.

The Case Continued…

On ERC, biliary obstruction because of a cystobiliary fistula was found. CE cyst content was removed from the common bile duct and the bile flow was restored. The patient's cholangitis was treated with ciprofloxacin and metronidazole. Once the inflammation settled, the patient was referred for surgery and partial cystectomy was performed on both cysts.

The patient has been followed up for 9 years after surgery and has had no recurrence. He is considered cured and further follow-up visits are not needed.

This case illustrates several learning points. In countries with low CE-endemicity provenance from a hyperendemic region is the single most important risk factor for CE in cystic liver lesions.

CE is generally a benign disease with the exception of complicated cysts; in this case a cyst with biliary fistula. CE cysts are currently classified by the WHO into six stages: CE1 and 2 (active), CE3a and 3b (transitional) and CE4 and 5 (inactive).

A very important question is which cysts can be left untreated and only observed ('watch and wait'). There is fairly solid evidence that inactive CE4 and CE5 cysts can be left untreated if they are not in critical sites.

In this patient the cyst walls of both cysts (CE1, CE3b) were calcified (Figs. 50.1 and 50.2). Previously, calcification was described only as a feature of CE5 cysts; this was later extended to CE4 cysts and has now been shown to occur in all cyst stages.

Retrospectively this case illustrates that surgical treatment was rightly offered to the patient at initial diagnosis.

Cystobiliary fistulas are some of the major reasons for complications in CE of the liver (as are cystobronchial fistulas in pulmonary CE). Fistulating cysts should be surgically treated before complications arise. The key question is how to identify fistulas early to prevent complications. Previously, endoscopic retrograde cholangiography (ERC) has been advocated as the method of choice. However, it has become evident that intracystic pressure may be too high for the contrast medium to enter. If available, MRI with magnetic resonance cholangiography (MRC) is an alternative option, with very good detection rates.

SUMMARY BOX

Cystic Echinococcosis

CE is an infection with the larval form of the dog tapeworm *Echinococcus granulosus*. It occurs worldwide with high endemicity in the Mediterranean basin, the Near and Middle East, North and East Africa, central Asia and Latin America.

Humans become infected by ingestion of eggs of *E. granulosus*.

Symptoms may occur months to years after infection because of mass effects of the growing cyst or because of complications. Liver (70%) and lung (15–30%) are the most commonly affected organs. Cyst complications include fistulas leading to biliary or bronchial obstruction, bacterial superinfection, cyst rupture leading to anaphylaxis, embolism of cyst content and compression syndromes.

Diagnosis of CE is based on imaging, mainly on ultrasound, which is crucial for the diagnosis and classification of disease activity. MRI or CT should be used when cysts are inaccessible by ultrasound.

Serology is hampered by a lack of sensitivity and specificity. In unclear cases, diagnostic cyst puncture and aspiration may be performed by experienced examiners. If CE is suspected, however, albendazole needs to be given peri-interventionally.

Generally, four treatment modalities are available: anthelmintic treatment, percutaneous sterilization techniques, surgery and a 'watch and wait' approach.

Management of CE patients in general depends not only on the individual case but also on local resources and expertise.

Long-term follow-up is important to detect recurrence of disease.

Further Reading

1. Stojkovic M, Gottstein B, Junghanss T. Echinococcosis. In: Farrar J, Hotez P, Junghanss T, Kang G, Lalloo D, White N, editors. Manson's Tropical Diseases. 23rd ed. London: Elsevier; 2013 [chapter 56].
2. Hosch W, Stojkovic M, Jänisch T, et al. The role of calcification for staging cystic echinococcosis (CE). Eur Radiol 2007;17:2538–45.
3. Stojkovic M, Zwahlen M, Teggi A, et al. Treatment response of cystic echinococcosis to benzimidazoles: a systematic review. PLoS Negl Trop Dis 2009;3(9):e524.
4. WHO Informal Working Group. International classification of ultrasound images in cystic echinococcosis for application in clinical and field epidemiological settings. Acta Trop 2003;85(2):253–61.
5. Stojkovic M, Rosenberger KD, Steudle F, et al. Watch and wait management of inactive cystic echinococcosis – does the path to inactivity matter – aalysis of a prospective patient cohort. PLoS Negl Trop Dis 2016;10(12):e0005243.

51

A 34-Year-Old HIV-Positive Woman from Malawi With Slowly Progressive Half-Sided Weakness

JURI KATCHANOV

Clinical Presentation

History

A 34-year-old Malawian woman presents to a neurology out-patient clinic in Malawi with slowly progressive weakness of the left arm and leg.

Her problems started approximately 3 months earlier when she first noticed a limp in her left leg. The weakness progressed, and over the following weeks she also realized that her left arm was becoming affected.

The patient is a poor historian and often has difficulty describing the onset and timing of sequential events, but from her story it appears likely that the problems started insidiously and have been slowly progressing since. She denies any head trauma, headache, recent episodes of fever, nausea, visual impairment or loss of weight. The review of systems is unremarkable.

The patient was diagnosed with smear-positive pulmonary tuberculosis 5 months earlier. At that time, she was also found to be HIV-reactive with a baseline CD4 count of 54/µL. She was started on antituberculous therapy, vitamin B_6, antiretroviral therapy and co-trimoxazole prophylaxis, all of which she is currently taking.

The patient works as a street vendor selling mobile phone vouchers. Despite her left-sided weakness she is still able to work sitting on a plastic chair and managing her vouchers and money with her right hand. She is divorced and does not have any children. She lives in an urban high-density area.

Clinical Findings

She is afebrile and her vital signs and general examination are normal apart from slightly pale conjunctivae. On fundoscopy her fundi are normal without any signs of papilloedema or retinitis.

The neurological examination reveals a spastic hemiparesis on the left with hyperreflexia. The power in the left leg is 2/5 (active movement with gravity eliminated) and in her left arm 3/5 (active movement against gravity). There is a pronator drift on the left (Fig. 51.1) indicating proximal weakness. Sensation of pain is reduced in her left leg and hand. The examination of her cranial nerves is normal.

Laboratory Results

Full blood count: WBC 3.8×10^9/L (reference range: 4–10), haemoglobin 9.9 g/dL (12–14), platelets 140×10^9/L (150–350).

Questions

1. What is your differential diagnosis?
2. What is your diagnostic approach in a resource-limited setting?

Discussion

A 34-year-old HIV-positive woman from Malawi presents with a 3-month history of progressive left-sided weakness of insidious onset. She was diagnosed with pulmonary

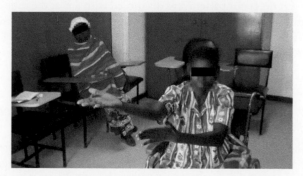

• **Fig. 51.1** Pronator drift on the left side as a sign of left upper limb weakness. The patient was asked to stretch out both arms and close her eyes.

tuberculosis (TB) and HIV 5 months before her presentation. She is on antiretroviral therapy (ART), co-trimoxazole prophylaxis and on antituberculous medication. On examination, there is a spastic hemiparesis on the left side with sensory involvement.

Answer to Question 1

What is Your Differential Diagnosis?

The combination of spastic hemiparesis with hyperreflexia and sensory impairment affecting one half of the body localizes the lesion to her brain. The onset appears subacute and the progression is slow. This makes ischaemic and haemorrhagic lesions ('strokes') unlikely causes because they present (hyper-)acutely and usually do not progress. Most likely the patient has one or several focal brain lesion(s).

The differential diagnosis of focal brain lesions (FBLs) in HIV-infected individuals in tropical countries is broad. Patients may suffer from HIV-related brain diseases such as cerebral toxoplasmosis, progressive multifocal leukoencephalopathy, CNS lymphoma, cryptococcoma and CMV encephalitis. *Mycobacterium tuberculosis* infection of the brain parenchyma can present as tuberculoma or tuberculous abscess.

Furthermore, HIV-positive individuals may suffer from conditions primarily unrelated to their HIV infection such as a brain tumour, brain metastases or a cerebral abscess.

Endemic 'tropical' diseases such as neurocysticercosis, neuroschistosomiasis or, in Latin America, Chagas' disease, can also present with focal brain lesions and should be considered according to the local epidemiological pattern.

In this particular case, the patient developed a focal brain lesion 2 months after starting ART. Central nervous system disorders are common after ART initiation. It is thought that the recovering immune system may 'unmask' or 'paradoxically deteriorate' pre-existing CNS infections. This phenomenon is called immune reconstitution inflammatory syndrome (IRIS) and, depending on the type, is termed 'unmasking' or 'paradoxical' IRIS.

Tuberculoma, progressive multifocal leukoencephalopathy (PML) and cryptococcoma have been well documented in the context of IRIS. Toxoplasmosis has been described after ART initiation, even in patients on co-trimoxazole prophylaxis.

Of note, our patient was diagnosed with TB at the time of ART initiation and CNS tuberculosis can deteriorate after ART introduction as well as after commencement of TB treatment.

Answer to Question 2

What is Your Diagnostic Approach in a Resource-Limited Setting?

The diagnostic work-up of FBLs in a resource-limited setting primarily depends on the availability of investigations. It often remains mainly clinical, guided by epidemiological evidence and by the degree of immunosuppression

in HIV-positive patients. Clinicians may often find themselves restricted to the pragmatic approach of 'treating the treatable'.

If the patient is HIV-positive, a CD4 count should be performed. Some FBLs are very unlikely if the CD4 count is above 200/μL, e.g. cryptococcoma or cerebral toxoplasmosis. Cerebral TB can occur at any CD4 count. PML mostly manifests in patients with advanced immunosuppression but has also been described in patients with higher CD4 counts.

Serum antitoxoplasma IgG and cryptococcal antigen (CrAG) are helpful, but may not be routinely available. Negative antitoxoplasma serology makes toxoplasmosis a very unlikely diagnosis, whereas a positive serological result documents past contact with the pathogen but fails to prove its relevance for the current illness.

Sensitivity of CSF examination in FBL is low, and both cryptococcoma and tuberculoma may present with a normal CSF. However, if XPert MTB/RIF or Ziehl-Neelsen stain, CrAg, India Ink or fungal cultures are available, these tests should be done and might help establish the diagnosis.

Chest radiography and abdominal ultrasound are useful because they may reveal tuberculous lesions, metastases or a primary neoplasm.

Cerebral imaging plays an important role in diagnosing FBLs; however, availability is extremely limited in resource-constrained settings. CT may at times produce non-specific results confirming the clinical diagnosis of an FBL but failing to assist the clinician in narrowing down the spectrum of differential diagnoses. MRI is more informative; however, it is practically unavailable as a routine investigation in tropical low- and middle-income settings. Cystic lesions on CT are indicative of neurocysticercosis. Cerebral oedema with mass effect and contrast enhancement would favour cerebral abscess, tuberculoma, toxoplasmosis and CNS lymphoma, whereas PML classically shows no mass effect and no enhancement. Meningeal enhancement is typical for tuberculosis.

The Case Continued...

Routine CSF examination was normal, India Ink stain and fungal cultures were negative. The patient was started on empirical antitoxoplasmosis treatment with high-dose co-trimoxazole. ART and antituberculous treatment were continued. Prednisolone 1 mg/kg bodyweight was added to cover for presumed IRIS. The patient was put on a waiting list for a cerebral MRI scan, which was available thanks to a local research project.

On 4-week follow-up her clinical status was unchanged. At 8 weeks there was further deterioration of power in her left hand. An MRI of her head was done which showed multifocal T2 hyperintense lesions exclusively affecting the white matter and more prominent in the right hemisphere (frontal and temporal lobes). Furthermore, there was a small area of demyelination in the left cerebellar peduncle. These radiological findings were deemed strongly suggestive of PML.

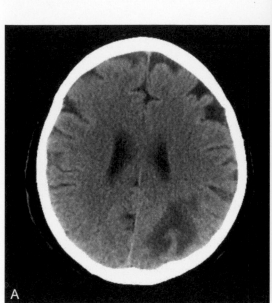
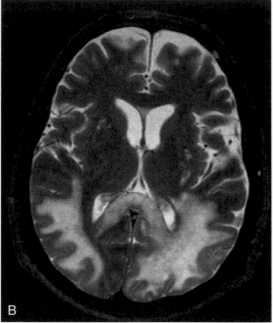

• **Fig. 51.2** (A) Cranial CT scan showing a hypodense lesion in the subcortical white matter in the left occipital lobe. (B) Cranial MRI showing bilateral T2 hyperintense (to grey matter) lesions in the subcortical white matter involving the so-called U-fibres resulting in a "scalloped appearance". (Courtesy Dr Eberhard Siebert, University Medical Center Charitè, Berlin, Germany)

A presumed diagnosis of PML was made. The patient was referred to a local rehabilitation centre for walking aids. The local palliative care team was involved.

<table>
<tr><td>SUMMARY BOX</td></tr>
</table>

Progressive Multifocal Leukoencephalopathy

PML is caused by a reactivation of the human JC polyomavirus. JC stands for 'John Cunningham', the first patient from whom the virus was isolated. JC polyomavirus is neurotropic, affecting oligodendrocytes.

PML always occurs as a result of virus reactivation because of immunosuppression. Primary infection usually takes place during childhood and the virus remains quiescent in the kidneys, bone marrow and lymphoid tissue. Upon reactivation, a productive infection of brain oligodendrocytes results in demyelination. The presenting symptoms include muscle weakness, sensory deficits, hemianopia, cognitive dysfunction, aphasia, and coordination and gait difficulties.

On imaging, multiple lesions are located in the subcortical white matter and cerebellar peduncles. The lesions look hypodense on CT (Fig. 51.2A), and hyperintense on T2-weighted MRI (Fig. 51.2B). There is no mass effect or contrast enhancement.

Besides its importance as an opportunistic infection in advanced HIV infection, PML in recent years has increasingly been described in other contexts of immunosuppression e.g. in transplant patients or patients treated with immune-modulatory drugs.

The only treatment showing benefit in PML patients with HIV is ART. Prognosis before introduction of ART was poor, and only 10% of PML patients survived for 1 year. However, in the ART era the 1-year survival rate has increased dramatically to 50%.

PML occurring within the first months of ART is often described as PML–immune reconstitution inflammatory syndrome (PML–IRIS). Of note, PML–IRIS possibly accounts for nearly 25% of all PML cases in HIV-positive patients. Steroids might have a beneficial effect in the management of PML–IRIS. However, in a setting with high prevalence of HIV-associated opportunistic infections and tuberculosis, it is probably advisable to apply steroids only if other common CNS infections are excluded or covered for.

Further Reading

1. Heckmann JE, Bhigjee AI. Tropical neurology. In: Farrar J, editor. Manson's Tropical Diseases. 23rd ed. London: Elsevier; 2013 [chapter 71].
2. Asselman V, Thienemann F, Pepper DJ, et al. Central nervous system disorders after starting antiretroviral therapy in South Africa. AIDS 2010;24(18):2871–6.
3. Grebenciucova E, Berger JR. Progressive multifocal leukoencephalopathy. Neurol Clin 2018;36(4):739–50.
4. Modi M, Mochan A, Modi G. Management of HIV-associated focal brain lesions in developing countries. QJM 2004;97 (7):413–21.

52

A 56-Year-Old Man from Peru With Prolonged Fever and Severe Anaemia

CIRO MAGUIÑA, CARLOS SEAS AND FREDERIQUE JACQUERIOZ

Clinical Presentation

History

A 56-year-old male Peruvian is admitted to a hospital in the capital, Lima, with a 2-week history of fever, jaundice and confusion.

Daily fever started 3 months after leaving a rural area in the highlands of northern Peru (altitude of 2400 m), where the patient spent 3 weeks on vacation. In the second week of illness the patient noticed dark urine and jaundice, and few days before admission his wife noticed confusion and somnolence. While in the rural area, the patient and his wife were bitten at night by tiny mosquitoes; no personal protection was used. Otherwise there has been no animal contact. The past medical history is unremarkable.

Clinical Findings

His blood pressure is 90/60 mmHg, pulse 110 bpm and regular, temperature 39.2°C (102.6°F), respiratory rate 22 breaths per minute. The patient appears confused and disorientated without any focal neurological findings or meningeal signs (GCS 14/15). Skin and conjunctivae are markedly pale and there is scleral jaundice. Cardiovascular and pulmonary examination are normal. The liver is slightly enlarged but there is no splenomegaly.

Laboratory Results

Creatinine, electrolytes and alkaline phosphatase are normal. His additional routine laboratory results are shown in Table 52.1. Coomb's test is negative. The CSF results are normal.

Further Investigations

A CT scan of the brain is normal. Abdominal ultrasound reveals hepatomegaly, but no focal lesions.

Questions

1. What are your differential diagnoses?
2. How would you approach this patient?

Discussion

A Peruvian man presents with a history of prolonged fever, altered neurological status and evidence of haemolysis after a stay in a rural area in the highlands of Peru.

Answer to Question 1
What Are Your Differential Diagnoses?

The most important differential diagnoses in this patient are malaria and bartonellosis.

Plasmodium vivax is the only species of *Plasmodium* prevalent in the highland regions of Peru. Interestingly, the patient presents with several features of severe and complicated malaria, including severe anaemia, jaundice and impaired consciousness. However, *P. vivax* is not

TABLE 52.1	Blood Results on Admission	
Parameter	Patient	Reference Range
WBC (× 10⁹/L)	14.9	4–10
Neutrophils (× 10⁹/L)	13.1	1.8–7.2
Lymphocytes (× 10⁹/L)	0.9	1.5–4
Band forms (%)	4	0–5
Haemoglobin (g/dL)	6	13–15
Reticulocytes (%)	8	0.5–1.5
Platelets (× 10⁹/L)	454	150–350
LDH (U/L)	1500	<250
Total bilirubin (µmol/L)	239	<19
Direct bilirubin (µmol/L)	103	<5

commonly associated with severe malaria. Bartonellosis is another important diagnosis to consider given the recent travel history in the highlands of Peru, where sandflies, the vectors of bartonellosis, are present. The patient also reported being bitten by tiny mosquitoes. Less common infections to include in the differential diagnosis are rickettsial diseases (both endemic and epidemic typhus are present in Peru), leptospirosis, typhoid fever, brucellosis and several viral diseases, including viral hepatitis and yellow fever. However, none of them produces significant haemolysis and some are not endemic in the highlands (yellow fever for instance). Non-infectious causes of haemolysis should also be considered.

Answer to Question 2

How Would You Approach This Patient?

The first step is to rule out malaria by performing a thick and thin smear or by using rapid diagnostic tests. Based on the exposure history and the high suspicion of bartonellosis, a thin film should be performed to calculate the differential leukocyte count and to look for the presence of *Bartonella bacilliformis* in red blood cells.

The Case Continued...

The patient progressed to shock. He was transferred to the intensive care unit (ICU) and required treatment with vasopressors. Blood films were negative for malaria. However, the thin film revealed massive red blood cell infestation by pleomorphic cocco-bacillary structures compatible with *B. bacilliformis* (Fig. 52.1). Blood cultures were negative, including cultures in special media for *Bartonella*. The patient was started on a combination of intravenous ciprofloxacin and ceftriaxone for 10 days. Altered mental status resolved after 3 days of antimicrobial treatment and fever subsided after 5 days. By day 4 the bacteria had disappeared from the blood smears. No further complications were observed during a 3-month follow-up period.

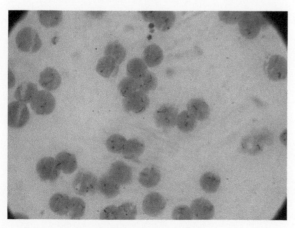

• **Fig. 52.1** Thin smear showing massive infestation of red blood cells with cocco-bacillary structures (Wright stain).

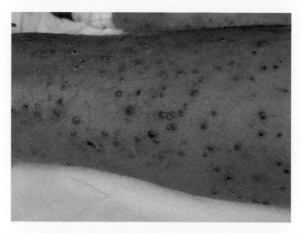

• **Fig. 52.2** Multiple erythematous-violaceous papules of different sizes characteristic of the chronic phase (verruga peruana).

SUMMARY BOX

Bartonellosis – Oroya Fever and Verruga Peruana

Bartonellosis, caused by *B. bacilliformis,* is a vector-borne disease mainly found in the Andean valleys of Peru at an altitude between 500 and 3200 metres, although transmission may occur at higher altitudes and in jungle areas as well. Colombia and Ecuador have also reported sporadic cases. The disease is transmitted by female sandflies, mostly *Lutzomyia verrucarum* or *L. peruensis,* which characteristically bite indoors at nighttime. Human beings are the only known reservoir. Non-vectorial *B. bacilliformis* transmission from mother to child or through blood transfusions has been described but remains scarce. Most infections are asymptomatic or oligosymptomatic. However, a minority of patients progress to severe disease ('Oroya fever') after a mean incubation period of 3 to 8 weeks (longer incubation periods up to 9 months have been observed). Oroya fever is characterized by high fever, malaise, myalgias and severe haemolytic anaemia with jaundice. Complications during this acute phase include heart failure, as well as pericardial and pleural effusions. CNS involvement, characterized by impaired consciousness, agitation and coma, occurs in approximately 20% of patients and is associated with higher case fatality rates. Secondary immunosuppression may occur during this phase and patients may present with opportunistic infections similar to those seen in advanced HIV-infection, e.g. salmonellosis, toxoplasmosis or *Pneumocystis jirovecii* pneumonia.

After acute Oroya fever, within 1 to 2 months a chronic angioproliferative cutaneous stage ('verruga peruana') may occur in approximately 5% of treated patients and in an unknown percentage of untreated individuals. Occasionally, verruga peruana is seen without noticeable acute-phase manifestations. It is mostly seen in children in endemic areas. Skin lesions are usually small (1–4 mm), red-violaceous, painless papules located on the face or the extremities, and can be single or multiple (Fig. 52.2). Nodular lesions can also be observed. The lesions resemble bacillary angiomatosis caused by *B. quintana* and *B. henselae.*

In the acute phase, diagnosis is made by proof of cocco-bacilli inside red blood cells. *B. bacilliformis* is a fastidious bacterium, and culture requires a specific medium incubated at 25 to 28°C for up to 2 weeks.

Recommended treatment of the acute phase includes ciprofloxacin alone or combined with ceftriaxone in severe cases. These antimicrobials also cover for *Salmonella* species, the commonest opportunistic infection observed in these patients. Increased antibiotic resistance of both *B. bacilliformis* and concomitant opportunistic pathogens has been observed and should be sought in the absence of a clinical response. Oral azithromycin is the drug of choice for verruga peruana. Alternatively, ciprofloxacin can be used.

Note: Oroya fever is also named Carrion's disease after a famous Peruvian medical student, Daniel Carrion, who in 1885 inoculated himself with fluid obtained of a wart from a patient with verruga peruana and developed acute bartonellosis (Oroya fever). He unfortunately died from the disease. However, his experiment demonstrated clearly that verruga peruana and Oroya fever were different clinical forms of the same infection.

Further Reading

1. Angelakis E, Raoult D. Bartonellosis, cat-scratch disease, trench fever, human Ehrlichiosis. In: Farrar J, editor. Manson's Tropical Diseases. 23rd ed. London: Elsevier; 2013 [chapter 30].
2. Gomes C, Ruiz J. Carrion's disease: the sound of silence. Clin Microbiol Rev 2017;31(1). e00056-17.
3. Maguina C, Garcia PJ, Gotuzzo E, et al. Bartonellosis (Carrion's disease) in the modern era. Clin Infect Dis 2001;33(6):772–9.

53

A 24-Year-Old Woman from Uganda With Fever and Shock

BENJAMIN JEFFS

Clinical Presentation

History

A 24-year-old woman presents to a small hospital in rural Uganda because of a 5-day history of a febrile illness. Apart from fever, the illness started with a sore throat and aching all over. She also developed some abdominal pain and diarrhoea. The patient has become increasingly unwell over the course of the past days. She is very weak and needs help to stand.

Her husband died of a severe febrile illness 6 days before she became ill. He had worked in a local gold mine and had previously been in good health. He had fallen ill about a week before his death. His wife had looked after him during his final illness and he had died at home.

Clinical Findings

The patient looks very unwell. Her blood pressure is 85/65 mmHg, pulse rate 105 bpm, temperature 38°C (100.4°F). She has bilateral conjunctivitis. There is no rash and no lymphadenopathy. The heart sounds are normal and her chest is clear. Her abdominal examination is normal.

Questions

1. What are your differential diagnoses?
2. How would you approach the patient and what tests would you do?

Discussion

A young Ugandan woman presents to a rural hospital with a severe febrile illness. She is hypotensive and has bilateral conjunctivitis. Her husband has recently died after a short febrile illness.

Answer to Question 1
What Are Your Differential Diagnoses?

The presentation is non-specific and a wide range of acute infectious diseases are possible.

Both malaria and typhoid fever present with non-specific symptoms and a septic picture, but neither would cause conjunctivitis. Other causes of bacterial sepsis, including invasive meningococcal disease have to be considered.

A severe viral infection with an adenovirus or influenza would be possible but the patient appears slightly too unwell for this. Measles commonly presents with pronounced conjunctivitis, but at this stage one would see a rash. Zika virus was discovered in Uganda and presents with conjunctivitis, but usually is a mild viral illness and does not cause shock.

The fact that the patient's husband has recently died of a similar severe febrile illness should raise the suspicion of a viral haemorrhagic fever (VHF). Marburg virus disease (MVD) has been associated with mines.

Answer to Question 2
How Would You Approach the Patient and What Tests Would You Do?

The patient should be treated with extreme caution because of the possibility of a viral haemorrhagic fever. Nosocomial spread of these diseases can cause hospital outbreaks with a high case fatality rate. The patient should ideally be isolated in a side room. Blood tests should be kept to a minimum to reduce the risk to laboratory staff. Protective clothing, such as gloves and a surgical gown, are recommended during procedures. The risk of transmission of VHF viruses from a malaria slide is very low once the blood spot is dry; therefore it would be reasonable to do a malaria slide or a rapid diagnostic test. However, the prevalence of *Plasmodium falciparum* parasitaemia in Uganda is high and a positive slide would not rule out VHF.

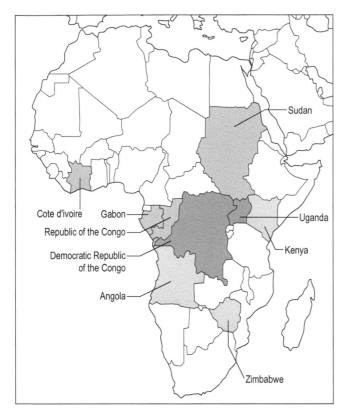

• **Fig. 53.1** Endemic areas for filoviruses. Only filoviruses known to cause haemorrhagic fever are shown. Countries where Ebola and Marburg haemorrhagic fevers have been seen are indicated in green and blue, respectively, with countries in red indicating documentation of both diseases. Incidence and risk of disease may vary significantly within each country. Filoviruses are likely to occur outside these countries but have not yet been recognised. (Reproduced from Farrar, J., Hotez, P., Junghanss, T., et al., 2013. Manson's Tropical Diseases. Farrar, J., Ed. London: Elsevier. Fig. 16.1.)

To protect laboratory staff all biochemical and haematological tests should be done using near-patient testing if possible.

The public health authorities should be alerted to the possibility of a case of viral haemorrhagic fever. Ideally testing for this should be organized, but samples are likely to need special shipping arrangements to be taken to a specialized laboratory.

The Case Continued...

A presumed diagnosis of Marburg virus disease was made. The malaria slide showed a low level of parasitaemia with *P. falciparum*. A sample for Marburg and Ebola PCR was sent in a sealed plastic container. The patient was isolated in a side room and all patient contact was carried out while wearing gloves. She was treated with IV artesunate and then artemether/lumefantrine. She was given empirical IV ceftriaxone to cover for possible sepsis and was resuscitated with IV fluids.

Over the next few days the patient remained very unwell, then she started to improve. Once she had recovered, she was kept in isolation for an additional 2 days and was then allowed to return home. The day after her discharge a

positive Marburg virus PCR result came back. Had this been known while she was in the hospital, stricter infection control procedures, including double gloves, a mask, goggles and a disposable (waterproof) surgical gown, would have been appropriate.

Her family members, close friends and medical staff were interviewed; anyone who had had physical contact with her, or her body fluids, was told to monitor their temperature for 21 days from the time of contact which is the maximum incubation period for MHF. Anyone who developed a fever or became unwell during this period was isolated.

SUMMARY BOX

Filoviral Diseases

Marburg virus disease (MVD) and Ebola virus disease (EVD) are both caused by filoviruses. They are clinically virtually indistinguishable and cause severe illnesses with a high case fatality rate. Symptoms are non-specific, and patients may present with fever, sore throat, general body ache, retrosternal chest pain and abdominal symptoms. Conjunctivitis is common. The most frequent cause of death is shock. Less than half of those who die develop haemorrhages because of disseminated intravascular coagulation.

Because symptoms are non-specific and testing is difficult in most of Africa, filoviral haemorrhagic fevers (FHF) are normally recognized only if a cluster of cases occurs. In particular, an outbreak in an endemic area in which health workers die should raise the suspicion towards FHF.

EVD and MVD have both been detected over wide areas of sub-Saharan Africa. Both are zoonoses of bats. Many cases of MHF have been linked to entering or working in caves or mines, whereas cases of EHF are associated with butchering and eating apes or monkeys.

Filoviruses can spread between people through direct physical contact or contact with infected body fluids. Large nosocomial outbreaks involving the death of large numbers of medical staff have been recorded. Therefore strict infection control measures should be followed while caring for anyone with a suspected viral haemorrhagic fever. Vaccines against MVD are under development but have not yet been tested on humans.

The preferred method of testing for MVD is with PCR, antigen detection tests are less sensitive and specific. The treatment of MVD is supportive. Treatments which have shown promise in EVD, such as antibody therapies e.g. ZMAPP or the antiviral drug favipiravir, have not been clinically tested in humans with MVD.

Further Reading

1. Blumberg L, Enria D, Bausch DG. Viral Haemorrhagic Fevers. In: Farrar J, editor. Manson's Tropical Diseases. 23rd ed. London: Elsevier; 2013 [chapter 16].

2. Emanuel J, Marzi A, Feldmann H. Filoviruses: Ecology, Molecular Biology, and Evolution. Adv Virus Res 2018;100:189–221 [chapter 9].

3. Bauer MP, Timen A, Vossen ACTM, et al. Marburg haemorrhagic fever in returning travellers: an overview aimed at clinicians. Clin Microbiol Infect 2019;21:e28–e31.

4. World Health Organization. Clinical management of patients with viral haemorrhagic fever, a pocket guide for front-line health workers, ISBN 978 92 4 154960 8 (NLM classification: WC 534). http://apps.who.int/medicinedocs/documents/s22501en/s22501en.pdf.

54

A 52-Year-Old Male Safari Tourist Returning from South Africa With Fever and a Skin Lesion

CAMILLA ROTHE

Clinical Presentation

History

A 52-year-old man presents to a tropical medicine clinic in Germany with a fever for the past 2 days. He is also complaining of night sweats and a frontal headache. There are no joint pains and he has not noticed a rash.

Ten days ago, he returned from a 2-week holiday trip to South Africa. He visited Cape Town and travelled the Garden Route and through KwaZulu–Natal. He went on safari in Kruger Park and several other game reserves. He did not take any antimalarial chemoprophylaxis. His past medical history is unremarkable.

Clinical Findings

Fair general condition. Tympanic temperature 37.5°C (99.5°F) (after taking 1g of paracetamol), pulse 80 bpm, blood pressure 130/70 mmHg.

No jaundice; neck supple. Enlarged lymph nodes in the left groin. You notice a small sticking plaster on the left upper thigh of the patient. He tells you that he has noted a skin lesion that he meant to show to a friend, who happens to be a surgeon, for advice. You ask the patient to take off the plaster (see Fig. 54.1).

Questions

1. What is the diagnosis?
2. How would you manage this patient?

Discussion

A 52-year-old German man presents with a short history of fever after a trip to South Africa. On examination there is a small necrotic skin lesion on his upper thigh with adjoining lymphangiitis and lymphadenitis.

Answer to Question 1
What is the Diagnosis?

The skin lesion is a typical eschar. Given the travel history, the clinical diagnosis is most likely African tick-bite fever. This rickettsial disease is a common cause of fever in safari tourists returning from Southern Africa.

Answer to Question 2
How Would You Manage This Patient?

The patient has travelled to KwaZulu–Natal, which is a malaria-endemic region, and he has not taken any antimalarial chemoprophylaxis. In any febrile traveller returning from a malaria-endemic region, malaria has to be ruled out, even if other diagnoses seem obvious.

The diagnosis of African tick-bite fever is primarily clinical.

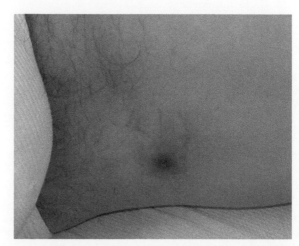

• **Fig. 54.1** Small necrotic skin lesion (about 0.7 cm in diameter) with surrounding inflammation and lymphangiitis on the left upper thigh of the patient.

TABLE 54.1 Overview of Rickettsial Infections and their Vectors

	Tick-borne	Mite-borne	Louse-borne	Flea-borne
Synonyms	Spotted fevers	Scrub typhus, Tsutsugamushi fever, Japanese river fever	Epidemic typhus	Murine typhus, Endemic typhus, Shop typhus
Classification	Spotted Fever (SF) Group	Scrub typhus Group	Typhus Group	Typhus Group
Pathogens	Many, e.g. *R. africae* (African tick bite fever) *R. conorii* (Mediterranean SF) *R. rickettsii* (Rocky mountain SF) *R. australis* (Queensland tick typhus)	*Orientia tsutsugamushi* *O. sp. nov. chuto* (UAE)	*R. prowazekii*	*R. typhi*
Vector	Ticks	Trombiculid mites (chigger mites, jungle mites)	*Pediculus humanus corporis* (human body lice)	*Xenopsylla cheopis* (rat flea)
Reservoir	Mammals Rodents Marsupials....	Mites (transovarian) Rodents	Humans	Rodents

A PCR from the eschar scab may confirm the diagnosis. For confirmative serology, paired samples would have to be taken and may be more of academic value in this case. African tick-bite fever is usually a mild, self-limiting disease. Doxycycline can be given to speed up recovery.

The Case Continued...

The malaria rapid diagnostic test, as well as thick and thin film for malaria, came back negative. The patient was prescribed doxycycline at 100 mg bid PO for 1 week. The fever settled within the next few days and the lymphadenopathy subsided. The eschar eventually healed after about 2 weeks.

SUMMARY BOX

African Tick-Bite Fever

African tick-bite fever (ATBF) is the second most common specific cause of fever after malaria in travellers returning from sub-Saharan Africa.

It belongs to the spotted fever group of rickettsioses, a large group of infections, which are mainly transmitted by ticks. An overview of rickettsial infections and their vectors is given in Table 54.1.

ATBF is caused by *Rickettsia africae* and transmitted by cattle ticks of the genus *Amblyomma,* which act both as reservoir and as vector.

Other reservoir hosts are wild and domestic animals, such as cattle, buffalos, rhinos, and hippos. ATBF is endemic in most of rural sub-Saharan Africa and in the West Indies.

ATBF commonly occurs in game hunters, safari tourists, cross-country runners and campers in veld areas or grasslands. ATBF is one of the most common causes of febrile presentations in international travellers to sub-Saharan Africa, and it is the most common rickettsial infection encountered in travel medicine. In contrast, fairly little is known about incidence and risk factors of ATBF in local indigenous populations.

The incubation period following the bite of an infected tick is about 6 to 10 days. Patients develop fever and flu-like symptoms such as myalgias and headache. There may be a characteristic inoculation eschar at the site of the bite with local lymphadenopathy. It may however take some time for the pathognomonic eschar to demarcate and early lesions may be non-specific erythematous papules, resembling mosquito bites. Multiple inoculation eschars are not uncommon, because *Amblyomma* ticks are known to aggressively attack their hosts.

Despite the fact that African tick-bite fever belongs to the group of 'spotted fevers', a rash is seen in less than half of cases. ATBF is usually a mild illness and no deaths have been reported so far.

However, neurological involvement has been described in ATBF, including encephalopathy and peripheral neuropathy. Also, retinitis and panuveitis have been described.

Diagnosis of ATBF is usually made clinically, but in febrile individuals living in or returning from tropical areas malaria should still be ruled out.

PCR from the eschar scab or even a skin swab is a non-invasive and sensitive way to confirm the diagnosis of acute infection. Serodiagnosis remains the gold standard for spotted-fever group rickettsial infections using seroconversion and fourfold antibody titre increases. Its use in clinical decision-making is however limited because of poor sensitivity during acute infection (antibodies are often not detectable within the first 10–14 days), the indirect nature of diagnostic evidence and cross-reaction with other *Rickettsiae.* The immunofluorescence assay (IFA) is currently considered the gold standard serological test

Treatment may not be necessary in mild cases. Doxycycline 100 mg bid PO may be given for 3 to 7 days. In pregnant women and in children younger than 8 years of age, macrolides are an alternative.

Preventive measures include appropriate clothing, which should be impregnated with pyrethroids, and topical insect repellents applied to the skin. Whether tetracyclines can be used as chemoprophylaxis against ATBF is still a matter of dispute.

Further Reading

1. Paris DH, Day NPJ. Tropical rickettsial infections. In: Farrar J, editor. Manson's Tropical Diseases. 23rd ed. London: Elsevier; 2013 [chapter 22].
2. Elden C, Parole P. Update on tick-borne bacterial diseases in travelers. Curr Inf Dis Rep 2018;20(17):1–9.
3. Jensenii M, Fournier PE, Raoult D. Rickettsioses and the international traveler. Clin Infect Dis 2004;39(10):1493–9.
4. Parole P, Paddock CD, Sokolowski C, et al. Update on tick-borne Rickettsioses around the world: a geographic approach. Clin Microbiol Rev 2013;26(4):657–702.
5. Paris DH, Dumper JD. State of the art of diagnosis of rickettsial diseases. Curr Opin Infect Dis 2016;29:433–9.

55

A 40-Year-Old Male Farmer from Peru With Chronic Cough and Weight Loss

FREDERIQUE JACQUERIOZ AND CARLOS SEAS

Clinical Presentation

History

A 40-year-old farmer from the Peruvian Amazon is referred to a hospital in the capital, Lima, with a 4-month history of chronic productive cough and chest pain. The patient reports dyspnoea on exertion and weight loss of about 20 kg. He denies diarrhoea, fever or night sweats.

Three and half months earlier, the patient was hospitalized at a regional hospital in the Peruvian Amazon for similar complaints. During the hospitalization, three sputum smears for acid-fast bacilli (AFB) were reported negative. No tuberculin skin test was performed. The chest radiograph was described as abnormal but no report is available and the patient does not have the film. A diagnosis of pulmonary tuberculosis (TB) was made based on clinical presentation and abnormal chest radiographic findings. The patient received first line TB therapy consisting of isoniazid, rifampicin, pyrazinamide and ethambutol.

In the following months, despite adherence to treatment, he showed no clinical improvement and reported persistence of productive cough with streaking of blood in the sputum. He was then referred to Lima with a suspected diagnosis of multi-drug resistant TB (MDR TB) for further work-up.

The patient had been found to be HTLV-1-positive 10 years previously. A recent HIV ELISA test was negative. The patient denies recent travels.

Clinical Findings

A 40-year-old man appears fatigued and cachectic. Temperature 37.2°C (98.96°F), blood pressure 120/75 mmHg, pulse 70 bpm regular, respiratory rate 15 breaths per minute. On inspection, few cervical and retroauricular lymph nodes are palpable, which are small, mobile, soft and non-tender. Lungs: crackles and rhonchi bilaterally. No hepatosplenomegaly. The rest of the physical examination is normal.

Laboratory Results

Platelets: 1093×10^9/L (reference range: 150–450); the rest of the full blood count is within normal limits.

Questions

1. What are your differential diagnoses?
2. How would you approach this patient?

Discussion

A male farmer from the Peruvian Amazon presents with a history of chronic cough and weight loss. After 3 months of TB treatment for a presumptive diagnosis of pulmonary tuberculosis, he shows no clinical improvement. The patient is cachectic with cervical lymphadenopathy and abnormal pulmonary auscultation. Laboratory investigations show thrombocytosis.

Answer to Question 1
What Are Your Differential Diagnoses?

The most important differential diagnoses in the given setting are MDR TB, histoplasmosis and paracoccidioidomycosis. TB is highly endemic in Peru and MDR TB is an increasing issue. TB and MDR TB almost always need to be considered when clinical symptoms and evolution, as in this case, are suggestive of the disease. What would be unusual about this patient is his origin from a rural area in the central Peruvian Amazon where MDR TB is still uncommon in comparison with underprivileged districts of Lima and other big cities of Peru.

Histoplasmosis can present with recurrent or progressive pulmonary symptoms that can mimic TB. However, his presentation would suggest a chronic form that is more often seen in individuals with preexisting chronic obstructive pulmonary disease, which this patient does not have. The patient's age, gender, occupation, origin and clinical symptoms with a pulmonary focus are all typical of the chronic form of paracoccidioidomycosis and make this diagnosis the most likely of the three. Co-infection of TB (non-MDR)

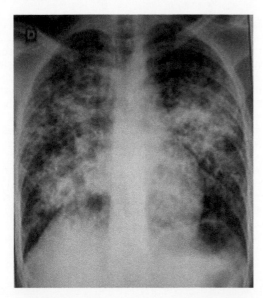

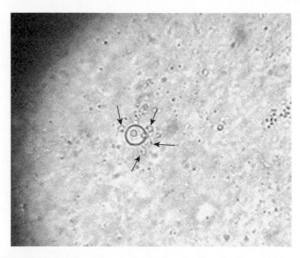

• **Fig. 55.2** Large budding yeast (range: 8–40 μm) with multiple surrounding smaller buds around (arrows) seen on KOH preparation of the patient's sputum.

• **Fig. 55.1** Chest radiograph showing bilateral confluent reticulonodular infiltrates predominantly in the central and upper zones of both lungs. Cavities are seen in the right lung. There is no hilar lymphadenopathy.

and paracoccidioidomycosis are not uncommon and should also be kept in mind as a possible differential. Parasitic infections such as paragonimiasis or pulmonary hydatid cyst are also possible diagnoses, though less common. Imaging (chest radiography and CT scan) will help identifying the typical lesions of these infections.

Answer to Question 2

How Would You Approach this Patient?

The first step in this patient is to evaluate him for MDR TB. Initial investigations should include chest radiography (the patient should also be asked to bring the initial chest x-ray and report for comparison), tuberculin skin test (PPD) and repeated AFB sputum smears and sputum-PCR (Xpert

MTB/RIF) for *M. tuberculosis*. Mycobacterial culture should complete the evaluation and, if positive, culture-based drug sensitivity testing should be added. Locally endemic fungal infections (e.g. histoplasmosis and paracoccidioidomycosis) should be evaluated by direct examination of sputum with wet mount potassium hydroxide (KOH) preparation and cultures. Depending on chest radiographic findings, local availability and costs, a CT scan of the chest could be considered as well as bronchoscopy with biopsy if less invasive diagnostic evaluation is unrevealing. The thrombocytosis should be confirmed on a smear.

The Case Continued...

The tuberculin skin test was negative as were two AFB smears. The chest x-ray showed bilateral confluent reticulonodular infiltrates and multiple cavities in the right lung (Fig. 55.1).

TABLE 55.1	Differences Between the Main Clinical Forms of Paracoccidioidomycosis	
Paracoccidioidomycosis	**Chronic (Adult) Form**	**Acute (Juvenile) Form**
Epidemiology	>90% of cases	<10% of cases
Infected Population	Men >30 years old (male:female ratio 14:1)	Children and young adults, both sexes HIV patients (rare)
Clinical Characteristics	Chronic Slow progression Reactivation years after initial exposure Lung (always) Dissemination to liver and lymph nodes can occur Mucocutaneous lesions (~70%) (face, nasal and oral cavity)	Acute or sub-acute Rapidly progressive Develops after recent exposure Systemic disease of reticuloendothelial system with dissemination from lung to liver, spleen, lymph nodes and bone marrow Mucosal lesions (rarely) *HIV patients: similar plus cutaneous lesions and severe pulmonary involvement*
Differential Diagnoses	Mimics other chronic fungal infections and pulmonary TB	Mimics leukaemia, lymphoma, severe disseminated TB
Treatment	Azoles (itraconazole) Co-trimoxazole	Azoles (itraconazole) Amphotericin B (HIV or severe disease)

Examination of his sputum (KOH preparation) revealed the characteristic yeast forms of *Paracoccidioides brasiliensis* (Fig. 55.2). Culture grew *P. brasiliensis.*

A diagnosis of chronic (adult) paracoccidioidomycosis was made. The thrombocytosis was considered reactive to the underlying chronic infection. Given the extensive pulmonary lesions and HTLV-1 co-infection, the patient was started on amphotericin B followed by itraconazole (as opposed to itraconazole alone). TB treatment was discontinued.

Our patient was HTLV-1 positive. His symptoms were confined to the lungs as in the chronic adult form of paracoccidioidomycosis (see Summary Box), but his pulmonary lesions were unusually extensive. His long-term prognosis depends on the extent of pulmonary fibrotic sequelae.

SUMMARY BOX

Paracoccidioidomycosis

Paracoccidioidomycosis is a systemic fungal infection endemic only to the moist tropical regions of Latin America. The infection is caused by the thermally dimorphic fungus *Paracoccidioides brasiliensis,* which grows as mould in the environment and as yeast in tissue and at 37°C. Humans are infected through the inhalation of aerosolized conidia (spores) from the soil. In endemic areas, initial exposure occurs in childhood and the majority of primary infections remain asymptomatic or subclinical. In those who develop disease, two main clinical forms are observed (Table 55.1). The chronic adult form is characterized by pulmonary symptoms that slowly develop over months, typically in middle-aged men living in rural endemic areas, which are often accompanied by mucosal lesions. Women of fertile age are rarely affected, probably because of a protective effect of oestradiol preventing the transformation of the fungus into the yeast stage. The acute juvenile form is seen in children and young adults of both sexes and presents as an acute systemic disease of the reticuloendothelial system. Adult patients with advanced HIV infection present a more aggressive acute disease similar to the juvenile acute form with extensive pulmonary involvement.

Diagnosis is confirmed by visualization of *P. brasiliensis* (yeast form) on wet preparation of specimen and/or isolation in fungal culture. The identification of *P. brasiliensis* is more difficult in sputum than in skin lesions or material from lymph nodes. The yeast is easily observed on KOH preparation but its isolation in culture is difficult and takes 20 to 30 days. Serological testing is useful for antibody detection and diagnosis, assessing disease severity and monitoring treatment response. Molecular methods could be used instead of culture to confirm the diagnosis but are not widely available in resource-limited endemic areas.

Treatment includes azoles for mild and moderate cases. Itraconazole (200 mg/day for 12 months) is considered the drug of choice. Voriconazole and co-trimoxazole are alternatives; the latter is commonly used in Brazil. Amphotericin B (cumulative dose of 1–2 g) is indicated for severe and extensive disease. However, the drug is not curative and should be followed by an azole or co-trimoxazole to complete 12 months' treatment.

Cure is determined based upon four criteria: clinical (i.e. absence of symptoms), mycological (i.e. negative testing), radiological (i.e. stability of lung lesions on x-ray for 1 year) and immunological (i.e. decrease of specific antibodies).

Recently case reports of severe and unusual extrapulmonary manifestations of paracoccidioidomycosis have been described in HTLV-1 infected patients and the two conditions might be associated.

Further Reading

1. Hay RJ. Fungal infections. In: Farrar J, editor. Manson's Tropical Diseases. 23rd ed. London: Elsevier; 2013 [chapter 38].
2. Morejon KM, Machado AA, Martinez R. Paracoccidioidomycosis in patients infected with and not infected with human immunodeficiency virus: a case-control study. Am J Trop Med Hyg 2009; 80(3):359–66.
3. León M, Alave J, Bustamante B, et al. Human T lymphotropic virus 1 and paracoccidioidomycosis: a probable association in Latin America. Clin Infect Dis 2010;51(2):250–1.
4. Mendes RP, Cavalcante RS, Marques SA, et al. Paracoccidioidomycosis: Current Perspectives from Brazil. Open Microbiol J 2017;11: 224–82.
5. Quieroz-Tellez F, Fahal AH, Falci DR, et al. Neglected Endemic Mycoses. Lancet Infect Dis 2017;17:e367–77.

56

A 21-Year-Old Pregnant Woman from The Gambia With a Rash

DAVID C.W. MABEY

Clinical Presentation

History

A 21-year-old woman comes to your clinic in The Gambia complaining of a generalized, non-itchy rash that she has had for 5 days. She is otherwise well and has no significant past medical history. She is 32 weeks pregnant. This is her first pregnancy.

Clinical Findings

She has a generalized rash (Fig. 56.1). Her mouth is normal, and there is no lymphadenopathy. She is not anaemic or jaundiced, and general examination is unremarkable.

Questions

1. What is the most likely diagnosis, and how might this affect the outcome of her pregnancy?
2. How would you manage the patient?

Discussion

A 21-year-old pregnant Gambian woman presents because of a generalized macular rash involving the palms of both hands. The rash is non-itchy and she is otherwise fine.

Answer to Question 1

What is the Most Likely Diagnosis, and How Might This Affect the Outcome of Her Pregnancy?

A generalized, non-itchy rash affecting the palms of the hands is syphilis until proven otherwise. Syphilis in pregnancy has a serious influence on pregnancy outcome. A study in Tanzania showed that, among women with latent syphilis and a rapid plasma reagin (RPR) titre of ≥1:8, 25% delivered a stillborn baby, and 33% a low-birth-weight baby.

The baby may be born with signs of congenital syphilis, including a generalized bullous rash, jaundice and hepatosplenomegaly. In this case the prognosis is bad, with a 50%

case fatality rate even with treatment. Alternatively, the baby may appear normal at birth, and present at the age of 3 to 4 months with failure to thrive and signs of congenital syphilis, usually including a generalized rash which affects the palms of the hands and soles of the feet (Fig. 56.2). Other common signs include hepatosplenomegaly, painful periostitis involving the long bones, and a persistent nasal discharge, which may be bloodstained (the 'syphilitic snuffles').

Answer to Question 2

How Would You Manage the Patient?

Intramuscular benzathine penicillin is the treatment of choice for syphilis. A single dose of 2.4 million units i.m. is recommended for primary, secondary and early latent syphilis (of less than two years' duration). A single dose, given before 28 weeks' gestation, has been shown to prevent adverse outcomes resulting from syphilis. Because this patient has not been treated before 28 weeks, her infant should receive a course of treatment for congenital syphilis (IM procaine penicillin 50 000 units/kg daily for 10–14 days)

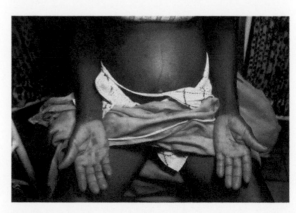

• **Fig. 56.1** Generalized, non-itchy macular rash in a pregnant Gambian woman.

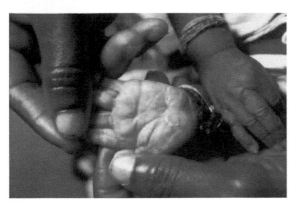

• **Fig. 56.2** Congenital syphilis in a 3-month-old infant: desquamating lesion of the palms.

The Case Continued...

The patient was treated with a single IM dose of benzathine penicillin and she made an uneventful recovery. She delivered a normal infant at term.

SUMMARY BOX

Syphilis in Pregnancy

Primary syphilis causes an ulcer or chancre, at the site of inoculation, which is usually painless. Women are often unaware of the lesion, because it may be on the cervix or vaginal wall. The secondary stage usually occurs 6 to 8 weeks later, causing a generalized rash that often affects the palms of the hands, and usually does not itch. There may be other manifestations, including jaundice or ocular involvement (uveitis). The clinical signs resolve over a few weeks in the absence of treatment, after which the patient enters the latent stage. A small minority develop tertiary lesions involving the cardiovascular or nervous system many years later. Progression may be more rapid in HIV-positive patients. Women with secondary syphilis, who have a

disseminated infection, are most likely to infect their foetus, but the infection can cross the placenta in pregnant women with latent syphilis.

According to current WHO estimates, syphilis in pregnancy causes 355,000 adverse pregnancy outcomes per year, including 143,000 early foetal deaths and stillbirths and 61,000 neonatal deaths. These could be prevented if all pregnant women were screened for syphilis, and treated with a single dose of penicillin if they test positive, before 28 weeks' gestation.

Serological tests for syphilis are either treponemal (e.g. TPHA, TPPA), or non-treponemal (e.g. RPR or VDRL). Treponemal tests remain positive for life, whereas non-treponemal tests usually revert to negative after successful treatment, and can therefore be used as a test of cure. They may give false-positive results because of other infections (e.g. malaria), or autoimmune diseases. Until recently it has not been possible to screen women attending antenatal clinics that do not have access to a laboratory. However, sensitive and specific treponemal point-of-care tests are now available at an affordable price (<$1) which can give a result in 15 minutes and require neither electricity nor laboratory equipment.

Further Reading

1. Richens J, Mayaud P, Mabey DCW. Sexually transmitted infections (excluding HIV). In: Farrar J, editor. Manson's Tropical Diseases. 23rd ed. London: Elsevier; 2013 [chapter 23].
2. Korenromp EL, Rowley J, Alonso M, et al. Global burden of maternal and congenital syphilis and associated adverse birth outcomes-Estimates for 2016 and progress since 2012. PLoS One 2019;14: e0211720. https://doi.org/10.1371/journal.pone.0211720.
3. Watson-Jones D, Changalucha J, Gumodoka B, et al. Syphilis in pregnancy in Tanzania. I. Impact of maternal syphilis on outcome of pregnancy. J Infect Dis 2002;186(7):940–7.
4. Watson-Jones D, Gumodoka B, Weiss H, et al. Syphilis in pregnancy in Tanzania. II. The effectiveness of antenatal syphilis screening and single-dose benzathine penicillin treatment for the prevention of adverse pregnancy outcomes. J Infect Dis 2002; 186(7): 948–57.

57

A 37-Year-Old Woman from Malawi With Haematemesis

CAMILLA ROTHE

Clinical Presentation

History

A 37-year-old woman from the Lower Shire Valley in southern Malawi is referred from a clinic on one of the local sugar plantations to the district hospital. She has vomited blood three times over the past 24 hours. The blood is bright red in colour. There is no epigastric pain and no previous history of vomiting. There is no history of fever or abnormal bleeding and her stool has been normal in colour. Before the onset of symptoms, she was fine. She has not taken any regular painkillers and does not drink any alcohol.

Her past medical history is unremarkable. She lives and works on a large sugar plantation in the area. She is married with three children, all are well. An HIV test done 3 months previously was negative.

Clinical Findings

37-year-old woman who is slim but not wasted. Conjunctivae are slightly pale, but there are no subconjunctival effusions and she is not jaundiced. Her blood pressure is 90/60 mmHg, pulse 110 bpm, respiratory rate 28 breath cycles per minute, and she is afebrile.

On examination of the abdomen there is no abdominal distension and no tenderness. The spleen is palpable at 10 cm below the left costal margin. The liver is slightly enlarged but there are no stigmata of chronic liver disease. There is no shifting dullness and no peripheral oedema. Her lymph nodes are not enlarged. The rest of the physical examination is normal.

Laboratory Results

Her laboratory results on admission are shown in Table 57.1.

Questions

1. What is the most likely cause of her haematemesis?
2. What further investigations would you like to do to establish the diagnosis?

Discussion

A Malawian woman presents with a first episode of haematemesis. She has neither taken NSAIDs nor alcohol. On examination she is afebrile, slightly pale, shocked and has an enlarged spleen. Her abdomen is non-tender. Her full blood count shows pancytopenia with normocytic anaemia.

Answer to Question 1

What is the Most Likely Cause of Her Haematemesis?

Splenomegaly and pancytopenia point towards the presence of portal hypertension and she is most likely to bleed from gastro-oesophageal varices. In one series from Malawi, the presence of splenomegaly in patients with upper gastrointestinal bleeding was the single most specific clinical criterion to distinguish between a variceal bleed and a haemorrhage of other origin.

Furthermore, portal hypertension is the most common cause of upper gastrointestinal bleeding in parts of sub-Saharan Africa, accounting for more than 50% of bleeds in some series. The reason for this remains only partly understood. The prevalence of chronic viral hepatitis or alcohol abuse is not higher in the affected regions than elsewhere in the tropical world.

However, Malawi and other countries in the region are highly endemic for schistosomiasis. Virtually all water bodies

TABLE 57.1 Laboratory Results on Admission

Parameter	Patient	Reference Range
WBC (× 10⁹/L)	2.8	4–10
Haemoglobin (g/dL)	8.3	12–14
MCV (fL)	88	80–99
Platelets (× 10⁹/L)	130	150–400

in the country are infested with both *Schistosoma mansoni* and *S. haematobium* and it is likely that a high prevalence of hepatosplenic schistosomiasis with periportal fibrosis may explain why portal hypertension is so common in the region.

Little is known about causes of liver cirrhosis other than hepatitis B and C and their contribution to the burden of disease (e.g. autoimmune hepatitis, primary biliary cirrhosis, primary sclerosing cholangitis, haemochromatosis or Wilson's disease).

Other aetiologies of gastrointestinal bleeding, such as peptic ulcer disease, erosive gastritis or a bleeding tumour are less likely and would not explain her splenomegaly. Notably though, in sub-Saharan Africa oesophageal cancer is strikingly common in young adults in their third and fourth decade of life. Risk factors remain poorly understood. Progressive dysphagia rather than haematemesis is usually the presenting symptom.

Patients with visceral leishmaniasis (VL) can present with splenomegaly and pancytopenia. However, in VL there is usually a history of fever, and the patient's platelet count is only slightly diminished, which cannot explain her bleed. VL, furthermore, is uncommon in Southern Africa, even though few sporadic cases have been described from the region.

Answer to Question 2

What Additional Investigations Would You Like to Do to Establish the Diagnosis?

In a resource-constrained setting, very limited options may be available to establish more than just a syndromic diagnosis.

The patient should be taken for gastroduodenoscopy without delay to detect and treat the source of bleeding. In case of oesophageal varices, an experienced ultrasonographer with a reasonable ultrasound machine would be able to distinguish between liver cirrhosis and periportal 'pipestem' fibrosis as seen in hepatic schistosomiasis (Fig. 57.1). Liver biopsy would be the most helpful tool to distinguish between cirrhosis and periportal fibrosis in case of schistosomiasis. It is usually unavailable, and it is risky in an environment where postinterventional monitoring is poor, and possible complications such as intra-abdominal bleeds are likely to go undetected.

Other investigations to diagnose schistosomiasis will lack sensitivity and/or specificity in the endemic setting. The demonstration of *Schistosoma* eggs in the stool is challenging in advanced disease and several samples would have to be examined which is commonly not feasible. The circulating cathodic antigen test (CCA) is a urine rapid diagnostic test based on antigens regurgitated by adult flukes. Its sensitivity decreases when the worm burden is low, as may be the case in advanced disease; but it is highly specific and – other than serology – the CCA test is able to distinguish between active and past infection.

Hepatitis B or C serologies should be done; other investigations for chronic liver disease are usually unavailable.

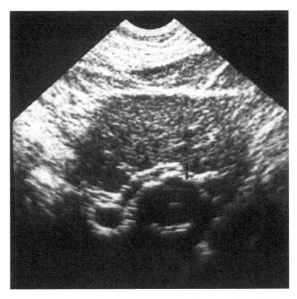

• **Fig. 57.1** Ultrasound of the liver showing pipestem fibrosis (Courtesy Prof. Joachim Richter).

The Case Continued...

The patient received IV fluids and was taken to the nearest central hospital for endoscopy. The presence of oesophageal varices was confirmed and banding was done. There was no other source of bleeding. Hepatitis B and C serologies were negative. One stool sample for *S. mansoni* ova was negative. However, on ultrasound of the liver a pattern typical of pipestem fibrosis was described. The patient received a single dose of praziquantel 40 mg/kg. She was discharged home.

SUMMARY BOX

Hepatosplenic Schistosomiasis

Hepatosplenic schistosomiasis is a complication of advanced infection with Schistosoma mansoni, S. japonicum or S. mekongi.

Only about 10% of people chronically infected with schistosomiasis develop late-stage disease. Risk factors for disease progression remain poorly understood. Apart from intensity and duration of infection, host genetic factors such as ethnic background and IFN-gamma polymorphism, variable degrees of semi-immunity and parasite strain differences may play a role.

Chronic infection with liver-pathogenic Schistosoma species results in periportal fibrosis and portal venous hypertension. One exception is S. intercalatum, which occurs focally in Central and West Africa and causes granulomatous inflammation of the liver without portal hypertension.

Patients may present with symptoms of hypersplenism, such as abdominal discomfort and fatigue secondary to progressive anaemia. Ascites is uncommon because of the preserved hepatocellular function but may occur in advanced disease or in coexisting liver cirrhosis.

The classical clinical signs of liver cirrhosis (e.g. gynaecomastia, palmar erythema, alterations in distribution of body hair) are absent in schistosomiasis.

A common, primary presenting sign of hepatosplenic schistosomiasis is upper gastrointestinal (GI) bleeding from gastro-oesophageal varices. In some endemic countries in sub-Saharan Africa half or more of upper GI bleeds are caused by portal hypertension.

The demonstration of *Schistosoma* eggs in the stool can be challenging in advanced disease because the adult flukes may have long died and egg production may have stopped.

Experienced ultrasonographers may be able to detect the typical pattern of 'pipestem fibrosis'. The term refers to the macroscopic aspect of the liver which shows wide bands of fibrosis around portal tracts resembling the stems of a clay pipe. If available, liver biopsy may show ova of *Schistosoma* species along with proliferation of fibrous tissue in and around the portal tract.

Praziquantel may have an effect in treatment of early fibrosis, but has little role to play in advanced disease. Nevertheless, a single dose treatment with praziquantel 40 mg/kg may be given to stop the progression of fibrosis and reduce the worm burden and further egg production.

Treatment of variceal bleeding includes endoscopic sclerotherapy, band-ligation and devascularization surgery. Splenectomy is not recommended in tropical settings, because of the increased susceptibility to malaria and bacterial infections.

Studies on the use of non-selective beta-blockers for prophylaxis of upper GI bleed in hepatic schistosomiasis have yielded controversial results.

A few reports from resource-rich settings seem to indicate that the placement of a transjugular intrahepatic portovenous shunt (TIPS) may be beneficial for the prevention of variceal bleeding in hepatic schistosomiasis.

Further Reading

1. Bustindy AL, King CH. Schistosomiasis. In: Farrar J, editor. Manson's Tropical Diseases. 23rd ed. London: Elsevier; 2013 [chapter 52].
2. Harries AD, Wirima JJ. Upper gastrointestinal bleeding in Malawian adults and value of splenomegaly in predicting source of haemorrhage. East Afr Med J 1989;66(2):97–9.
3. Wolf LL, Ibrahim R, Miao C, et al. Esophagogastroduodenoscopy in a public referral hospital in Lilongwe, Malawi: spectrum of disease and associated risk factors. World J Surg 2012;36(5):1074–82.
4. Colley DG, Bustinduy AL, Secor WE, et al. Human schistosomiasis. Lancet 2014;383(9936):2253–64.
5. Richter J, Bode JG, Blondin G, et al. Severe liver fibrosis caused by Schistosoma mansoni: management and treatment with a transjugular intrahepatic portosystemic shunt. Lancet Infect Dis 2015;15: 731–7.

58

A 25-Year-Old Woman from Egypt With Severe Chronic Diarrhoea and Malabsorption

THOMAS WEITZEL AND NADIA EL-DIB

Clinical Presentation

History

A 25-year-old woman from Bani Suwaif in Upper Egypt (115 km south of Cairo) presents to a hospital in Cairo complaining of severe diarrhoea for 2 months accompanied by weight loss of about 15 kg and amenorrhoea. The symptoms started with stomach rumbles and colicky abdominal pain; later on, she suffered anorexia and vomiting. The diarrhoea is voluminous, not related to meals, and occurs both during the day and at night (five to ten times in 24 hours).

She received various antibiotics, including metronidazole, as well as antidiarrhoeal drugs, without any improvement. During the last month she has developed lower limb swelling and severe prostration.

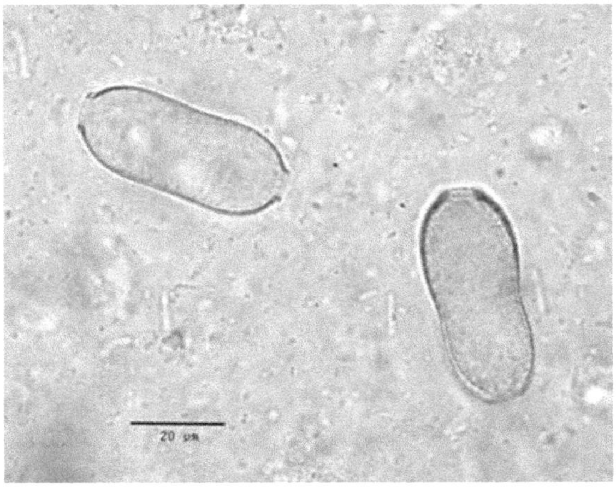

Clinical Findings

The patient appears generally unwell; she is pale and has angular stomatitis. She is afebrile, heart rate 100 bpm, blood pressure 100/60 mmHg, scaphoid abdomen with borborygmi, pitting oedema of the lower limbs, and decreased skin turgor.

Laboratory Results

Laboratory results are summarized in Table 58.1. D-xylose test shows evidence of malabsorption. On stool microscopy, numerous helminth ova are detected (Fig. 58.1).

Questions

1. Which helminth is causing the patient's clinical problems and why is it able to cause such severe infections?
2. Where does this parasite occur and how is it transmitted?

• **Fig. 58.1** Helminth ova in a stool sample of a 25-year-old woman from Egypt with chronic diarrhoea.

TABLE 58.1	Laboratory Results on Admission	
Parameter	Patient	Reference
Potassium (mmol/L)	2.8	3.5–5
Sodium (mmol/L)	127	136–145
Calcium, total (mmol/L)	2.1	2.25–2.63
Albumin (g/L)	23	35–55
Haemoglobin (g/dL)	10.8	11.5–15.5
WBC (× 10^9/L)	6.6	3.8–11
Eosinophil count (× 10^9/L)	0.53	<0.45
Platelets (× 10^9/L)	350	150–350
Creatinine (µmol/L)	115	53–106

Discussion

A 25-year-old woman from Upper Egypt presents with severe chronic diarrhoea and colicky abdominal pain. She is afebrile but shows clinical signs of chronic malabsorption. Full blood count reveals mild eosinophilia, blood chemistry shows electrolyte derangement and hypoalbuminaemia. Stool samples yield peanut-shaped helminth eggs.

Answer to Question 1

Which Helminth is Causing the Patient's Clinical Problems and Why is it Able to Cause Such Severe Infections?

The peanut-shaped eggs spotted on stool microscopy are typical ova of *Capillaria philippinensis*. The patient's complaints are very compatible with intestinal capillariasis, and she resides in an endemic area. In contrast to most other intestinal helminths, *C. philippinensis* is able to multiply within the intestine of its final host causing long-lasting infection and severe clinical manifestations.

Answer to Question 2

Where Does this Parasite Occur and How is it Transmitted?

C. philippinensis is endemic in various East and South-east Asian countries such as The Philippines, Thailand, Laos, China, Korea, Japan and Taiwan. Furthermore, cases have been reported from Egypt, Iran and India. Sporadic cases may occur elsewhere. One indigenous case has been reported from Cuba and another patient acquired the infection most probably in Colombia. Capillariasis is transmitted through consumption of raw or undercooked fish.

The Case Continued…

The patient was admitted to hospital. Albendazole was initiated at a dose of 400 mg bd and continued for 3 weeks. Oral and parenteral fluids and electrolytes were given for resuscitation, and she received a high protein diet and vitamins. During the first days of treatment, numerous adult helminths (length 3–5 mm) were found in more stool samples (Fig. 58.2). The patient's general condition improved significantly within the first week and vomiting stopped. Diarrhoea subsided after 2 weeks of treatment.

SUMMARY BOX

Intestinal Capillariasis

Intestinal capillariasis is a zoonotic disease caused by *C. philippinensis*, a tiny nematode usually infecting fish-eating birds, which

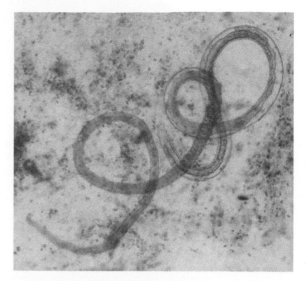

• **Fig. 58.2** Adult *C. philippinensis* in the patient's stool sample during treatment with mebendazole.

recently has been transferred to the genus *Paracapillaria*. Humans are accidentally infected when eating raw or under-cooked small fresh- or brackish-water fish harbouring infective larval stages of the parasite. Adult parasites invade the wall of the small intestine and live partially embedded in the mucosa of jejunum and ileum. The unique life cycle includes an alteration of oviparous and larviparous females. Oviparous females shed thick-shelled eggs, which exit the body with the stool and, after being eaten by small fish, develop into the infective larvae. Larviparous females contain thin-shelled eggs, which mainly hatch *in utero* and permit an internal autoinfection and multiplication cycle, i.e. larvae develop into adults within the intestinal mucosa without leaving the host. This leads to a gradual increase of both worm burden and severity of clinical manifestations. With its autoinfection cycle, the parasite is one of the few intestinal helminths causing chronic and life-threatening infections. Patients present with colicky abdominal pain and intermittent or chronic diarrhoea accompanied by anorexia, vomiting and dehydration. Without treatment, infection progresses to severe enteropathy with crypt atrophy and flattening of villi. Chronically infected patients suffer cachexia and pitting oedema of the lower limbs. Untreated, they may eventually die of severe protein loss, electrolyte imbalance and concomitant bacterial infections. Parasitological diagnosis relies on the demonstration of typical peanut-shaped eggs in stool samples, which have protruding polar plugs on both ends and measure 36 to 42 × 20 μm. Treatment is with mebendazole or albendazole for 20 or 10 days, respectively.

Further Reading

1. Jones MK, McCarthy JS. Medical helminthology. In: Farrar J, editor. Manson's Tropical Diseases. 23rd ed. London: Elsevier; 2013 [Appendix 3].
2. El-Dib N, Weitzel T. Capilariasis intestinal. In: Apt W, editor. Parasitología Humana. McGraw-Hill; 2013 [chapter 36].
3. Attia RAH, Tolba MEM, Yones DA, et al. Capilaria philippinensis in Upper Egypt: has it become endemic? Am J Trop Med Hyg 2012;86(1):126–33.
4. Cross JH. Intestinal capillariasis. Clin Microbiol Rev 1992;5(2):120–9.

59

A 24-Year-Old Man from Malawi With Skin Lesions and Breathlessness

M. JANE BATES

Clinical Presentation

History

A 24-year-old Malawian businessman presents to your clinic having noticed dark spots on his arm and leg for the last month. The lesions are progressing and he is now getting facial swelling.

On questioning, he also reports a 3-month history of cough and worsening shortness of breath. He has no constitutional symptoms of weight loss, fevers or night sweats. His cough is productive of white sputum. He has no history of previous tuberculosis. He tested positive for HIV a week before coming to your clinic and has not yet started antiretroviral medication.

Clinical Findings

The patient appears comfortable at rest with moderate facial oedema (Fig. 59.1). His temperature is 36°C (96.8°F), respiratory rate 32 breath cycles per minute and pulse 102 bpm. Widespread dark-purplish plaques are noted on the skin (Fig. 59.1) and palate. On respiratory examination, he has decreased air entry and dullness at the right lung base. He has swelling of his right leg from the foot to the knee, with prominent dark plaques which are coalescing (Fig. 59.2). The rest of the physical examination is normal.

Questions

1. What are your most important differential diagnoses?
2. How would you approach this patient?

Discussion

A young Malawian man presents with widespread dark purplish cutaneous and mucosal lesions. He also reports cough and shortness of breath for 3 months and there are some chest findings on examination of his right lung. He has recently been found to be HIV-positive.

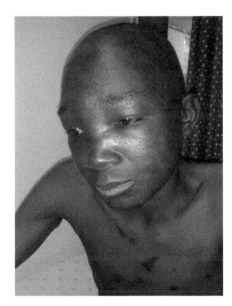

• **Fig. 59.1** Facial swelling and dark-purplish skin lesions on chest and nose of the patient.

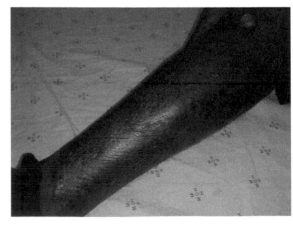

• **Fig. 59.2** Swollen right leg with prominent coalescing dark plaques.

Answer to Question 1

What Are Your Most Important Differential Diagnoses?

In a newly diagnosed HIV-infected patient with a chronic history of cough, the diagnosis of tuberculosis should always be considered and vigorous attempts made to exclude it. The skin lesions are typical for Kaposi's sarcoma (KS). The presence of palatal lesions supports this possibility and increases your suspicion of pulmonary involvement.

Answer to Question 2

How Would You Approach This Patient?

The patient should be assessed for possible pulmonary tuberculosis, which should include a urine LAM, sputum microscopy for acid-fast bacilli (AFB), Xpert MTB/RIF and chest radiograph where necessary. Where available, bronchoscopy remains the gold standard investigation for endobronchial KS. Dual pathology of pulmonary KS and TB is not uncommon, and a high index of suspicion for TB should be maintained, particularly as TB remains responsible for many HIV-related deaths.

The main concern of the patient and primary caregiver should be recorded to assist with prioritizing interventions that promote quality of life. These concerns may be physical, psychological, social or spiritual. General positive living advice, including safe sexual practice, screening for STIs and partner(s) and children testing for HIV, may also be addressed. The diagnosis should be explained to the patient in a style and language which is supportive and understandable. The practitioner should allow time for questions and exploration of relevant issues, which can assist with planning. Such communication can facilitate the development of realistic expectations from the start of the therapeutic process.

The patient should be started on antiretroviral therapy (ART) as soon as possible both to control HIV and as part of the therapeutic response to KS. There is a small possibility of KS immune reconstitution inflammatory syndrome, recognizable as worsening disease some weeks after commencement of ART.

Adjuvant palliative chemotherapy is indicated for patients with pulmonary KS.

The Case Continued...

His main concern was shortness of breath. His wife was also HIV-positive but not on ART, and his two children 6 and 4 years old had not yet been tested. His CD4 count was 134 cells/μL, HB 10.2 g/dL and MCV 88.4 fL. Other parameters were normal.

His chest radiograph showed bilateral patchy opacifications in the lower and mid zones of the lungs (Fig. 59.3). Peribronchovascular changes are typically seen in patients with pulmonary KS.

Sputum and GeneXpert tests were negative for the presence of tuberculosis. A bronchoscopy was attempted but failed because of technical difficulties. The patient made no improvement with a short course of oral antibiotics.

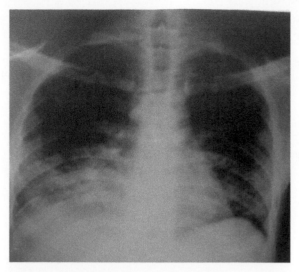

• **Fig. 59.3** Chest radiograph showing bilateral peribronchovascular infiltration in the lower and mid lung zones.

He was referred to start antiretroviral medication and palliative chemotherapy.

SUMMARY BOX

Kaposi's Sarcoma

KS is an incurable HIV-associated malignancy. The incidence of KS is on the decline globally as a result of prevention of disease because of early initiation of ART. KS is caused by human herpesvirus-8 (HHV-8), also known as Kaposi's sarcoma-associated herpes virus (KSHV). KS commonly affects the skin but may also involve lymph nodes, lungs and the gastrointestinal tract. Diagnosis of cutaneous disease is often made by clinical appearance though biopsy is recommended.

Endemic KS does occur in HIV-uninfected individuals, typically with a more indolent course. All HIV infected patients with KS should be started on ART. For those with more extensive cutaneous disease or visceral involvement, combining antiretroviral medication with chemotherapeutic agents promotes optimal tumour regression. Agents such as liposomal doxorubicin, paclitaxel, bleomycin, vincristine, vinblastine and etoposide can be considered. Drug availability, access to safe chemotherapy administration, contraindications and side effects of particular agents should be considered with reference to the patient and the setting. Tumour response to immunomodulating agents has been demonstrated in a small study in the USA. Outcomes remain poor for patients with extensive visceral disease (AIDS Clinical Trials Group stage T1). In these situations, quality of life remains the goal of care, involving patient and supportive family members to provide holistic palliative care, which should be initiated long before the end of life.

Pain and other symptoms should be assessed and managed. Low-dose liquid morphine has an established role for symptom relief of breathlessness once all other causes have been excluded and/or treated optimally. Non-drug measures to improve breathlessness, such as positioning and companionship to reduce distress and anxiety are also indicated.

Further Reading

1. Wood R. Clinical features and management of HIV/AIDS. In: Farrar J, editor. Manson's Tropical Diseases. 23rd ed. London: Elsevier; 2013 [chapter 10].

2. Malawi Guidelines for the Clinical Management of HIV in Children and Adults 3rd ed. Available from: https://aidsfree.usaid.gov/sites/default/files/malawi_art_2016.pdf.

3. Gonçalves PH, Uldrick TS, Yarchoan R. HIV associated Kaposi's Sarcoma and related diseases, AIDS 2017;31(14):1903–16. https://www.ncbi.nlm.nih.gov/pmc/articles/PMC6310482/.

4. Chin C, Booth S. Managing breathlessness: a palliative care approach. Postgrad Med J 2016;92:393–400. https://doi.org/10.1136/postgradmedj-2015-133578.

5. Caesarman E, Damania B, Known SE, et al. Kaposi Sarcoma. Nat Rev Dis Primers 2019;5:9. https://doi.org/10.1038/s41572-019-0060-9.

60

A 6-Year-Old Boy from Malawi With Proptosis of the Left Eye

ELIZABETH M. MOLYNEUX

Clinical Presentation

History

A 6-year-old Malawian boy from the lakeshore of Lake Malawi presents with a painless, proptosed left eye that his family first noticed 3 weeks ago. It has worsened rapidly though his vision is still normal. He denies any pain.

Clinical Findings

On examination he is afebrile, the right eye is normal, the left eye is proptosed but non-pulsating (Fig. 60.1). The pupil is round and clear and responds well to light. When he is asked to follow an object with his eyes the left eyeball hardly moves. He has no other swellings or abnormalities; and though he is thin, he is not malnourished.

Questions

1. What are the three most likely diagnoses?
2. What investigations would you do to confirm the diagnosis and direct your treatment plan?

Discussion

A young Malawian boy presents because of a progressive painless proptosis of his left eye for the past 3 weeks. His vision is not impaired. Apart from being proptosed, the eye on examination looks normal.

The boy resides in an area endemic for malaria and schistosomiasis.

Answer to Question 1

What Are the Three Most Likely Diagnoses?

This is a rapidly developing proptosis in a boy who lives in a malaria-endemic area; the most likely diagnosis is Burkitt's lymphoma.

The second possibility is that it is another type of B cell lymphoma; and the third possibility is rhabdomyosarcoma.

It is not a retinoblastoma, which starts in the eye and usually, but not always, presents at an earlier age. The process is painless, which excludes infection, and it is non-pulsating which makes the diagnosis of an arteriovenous malformation unlikely. Lachrymal gland tumours are more anteromedial than this mass.

Answer to Question 2

What Investigations Would You Do to Confirm the Diagnosis and Direct Your Treatment Plan?

There are three questions to ask: what is it, where is it and is it safe to treat?

What is it? A thorough history and physical examination will narrow the field. Is this a multifocal or localized lesion? Knowing the age will rule in some more likely diagnoses and rule out others. Are there any systemic or neurological signs and symptoms? A fine-needle aspirate (FNA) or biopsy will confirm the diagnosis.

Where is it? Again, the examination will assist. An abdominal ultrasound scan will demonstrate any intra-abdominal masses and organ involvement. A cytospun sample of cerebrospinal fluid (CSF) should be examined for malignant cells; a full blood count (FBC) should also be done and bone marrow aspirate (BMA) examined. A chest radiograph is useful if intrathoracic pathology is suspected.

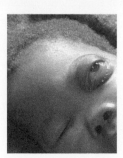

• **Fig. 60.1** The boy before four courses of chemotherapy.

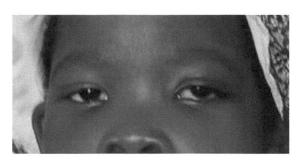

• **Fig. 60.2** The boy after four courses of chemotherapy.

Is it safe to treat? Anaemia (<7 g/dL) and thrombocytopenia (<50 × 10^9/L) should be corrected before giving chemotherapy. A blood film and stool and urine samples should be examined to exclude or treat malaria or any other invasive parasitic infections such as schistosomiasis or strongyloidiasis. The abdominal ultrasound scan will demonstrate any renal involvement and forewarn of possible complications when treatment is given. Baseline renal function and liver function tests are useful but not essential. HIV status will not affect the treatment; but if positive, infections and anaemia should be anticipated during chemotherapy.

The Case Continued...

The boy was admitted and a full work-up was done as a matter of urgency (FNA, BMA, FBC, lumbar puncture (LP), HIV antibody test, stool and urine microscopy) and an abdominal scan was carried out. This was to enable treatment for presumed Burkitt's lymphoma to start as soon as possible to prevent further proptosis and irreversible damage to the eye. Delay could mean the eye losing its blood supply and 'melting', leaving the boy sightless in that eye.

When the LP was done, intrathecal methotrexate and hydrocortisone were given as prophylaxis against CNS involvement. Oral allopurinol and hyperhydration were commenced; chemotherapy was given the next day. The eye looked less proptosed within 48 hours and was back to normal within a week. He had four courses of chemotherapy in the next 30 days (Fig. 60.2). A year later he was free of disease and pronounced cured.

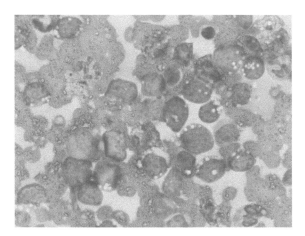

• **Fig. 60.3** Histology of Burkitt's lymphoma (H&E stain) showing monomorphic tumour cells of intermediate size, indistinct nuclei with coarse chromatin and vacuoles in the cytoplasm (×100 high-power field).

SUMMARY BOX

Burkitt's Lymphoma

Endemic Burkitt's lymphoma is a highly aggressive B-cell non-Hodgkin's lymphoma. It is the fastest-growing tumour known in man and doubles its cells' numbers every 24 to 48 hours (Fig. 60.3). It is causally associated with the Epstein–Barr virus (EBV) and malaria, and has a chromosomal translocation that activates the c-myc oncogene. It is the most common childhood cancer (about 50%) in areas where malaria is holoendemic. It is twice as common in boys as girls and the peak age of presentation is 6 to 7 years. Outcome with early diagnosis and intensive chemotherapy in children is excellent. In resource-constrained settings, treatment intensity has to be balanced with good supportive care, the child's nutritional status and stage of the disease. This means that less aggressive treatment often has to be given with less successful outcomes. Nevertheless, with stage-adjusted therapies, designed by oncologists of the Paediatric Oncology in Developing Countries group (PODC), which is an arm of the International Society of Paediatric Oncology (SIOP), and by common consensus and studies done in low-income settings, 60% cure at 1 year can be achieved at a very low cost and manageable toxicity.

Further Reading

1. Newton R, Wakeham K, Bray F. Cancer in the tropics. In: Farrar J, editor. Manson's Tropical Diseases. 23rd ed. London: Elsevier; 2013 [chapter 64].
2. Molyneux EM, Rochford R, Griffin B, et al. Burkitt's lymphoma. Lancet 2012;379(9822):1234–44.
3. Hesseling P, Israels T, Harif M, et al. Practical recommendations for the management of children with endemic Burkitt's lymphoma (BL) in a resource limited setting. Pediatr Blood Cancer 2013;60(3): 357–62.
4. Gopal S, Thomas G. Gross. How I treat Burkitt lymphoma in children, adolescents and young adults in Sub-Saharan Africa. Blood 2018;132(3):254–63.

61

A 48-Year-Old Woman from Thailand With Fever and Disseminated Cutaneous Abscesses

SABINE JORDAN

Clinical Presentation

History

A 46-year-old Thai woman is transferred to a German clinic for tropical diseases with a 2-month history of recurrent cutaneous and subcutaneous abscesses, progressive lymphadenopathy and weight loss.

Despite various antibiotic therapies, clinical symptoms and inflammatory markers had deteriorated, resulting in hospital admission. Pus and blood cultures did not yield any growth, and histopathology of a lymph node biopsy showed non-specific lymphadenitis. The symptoms started 6 to 8 weeks after her return from a family visit to northern Thailand. During her stay the patient had suffered from high fever, dry cough and fatigue.

Clinical Findings

A 46-year-old woman, 158 cm, 65 kg (BMI 26 kg/m^2), afebrile, blood pressure 130/80 mmHg, pulse 80 bpm.

Enlarged, tender cervical, nuchal, inguinal and axillary lymph nodes. Massive, tender swelling of the upper eyelids. Disseminated fluctuant cutaneous and subcutaneous abscesses with surrounding erythema (Fig. 61.1), discharge of pus on slight pressure. Painful swelling of the left elbow. Otherwise normal physical examination.

Laboratory Results and Imaging

Lab results on admission are shown in Table 61.1.

A radiograph of the patient's left elbow is shown in Figure 61.2.

Questions

1. What are your most important differential diagnoses?
2. What investigations would you like to do?

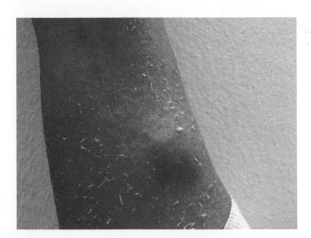

• **Fig. 61.1** Subcutaneous abscess on the left forearm.

TABLE 61.1	Laboratory Results on Admission	
Parameter	Patient	Reference
WCC (× 10^9/L)	30.8	3.8–11
Haemoglobin (g/dL)	8.2	12.3–15.3
MCV (fL)	88	80–94
Platelets (× 10^9/L)	592	150–400
CRP (mg/L)	267	<5
ESR (mm/h)	>110	<20

Discussion

A 46-year-old woman from Thailand presents with a 2-month history of recurrent and treatment-refractory cutaneous and subcutaneous abscesses, progressive lymphadenopathy and weight loss. Her symptoms started 6 to

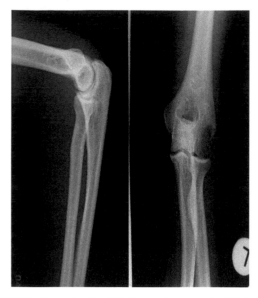

• **Fig. 61.2** Radiograph of the left elbow, showing osteolytic lesions of the radial epicondylus, osteomyelitis and articular effusion.

8 weeks after returning from a visit to northern Thailand. On examination, multiple cutaneous and subcutaneous abscesses and a generalized lymphadenopathy are noted. Laboratory findings show elevated systemic markers of inflammation. A radiograph of the swollen elbow reveals osteomyelitis.

Answer to Question 1

What Are Your Most Important Differential Diagnoses?

The clinical picture and the laboratory and radiological findings are highly suspicious of a systemic infection. As previous antibiotic treatment courses were ineffective and microbiological tests were negative, fungal infections, such as histoplasmosis, and mycobacterial infections should be considered. Furthermore, bacterial infections with special requirements for cultivation and/or limited antibiotic susceptibility such as *Burkholderia pseudomallei*, *Brucella* species, *Francisella tularensis* or *Actinomyces* species could have been misdiagnosed before.

As a result of the extensive disease, underlying immunodeficiency, such as HIV infection, diabetes mellitus, antibody deficiency or impaired granulocyte function, have to be ruled out.

If further microbiological investigations remain negative, rare autoimmune syndromes such as idiopathic nodular panniculitis (Weber–Christian disease) or aseptic abscesses syndrome have to be taken into account.

Answer to Question 2

What Investigations Would You Like to Do?

Additional microbiological and histopathological investigations seem to be crucial in this case. Biopsies of skin, abscesses and lymph nodes should be sent for culture and histopathological studies. Testing should focus on fungal and mycobacterial infections. PCR (polymerase chain reaction)

methods – where available – can help accelerate the diagnosis, because isolation of the pathogen from culture might take several weeks. For histoplasmosis, serological antigen and antibody tests are available. These may also help speed up the diagnostic process, but negative results do not rule out infection; antibody testing lacks sensitivity in immunocompromised patients. Furthermore, the patient should be tested for HIV, and a fasting blood glucose level can help rule out diabetes mellitus.

The Case Continued...

Initially, the clinically suspected diagnosis was melioidosis, which is a common cause of disseminated abscesses in patients from north-eastern Thailand. The patient received imipenem, which led to a slight improvement of her skin manifestations but inflammation parameters remained grossly elevated.

Once various cultures from skin and lymph node biopsies remained sterile, a submandibular lymph node was extirpated. Histologically, this lymph node showed fungal cells that were identified as *Histoplasma capsulatum* by PCR. This was later confirmed by culture. Serology for histoplasmosis remained negative.

In retrospect, the febrile illness the patient had suffered whilst in Thailand may have been acute pulmonary histoplasmosis (see Summary Box).

While on antifungal treatment with liposomal amphotericin B (3 mg/kg per day, total dose 3 g) the patient developed a generalized seizure. CSF analysis revealed lymphocytic pleocytosis, which, despite the absence of direct pathogen detection, may have been a cerebral manifestation of histoplasmosis.

On treatment with liposomal amphotericin B the patient's clinical state and the laboratory findings improved dramatically. The patient was started on itraconazole maintenance therapy for an additional 6 months.

No evidence of immunosuppression was found in the diagnostic work-up.

On follow-up the patient presented in a fair general condition. Some of the former abscess sites showed post-inflammatory hyperpigmentation, enlarged lymph nodes were no longer present and the osteolytic lesions were partly recalcified. Repeat histoplasma serology remained negative.

SUMMARY BOX

Histoplasmosis

Histoplasmosis is caused by *H. capsulatum,* a dimorphic fungus that remains in a mycelial form at ambient temperatures and grows as yeast at body temperature in mammals. The fungus can be found in temperate climates throughout the world, predominantly in river valleys in parts of the USA, the West Indies, Central and South America, Africa, India, South East Asia and Australia. The soil in areas endemic for histoplasmosis provides an acidic damp environment with high organic content that favours mycelial growth. Highly contaminated soil is found near areas inhabited by bats and birds. Birds cannot be infected by the fungus and do not transmit the disease; however, bird excretions contaminate the soil, thereby enriching the growth medium for the mycelium. In contrast, bats can become infected, and they transmit histoplasmosis through their droppings. Contaminated soil can be potentially infectious for years. Outbreaks of histoplasmosis have been associated with construction and renovation activities that disrupt soil contaminated with *Histoplasma* species.

Inhalation of fungal spores may lead to acute pulmonary histoplasmosis; however, approximately 90% of individuals with acute infection remain asymptomatic. In patients with underlying lung pathology, chronic pulmonary disease can occur. Patients develop cavities that may enlarge and result in necrosis. Untreated histoplasmosis may lead to progressive pulmonary fibrosis that leads to recurrent infections and respiratory and cardiac failure.

In children, older individuals and immunocompromised patients, dissemination of the infection may occur. The symptoms of disseminated histoplasmosis typically include fever, malaise, anorexia and weight loss. Physical examination will often show hepatosplenomegaly and lymphadenopathy, some patients may present with mucous membrane ulcerations as well as skin ulcers, nodules or molluscum-like papules. Rarely, disseminated infection can also occur in immunocompetent patients.

In disseminated disease, culture of tissue samples or body fluids and histopathology should be obtained. PCR can help speed up the diagnostic process because isolation from fungal cultures takes up to 3 weeks. Serology lacks sensitivity, especially in immunocompromised patients. In these cases, blood and urine antigen testing should be performed.

In patients with disseminated infection, initial treatment with liposomal amphotericin B (3–5 mg/kg daily) is highly effective. Itraconazole (400 mg daily) is favoured for maintenance therapy. The duration of treatment depends on the severity of infection and the immune status of the patient. IDSA (Infectious Diseases Society of America) guidelines recommends 6 to 18 months in total.

Further Reading

1. Hay RJ. Fungal infections. In: Farrar J, editor. Manson's Tropical Diseases. 23rd ed. London: Elsevier; 2013.
2. Kauffman CA. Histoplasmosis: a clinical and laboratory update. Clin Microbiol Rev 2007;20:115–32.
3. Wheat LJ, Freifeld AG, Kleiman MB, et al. Clinical practice guidelines for the management of patients with histoplasmosis: 2007 update by the Infectious Diseases Society of America. Clin Infect Dis 2007;45:807–25.
4. Wheat LJ, Azar MM, Bahr NC, Spec A, Relich RF, Hage C. Histoplasmosis. Infect Dis Clin North Am 2016;30(1):207–27.
5. Azar MM, Hage CA. Laboratory diagnostics for histoplasmosis. J Clin Microbiol 2017;55(6):1612–20.

62

A 28-Year-Old Man from Ghana With a Chronic Ulcer on His Ankle

FREDERICKA SEY AND IVY EKEM

Clinical Presentation

History

A 28-year-old West African man presents to a clinic in Ghana complaining of a painful ulcer on his left ankle. The ulcer has been present for the past 4 months and is not healing (Fig. 62.1). There is no history of prior trauma; however, he had a previous ulcer on his right ankle some years ago which took about a year to heal. He also complains of pain in his right thigh and in both knees.

Clinical Findings

The patient is short for an adult; he is pale and has a tinge of jaundice. The ulcer is on his left ankle, next to the medial malleolus; the skin surrounding it is hyperpigmented. There is tenderness in both knee joints and in his right thigh. The rest of the physical examination is normal. Vital signs: Temperature 36.6°C, pulse 88 bpm, blood pressure 110/70 mmHg.

Questions

1. What is your differential diagnosis?
2. How would you confirm the diagnosis?

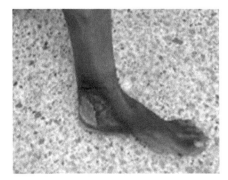

• **Fig. 62.1** The patient's left leg showing an ulcer surrounded by hyperpigmented skin on the medial malleolus.

Discussion

A 28-year-old West African man presents with a chronic, painful ankle ulcer. He had a similar ulcer on the other foot a few years prior. He also complains of bone pains. He is short for an adult, pale and mildly jaundiced.

Answer to Question 1

What is Your Differential Diagnosis?

The chronic nature of the ulcer, its site and the surrounding hyperpigmentation make a venous ulcer likely. The patient's bone pain, jaundice and pallor could point to a haemolytic anaemia. Various hereditary haemolytic anaemias may be complicated by chronic leg ulceration, e.g. haemoglobinopathies (thalassaemia and sickle cell disease), spherocytosis and pyruvate kinase deficiency. In the West African context, sickle cell disease is the most likely diagnosis.

Further differentials would be tropical ulcer, diabetic ulcer or chronic osteomyelitis with a discharging sinus. Buruli ulcer, caused by *Mycobacterium ulcerans,* is usually painless. Other mycobacterial infections can also present with chronic skin ulcers. Pyoderma gangrenosum and malignant diseases also need to be considered.

Answer to Question 2

How Would You Confirm the Diagnosis?

A full blood count and a peripheral blood film should be done. In sickle cell disease, during an acute crisis, abundant sickled red cells can be seen on a blood film. Other characteristic but non-specific features include target cells, Howell–Jolly bodies, polychromasia and nucleated red cells. The presence of HbS can be demonstrated by using a simple sickle slide or solubility test. Blood is mixed with sodium metabisulphite, which will provoke sickling of cells containing HbS; this can be demonstrated on a slide. If resources allow, confirmation is by haemoglobin electrophoresis, liquid chromatography or isoelectric focusing.

Fasting blood sugar and wound swab for culture and sensitivity as well as a radiograph of the left leg should be done to rule out other differential diagnoses and osteomyelitis.

The Case Continued...

Blood was taken and the available results are shown in Table 62.1. The patient's blood film is shown in Figure 62.2. The sickling test was positive and haemoglobin electrophoresis showed a homozygous HbSS-type. The wound swab grew *Pseudomonas* species sensitive to levofloxacin. Radiography showed a periosteal reaction with slightly sclerotic bones.

TABLE 62.1	Laboratory Results		
Parameter	Patient initial visit	Patient 6 years later	Reference Range
WBC ($\times 10^9$/L)	17.6	9.2	4–10
Haemoglobin (g/dL)	6.9	8.3	13–15
Platelet ($\times 10^9$/L)	Adequate	364	150–400
Fasting blood glucose (mmol/L)	4.8	Not done	4.4–6.1

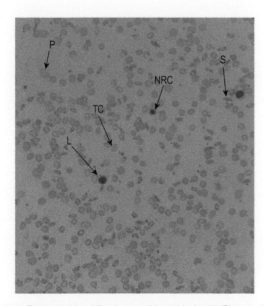

• **Fig. 62.2** Patient's blood film: irreversibly sickled cells (S), polychromasia (P), target cells (TC), nucleated red cells (NRC) – note similarity with lymphocyte (L). Adequate platelets.

The diagnosis made was sickle cell disease with a chronic ankle ulcer. The patient was managed with alternate daily wound dressing using normal saline irrigation and povidone-iodine. High white cell counts are commonly seen in sickle cell disease. They may be the result of bone marrow stimulation and do not necessarily indicate systemic infection. However, in view of the patient's generally poor condition and the *Pseudomonas* grown from his wound swab, it was decided to give him systemic antibiotic treatment.

Strict bed rest was difficult to enforce because the young man was self-employed and could not afford to take the required time off work. His recurrent bone pain was managed conservatively with good hydration, prompt treatment of infections and relief of other identifiable precipitants of crises. He received daily folic acid supplementation. Pain relief was achieved with paracetamol and tramadol.

However, on follow-up 3 years later, the ulcer was still not healed. Grafting was under consideration, when healthy granulation tissue would be achieved.

Six years later, the wound had still not healed and the patient could not afford a skin graft. He had 3 times weekly dressing and felt well in himself. His WBC was normal and his Hb had slightly increased (see Table 62.1).

SUMMARY BOX

Leg Ulcers in Sickle Cell Disease

Sickle cell disease (SCD) is a collection of autosomal-codominant genetic disorders characterized by the production of abnormal sickle haemoglobin S (HbS). Homozygous HbSS leads to sickle cell anaemia, the most severe form of SCD. Sickle cell disease is the commonest hereditary haematological disorder.

HbS has the tendency to polymerize during hypoxia. This leads to a reduction of the flexibility of the erythrocyte and to the typical sickle shape of the affected cell. Sickled red blood cells lead to haemolysis and vaso-occlusion.

The disease is characterized by episodes of acute illness against a background of progressive organ damage. Any organ can be affected by SCD at any age; however, certain features tend to predominate in certain age-groups. Leg ulcers tend to manifest in adulthood. Pathophysiology is complex and remains incompletely understood. Ulcers in SCD occur in areas with thin skin and little subcutaneous fat, most commonly on the ankles. They are notoriously difficult to treat. The ulcers are slow to heal and are characterized by unexplained relapses. They are commonly very painful and patients may occasionally require opioids for pain control. Colonization with pathogenic bacteria is common. Periosteal reaction is usually seen in the underlying bones but osteomyelitis is uncommon.

Of the many treatments, the most certain to aid healing is complete bed rest with leg elevation. Oral zinc sulphate tablets (200 mg tid) have been shown to be helpful. Systemic antibiotic therapy is given in acute sepsis. The use of hydroxyurea in leg ulcers is controversial. Chronic transfusion regimens to maintain the haemoglobin level above 10 g/dL may help when conservative therapy fails. Skin grafting for clean wounds is recommended, especially when the defect is large. The relapse rate is high, however. Poor nutrition which has not been given much attention may be a crucial factor and needs to be investigated on a wide scale in sickle cell disease.

Further Reading

1. Thachil J, Owusu-Ofori S, Bates I. Haematological diseases in the tropics. In: Farrar J, editor. Manson's Tropical Diseases. 23rd ed. London: Elsevier; 2013 [chapter 65].
2. Ware RE, de Montalembert M, Tshilolo L, Abboud MR. *Sickle cell disease*. Lancet 2017;390:311–23.
3. Delaney KM, Axelrod KC, Buscetta A, et al. Leg ulcers in sickle cell disease: current patterns and practices. Hemoglobin 2013;37(4): 325–32.
4. Halabi-Tawil M, Lionnet F, Girot R, et al. Sickle cell leg ulcers: a frequently disabling complication and a marker of severity. Br J Dermatol 2008;158(2):339–44.
5. Serena TE, Yaakov RA, DeLegge M, Mayhugh TA, Moore S. Nutrition in patients with chronic non-healing ulcers: a paradigm shift in wound care. Chronic Wound Care Manage Res 2018;5:5–9. Available from: https://doi.org/10.2147/CWCMR.S155114. Accessed 11 April 2019.

63

A 38-Year-Old European Expatriate Living in Malawi With Difficulty Passing Urine

JOEP J. VAN OOSTERHOUT

Clinical Presentation

History

A 38-year-old European expatriate presents at the medical outpatient clinic in a tertiary hospital in Malawi with progressive constipation and difficulty passing urine for the past 3 weeks. He noticed that he had to use increasing abdominal pressure to pass urine and eventually became only able to pass small amounts at a time. This is associated with increasing lower abdominal discomfort, abnormal sensations in the groins and around the genitals and some erectile dysfunction. He has no weakness and there is no dysaesthesia and no loss of sensation in his legs. However, he mentions that walking did not feel normal, although he cannot fully explain what the abnormality is. He has no backache.

Over the past 2 months he has experienced unintentional weight loss of 8 kg and fatigue without fever or night sweats. He blames this on stressful circumstances at work. He has sexual contact with his wife only, to whom he has been married for several years.

One week prior to presentation he had noticed reddish discoloration of his urine. He had no painful micturition or fever at that time. He visited a local clinic and was prescribed four different types of medication, which he completed. There is no history of trauma and the rest of his previous medical history is unremarkable.

Physical Examination

He looks healthy and has normal vital signs. There are no abnormalities on general examination, except for a palpable bladder. The rectal examination reveals a low anal sphincter tone and the genital examination is normal. He has lively, symmetrical tendon reflexes in the legs without clonus or pathological plantar reflexes, and no abnormalities in the rest of the neurological examination.

Questions

1. Which important pieces of information are missing?
2. What are possible diagnoses and which investigations would you order?

Discussion

A 38-year-old European expatriate living in Malawi presents with constipation, bladder retention, an episode of probable haematuria, erectile dysfunction, genital paraesthesia, significant weight loss and fatigue. There are no abnormal neurological findings on examination, however most of the complaints are compatible with a conus syndrome because of a lesion within the conus medullaris or because of compression. The constitutional symptoms suggest an underlying chronic infection or malignancy.

Answer to Question 1

Which Important Pieces of Information Are Missing?

The important missing pieces of information are details of the recent visit to the local clinic and exposure to fresh water in Malawi. On physical examination, the anal reflex should have been tested.

Answer to Question 2

What Are Possible Diagnoses and Which Investigations Would You Order?

The most important differential diagnosis for a conus medullaris syndrome in a young, otherwise healthy man living in tropical Africa is spinal cord schistosomiasis. Other important infections to consider are spinal tuberculosis, a spinal abscess and neurosyphilis. A tumour or metastases impinging on the conus medullaris should be ruled out.

Urine and stool microscopy for ova of *Schistosoma haematobium* and *S. mansoni*, respectively, should be ordered. A full blood count should be done, including a white cell differential count to look for eosinophilia. Creatinine and C-reactive protein should be tested.

Schistosomiasis serology would be useful in this expatriate.

A VDRL and an HIV test should be done. An ultrasound of the abdomen assessing bladder volume before and after micturition and imaging of the spinal cord should be requested.

The Case Continued...

The patient was able to retrieve details of his urine microscopy from the local clinic. *Schistosoma haematobium* eggs had been identified in his urine and he had been treated with a full dose of praziquantel, a course of ciprofloxacin, buscopan and bisacodyl.

He had swum regularly in Lake Malawi.

An abdominal ultrasound scan after attempted micturition showed a large bladder residue without further abnormalities.

Full blood count showed a normal absolute WBC of 9×10^9/L with a relative eosinophilia of 21.8% (reference range: 1–6%) and an absolute eosinophil count of 1.15×10^9/L (reference: $<0.45 \times 10^9$/L). ALT was slightly elevated. Creatinine and CRP were normal.

An HIV test and the VDRL were negative and microscopy of a stool and urine sample were normal. Serological tests for schistosomiasis were not available.

An MRI scan of the spinal cord was performed (Fig. 63.1). An enhancing 1 cm large lesion was seen at the anterior aspect of the conus, with associated high T2 signal representing oedema extending from the lower end of the conus to the level of T9. In addition, there was nodular

thickening of the urine bladder wall at the base and the posterior aspect.

The diagnosis of an infection with *Schistosoma haematobium* was made as evidenced by the urine findings and supported by the eosinophilia and the abnormalities seen in the bladder wall on MRI scanning. This was complicated by spinal cord schistosomiasis (see Summary Box) with lesions in the conus medullaris, causing a conus syndrome. A dual infection with *S. haematobium* and *S. mansoni* is possible, because *S. mansoni* is the more common pathogen causing spinal cord schistosomiasis, and both pathogens are endemic in Malawi. Theoretically, the spinal cord abnormalities could have been caused by other conditions, such as tuberculosis and metastatic cancer, for instance from a bladder carcinoma. Although it has been argued that *S. haematobium* infection is a risk factor for bladder carcinoma, this is mainly observed in long-term heavy infections, which are uncommon in expatriates. Further tests to rule out such distinct possibilities are not readily available in Malawi and were not deemed necessary.

The patient required urinary catheterization for 2 weeks. He made a full recovery after a second course of praziquantel and a course of high-dose prednisolone, tapered off over 2 months. He was well after more than 2 years of follow-up.

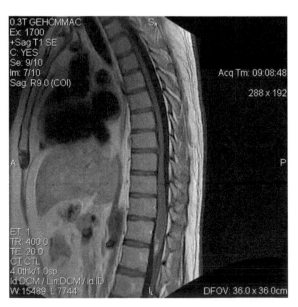

• **Fig. 63.1** T2-weighted MRI scan of the spinal cord.

SUMMARY BOX

Neuroschistosomiasis

Neuroschistosomiasis can occur in the brain and more frequently in the spinal cord. Cerebral schistosomiasis can be asymptomatic or present with seizures, lateralizing signs and meningo-encephalitis. Spinal cord schistosomiasis (SCS) is more frequent in *S. mansoni* than in *S. haematobium* infections and often causes severe disability because of paraparesis and bladder dysfunction. It is also the most important severe complication of schistosomiasis in travellers.

Our understanding of the pathophysiology of neuroschistosomiasis is limited. For unknown reasons, ectopic worms lodge in the venous plexus around the CNS instead of their normal habitat. Laminectomy with biopsy of the nervous tissue is the only method that gives a definite diagnosis of SCS. However, this procedure should be avoided because of its risks. Diagnosis is based upon spinal cord imaging and proof of exposure to the parasite. Urine should be examined for *S. haematobium* eggs; for *S. mansoni*, stool microscopy may be attempted but lacks sensitivity, which is much higher for rectal biopsies. The circulating cathodic antigen (CCA) test is a urine antigen test, which may prove *S. mansoni* infection. It detects an antigen regurgitated by adult worms of *S. mansoni*. It is less sensitive for *S. haematobium* and generally works better if the parasite burden is high. A novel test for the circulating anodic antigen (CAA) is under development and seems to be more promising for proof of both parasite species in urine and blood. Serological tests are useful in patients from non-endemic countries. They lack sensitivity and specificity in endemic populations. Detection of schistosomal antibodies in the CSF is specific but not widely validated. Eosinophils are present in the CSF in about 50% of patients.

Other causes of myelitis should be ruled out, which is often impossible in low-resource settings where pragmatic treatment for suspected neuroschistosomiasis may be justified.

Treatment of neuroschistosomiasis is with antischistosomal drugs (praziquantel) plus corticosteroids and is based on case series and expert opinion. The pathology is caused by inflammation around *Schistosoma* eggs. Praziquantel kills adult flukes only and thereby stops additional eggs being shed into the spinal cord. Most early improvement of the neurological presentation is thought to result from the antiinflammatory effects of corticosteroids. The optimal dose and duration are not well known. Up to 6 months of high-dose corticosteroids is recommended; however, data from randomized controlled trials are lacking.

Laminectomy should be considered in patients with severe spinal cord compression.

About 65% of patients with spinal cord schistosomiasis who are treated early, recover completely or are left with negligible deficits that do not cause any functional limitations; the remaining patients are left with sequelae that vary from mild to severe.

Further Reading

1. Bustinduy AL, King CH. Schistosomiasis. In: Farrar J, editor. Manson's Tropical Diseases. 23rd ed. London: Elsevier; 2013 [chapter 52].
2. Ferrari TC, Moreira PR. Neuroschistosomiasis: clinical symptoms and pathogenesis. Lancet Neurol 2011;10(9):853–64.
3. Colley DG, Bustinduy AL, Secor WE, King CH. Human schistosomiasis. Lancet 2014;383(9936):2253–64.
4. Silva LC, Maciel PE, Ribas JG, et al. Treatment of schistosomal myeloradiculopathy with praziquantel and corticosteroids and evaluation by magnetic resonance imaging: a longitudinal study. Clin Infect Dis 2004;39(11):1618–24.
5. Bonnefond S, Cnops L, Duvignaud A, et al. Early complicated schistosomiasis in a returning traveller: key contribution of new molecular diagnostic methods. Int J Infect Dis 2019;79:72–4.

64

A 40-Year-Old Woman from Thailand and Her Brother-in-Law With Severe Headache

CAMILLA ROTHE AND JURI KATCHANOV

Clinical Presentation

History

A 40-year-old Thai woman presents to an outpatient clinic in Germany with a history of severe headache for the past 8 days. The headache was of gradual onset and did not respond to any painkillers. There is no fever and no chills. She denies any visual problems, any weakness of her limbs or memory problems.

Ten days earlier she had returned from a 4-week journey to north-east Thailand, where she visited friends and relatives. During her visit she ate traditional regional dishes, including freshwater fish, seafood, snails and frogs. She reports that her brother-in-law, with whom she had shared several traditional meals, has also fallen ill with a severe headache.

She presented to a municipal hospital 3 days earlier. A CT scan of her brain was performed and reported to be normal. Her blood count was also normal. A differential white cell count has not been done.

Her past medical history is unremarkable. The patient is married, she is a housewife and has lived in Germany for the past 13 years.

Clinical Findings

On examination, she is afebrile, her neck is supple and Lasègue's sign (straight leg raise) is negative. Pupils are equal, round and react to light and accommodation, and there are no cranial nerve palsies. The remainder of the neurological examination, including the assessment of higher cortical functions such as language, memory and praxia, is unremarkable. There is no rash, no oral thrush and there are no subcutaneous swellings. Cardiopulmonary examination is normal. Liver and spleen are not enlarged, and there is no lymphadenopathy.

Laboratory Results

Her laboratory results at presentation in the clinic are shown in Table 64.1.

Questions

1. What is your presumptive diagnosis?
2. Which investigation would you perform to substantiate your diagnosis?

Discussion

A 40-year-old Thai woman presents with a history of severe intractable headache after a stay in north-east Thailand where she enjoyed traditional regional dishes. Her brother-in-law in Thailand is suffering from the same severe headache.

TABLE 64.1	Laboratory Results at Presentation in the Clinic	
Parameter (units)	Patient	Reference
WBC ($\times 10^9$/L)	12.3	4–10
Eosinophils ($\times 10^9$/L)	2.34	<0.5
Haemoglobin (mg/dL)	11.7	12–14
MCV (fL)	70	83–103
Platelets ($\times 10^9$/L)	330	150–350
ESR (mm/h)	20	≤10
IgE (U/mL)	944	<100
Creatinine (µmol/L)	62	<80
ALT (U/L)	28	<30
GGT (U/L)	35	<40
C-reactive protein (mg/L)	<5	<5

On examination, she is afebrile with no meningism and no focal neurological deficits. Her blood results reveal peripheral eosinophilia and elevated IgE levels. A CT scan of her brain done elsewhere showed no abnormalities.

Answer to Question 1

What is Your Presumptive Diagnosis?

The most likely diagnosis is a food-borne parasitic infection of the meninges. The key points from the history which support a food-borne infection are: (1) temporal relationship with travelling to north-east Thailand, where food-borne nematodes are prevalent; (2) consumption of traditional Thai food, including raw or undercooked freshwater fish, seafood, snails and frogs; and (3) the occurrence of similar symptoms in a relative who participated in the same meals (cluster).

Headache is a typical symptom of meningitis, therefore infestation of the meninges is very likely. The diagnosis of a parasitosis is strongly supported by the presence of considerable blood eosinophilia and elevated IgE levels in serum.

Answer to Question 2

Which Investigation Would You Perform to Substantiate Your Diagnosis?

Parasitic infection of the meninges typically results in eosinophilic meningitis. The next investigation to perform is a lumbar puncture to confirm meningitis and to look for a possibly eosinophilic profile of inflammation. Eosinophilic meningitis in an otherwise healthy person with positive history of exposure to helminths and features of an outbreak is almost always attributable to a parasitic infestation.

The main differential diagnoses are fungal meningitis with *Coccidioides immitis* (in North and Central America), lymphoma, eosinophilic leukaemia, sarcoid and idiopathic hypereosinophilic syndrome.

It is important to measure the CSF opening pressure. If it is elevated, serial spinal taps might relieve the symptoms.

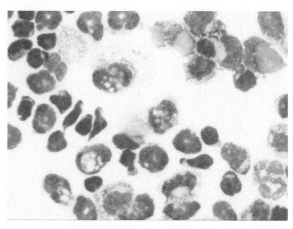

• **Fig. 64.1** Romanowski–Giemsa stain of the CSF sample revealing large numbers of eosinophils with red (eosinophilic) cytoplasm. (Courtesy Prof. Thomas Schneider)

The Case Continued...

A lumbar puncture was performed. The cerebrospinal fluid showed 1877 leukocytes/μL (reference value <5), with 42% eosinophils, 39% lymphocytes, 18% monocytes and 1% neutrophils (Fig. 64.1). CSF protein levels were elevated at 1.59 g/L (reference value <0.45), glucose was 1.85 mmol/L (reference range: 2.2–3.9).

On microscopic examination of the CSF, no larvae could be detected. Ziehl–Neelsen stain as well as cryptococcal antigen were negative. There were no suspected malignant cells. CSF culture did not yield any bacterial or fungal growth. Urine and stool microscopy did not show any ova of *Schistosoma* species. *Taenia solium* serology was negative, as were *Fasciola hepatica* and *Paragonimus* serologies. *Toxocara canis* serology was weakly positive but did not show any change of titre on follow-up. HIV serology was negative.

The initial CSF opening pressure was elevated, at 34 cmH$_2$O (reference range 12–20). Lumbar puncture relieved the patient's headache and was therefore repeated

TABLE 64.2	Main Causes and Characteristics of Parasitic Eosinophilic Meningitis				
Pathogen	Incubation Period	Source of Infection	Geography	Clinical Features	Serology
Angiostrongylus cantonensis	2–35 days	Consumption of infected crustaceans, snails, prawns, crabs, frogs, and/or contaminated vegetables	South-east Asia, Pacific basin, Australia, Caribbean	Paraesthesia of trunk, limbs, or face	Western blot of antibodies against 31 kD antigen*
Gnathostoma spinigerum	Days to months	Consumption of infected poultry or fish, snakes, frogs	South-east Asia (mainly Thailand), emerging in sub-Saharan Africa	Migrating subcutaneous swellings, creeping eruption, sharp radicular pain at onset	Western blot of antibodies against 24 kD antigen*

*Serology can be negative in acute state and a paired convalescence sample should be taken after 4 weeks.

twice, whereupon the patient felt markedly better. No further specific treatment was prescribed. She received iron tablets for a mild microcytic anaemia. The patient was discharged significantly improved after a 1-week hospital stay. After her discharge, serology results came back and Western Blot showed specific antibodies against 31kD *Angiostrongylus cantonensis* antigen. Since the patient hat no symptoms any more no further treatment was prescribed. At 4-week follow-up she had fully recovered and her peripheral eosinophil count had returned to normal.

SUMMARY BOX

Eosinophilic Meningitis

Eosinophilic meningitis is defined as the presence of ten or more eosinophils per microlitre of CSF, or eosinophilia of at least 10% of the total CSF leukocyte count. Invasion of the central nervous system by the food-borne nematodes *Angiostrongylus cantonensis,* and less frequently, *Gnathostoma spinigerum,* are the most common causes (Table 64.2). Rarely, neurocysticercosis, neuroschistosomiasis, paragonimiasis, fascioliasis, toxocariasis, baylisascariasis and trichinellosis can be associated with eosinophilic meningitis; however, the meningeal involvement is usually not prominent.

Angiostrongylus cantonensis, the rat lungworm, is the most common infectious cause of eosinophilic meningitis. Humans are infected by ingestion of *Angiostrongylus* larvae in intermediate hosts such as fresh water snails and slugs; or transport (paratenic) hosts, such as prawns, crabs and frogs; or salad and vegetables contaminated with slime of infected snails. Once ingested, the third stage larvae (L3) penetrate the intestinal wall, reach the portal vein and from there enter the systemic circulation. *A. cantonensis* is a truly neurotropic helminth. Humans are dead-end hosts, the larvae die in the human subarachnoid space, causing an eosinophilic inflammatory response.

To date, no standard of care treatment regimen for CNS angiostrongyliasis exists. Mild cases may be managed symptomatically with serial lumbar punctures and analgesics. More severe cases may be treated with corticosteroids alone or in combination with anthelmintic drugs. Corticosteroids (eg prednisolone 1 mg/kg/day) reduce the duration and intensity of headache. The use of antiparasitic drugs (eg albendazole) is controversial and the benefit of antipararasitic treatment compared to steroid use alone is marginal. If antiparasitic drugs are administered, they should be given with steroid cover.

Further Reading

1. Heckmann JE, Bhigjee AI. Tropical neurology. In: Farrar J, editor. Manson's Tropical Diseases. 23rd ed. London: Elsevier; 2013 [chapter 71].
2. Graeff-Teixeira C, da Silva AC, Yoshimura K. Update on eosinophilic meningoencephalitis and its clinical relevance. Clin Microbiol Rev 2009;22(2):322–48.
3. Wang QP, Lai DH, Zhu XQ, et al. Human angiostrongyliasis. Lancet Infect Dis 2008;8(10):621–30.
4. Martins YC, Tanowitz HB, Kazacos KR. Central nervous system manifestations of Angiostrongylus cantonensis infection. Acta Tropica 2015;141:46–53.
5. McAuliffe L, Ensign SF, Larson D, et al. Severe CNS angiostrongyliasis in a young marine: a case report and literature review. Lancet Infect Dis 2019;19:e132–42.

65

A 4-Year-Old Girl from Bolivia With a Dark Nodule on Her Toe

THOMAS WEITZEL

Clinical Presentation

History

A 4-year-old girl presents with a history of several days of a slowly growing nodule on the fifth toe of her right foot that is moderately painful when wearing shoes. The family moved from Chile to the Cochabamba region in Bolivia about 6 months ago, where they live on a farm. Her 9-year-old brother has similar lesions on two toes.

Clinical Findings

4-year-old girl in good general health. Close to the root of the fifth toenail of the right foot there is a dark-brown small nodule with a tiny central ulceration, surrounded by minimal inflammatory reaction (Fig. 65.1). The parents report that when they had tried to squeeze the lesion, they observed white oval granules emerging from the nodule.

Questions

1. How would you diagnose this disease?
2. How would you treat the patient?

Discussion

A 4-year-old girl who lives on a farm in Bolivia presents with a slowly growing nodular lesion on her toe. Her brother has similar lesions on his feet.

Answer to Question 1
How Would You Diagnose This Disease?

The macroscopic presentation and localization of this lesion allows the clinical diagnosis of tungiasis. Physicians who are not familiar with the disease might send a sample for microscopic confirmation. Fig. 65.2 shows parts of the parasite and an egg in a tissue sample. The female flea is usually destroyed during the process of removal, but parts of the body as well as eggs can still be found.

Answer to Question 2
How Would You Treat the Patient?

The parasite should be completely removed using a sterile needle and/or curette. The resulting round lesion must be disinfected and dressed. The patient's tetanus vaccination

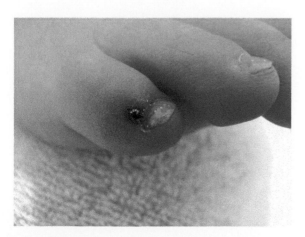

• **Fig. 65.1** Small nodule on the fifth toe of right foot. (Toenails with leftovers of glitter nail polish.)

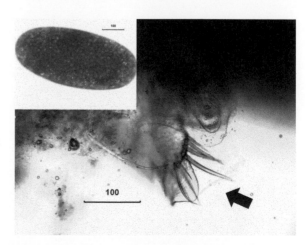

• **Fig. 65.2** Microscopic examination of removed tissue containing parts of female flea (arrow) and typical eggs (size 600 × 280 µm).

status should be checked and the wound should be observed; and if necessary, treated for superinfection.

The Case Continued...

The skin lesion healed within a week without complications.

SUMMARY BOX

Tungiasis

Tungiasis is caused by the female *Tunga penetrans* (syn. sand flea, jigger, bicho do pé), which burrows into the epidermis of humans and various animals before oviposition. There, the parasite engorges to a size of approximately 1 cm, causing a slowly growing nodular skin lesion. The flea is completely embedded into the skin, except for the tip of the posterior end, through which the respiration, defecation and oviposition occurs.

Typical localizations are the periungual regions of the feet, interdigital spaces and soles. However, other parts of the body might be affected after contact with contaminated soil.

Clinically, the flea together with the surrounding inflammatory reaction initially presents as a pale nodule with a dark centre; later the lesion might turn brown with a dark scab. It often causes local itching or pain. Symptoms are usually mild in patients visiting endemic areas and start after several days in cases of first infestation. Individuals living in endemic regions may suffer massive and repeated infestations leading to superinfection with complications such as gangrene, bacteraemia or tetanus.

The parasite is endemic in Latin America from Mexico to northern Argentina and the Caribbean. From there it was introduced into sub-Saharan Africa, probably around 150 years ago. Tungiasis belongs to the category of neglected and poverty-related infectious disease. In poor communities of endemic countries, constant re-infection causes severe morbidity including deformation and permanent disability. Important zoonotic reservoirs for human infections include pigs, dogs and rats. In travellers, tungiasis is found in about 1% of those presenting with dermatological problems.

The diagnosis is usually based on the clinical presentation. In non-endemic regions, the parasite and its eggs may be demonstrated in tissue samples and histopathological sections. Treatment consists of removing the flea with a sterile needle or curette with or without local anaesthesia, disinfection and prevention or treatment of concomitant bacterial infections.

To prevent the disease, contact with contaminated sand or soil should be avoided, e.g. by using solid footwear. The effect of commonly used repellents has not been studied. Another strategy is to daily inspect the feet and extract sand fleas at an early stage of penetration.

Further Reading

1. Vega-Lopez F, Ritchie S. Dermatological problems. In: Farrar J, editor. Manson's Tropical Diseases. 23rd ed. London: Elsevier; 2013 [chapter 68].
2. Mumcuoglu KY. Other ectoparasites: leeches, myiasis and sand fleas. In: Farrar J, editor. Manson's Tropical Diseases. 23rd ed. London: Elsevier; 2013 [chapter 60].
3. Feldmeier H, Keysers A. Tungiasis - A Janus-faced parasitic skin disease. Travel Med Infect Dis 2013;11:357–65.
4. Heukelbach J. Revision on tungiasis: treatment options and prevention. Expert Rev Anti Infect Ther 2006;4(1):151–7.
5. Walker SL, Lebas E, De Sario V, et al. The prevalence and association with health-related quality of life of tungiasis and scabies in schoolchildren in southern Ethiopia. PLoS Negl Top Dis 2017; 11(8):e0005808.

66

A 32-Year-Old Man from Malawi With Pain in the Right Upper Abdomen and a Feeling of Faintness

ANTHONY D. HARRIES

Clinical Presentation

History

A 32-year-old man from Malawi presents to a local hospital with a history of pain in his right upper abdomen and a feeling of faintness, especially when standing up and walking. He was well until 1 month previously, when he began to experience a feeling of fullness in his upper abdomen. In the week before admission he developed pain in the right upper abdomen that was particularly apparent when sleeping on his right side. He has recently started to feel breathless on lying down and feels faint, especially on standing up. His past medical history is unremarkable, except for an episode of a blistering and painful skin lesion 3 years previously that affected the right side of his abdomen around the level of the umbilicus – this had healed spontaneously after several weeks.

Clinical Findings

He is thin and slightly breathless in the supine position. His pulse is regular at 130 bpm with pronounced pulsus paradoxus measured at 15 mmHg. Blood pressure in the supine position is 90/60 mm Hg. The jugular venous pulse is difficult to visualize but appears elevated. The apex beat is impalpable. The heart sounds are quiet but audible; no triple rhythm and no heart murmurs are heard. Auscultation of the chest is normal. There is an enlarged tender palpable liver measured at 8 cm below the right costal junction and evidence of mild peripheral oedema of the legs and sacral area.

Laboratory Results

Haemoglobin 10.5 g/dL; WBC 9.8 G/L (4–10). Chest radiography shows an enlarged globular heart with clear lung fields (see Fig. 66.1).

Questions

1. Based on the clinical history, examination and investigations done, what is the most likely pathology to explain this man's illness and what would be the most frequent cause of the problem?
2. What other investigations should be carried out? Outline the immediate and long-term management of his condition.

Discussion

This young African man presents with a history of right upper abdominal pain, breathlessness and syncope. On physical examination, he has signs of cardiac decompensation associated with right heart failure. It is likely that his skin lesion 3 years previously was herpes zoster.

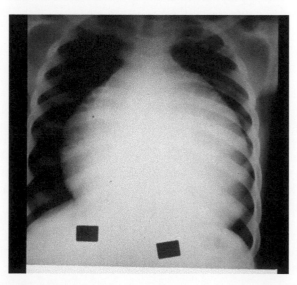

• **Fig. 66.1** Chest radiograph of the patient showing an enlarged globular cardiac silhouette with clear lung fields.

Answer to Question 1

What is the Most Likely Pathology to Explain This Man's Illness and What Would be the Most Frequent Cause of the Problem?

The history, physical examination and chest radiograph findings all point to a diagnosis of pericardial tamponade caused by a large pericardial effusion. The cardiovascular manifestations of tachycardia, pulsus paradoxus, hypotension, impalpable apex beat, raised jugular venous pressure and quiet heart sounds are indicative of pericardial effusion. The presence of syncope, pulsus paradoxus and hypotension are signs of cardiac tamponade indicating the need for a therapeutic pericardial aspiration. In Africa there are several causes of pericardial effusion that include tuberculosis, other bacterial infections, malignancy and HIV-related Kaposi's sarcoma. The presence of a previous attack of herpes zoster is a strong pointer to HIV infection, and in this case the most likely diagnosis is HIV-associated tuberculosis.

Answer to Question 2

What Other Investigations Should be Carried Out? Outline the Immediate and Long-Term Management of His Condition.

The most important investigation that should be carried out immediately is an ultrasound of the heart, which should show the presence of pericardial fluid and sometimes fibrous strands that are strongly suggestive of tuberculosis, especially in highly endemic areas. An electrocardiogram is useful in showing low-voltage QRS complexes and in occasional cases there may be electrical alternans. If there is pericardial fluid on ultrasound, the patient requires a therapeutic pericardial aspiration to relieve the pressure on the heart and restore cardiac output. Once fluid is aspirated and the cardiac output is restored, the patient should be started on antituberculous treatment and corticosteroids. An HIV test should be carried out with appropriate counselling, and consideration given to starting antiretroviral therapy after a few weeks if the HIV test is positive.

The Case Continued...

The patient underwent therapeutic pericardial aspiration and 500 mL of bloodstained pericardial fluid were aspirated. The blood pressure increased to 120/80 mmHg almost immediately. The patient was started on standard first-line antituberculous treatment with rifampicin (R), isoniazid (H), pyrazinamide (Z) and ethambutol (E) and also on prednisolone at a dose of 60 mg daily. HIV testing was carried out and the patient was found to be HIV positive.

The patient received a full 6-month course of antituberculous treatment consisting of a 2-month initial phase of four drugs given daily (2RHZE) and a 4-month continuation phase of two drugs given daily (4RH), prednisolone in tapered doses for ten weeks, and antiretroviral therapy which was started at 4 weeks after commencing antituberculous treatment. He made a full and uneventful recovery.

SUMMARY BOX

Tuberculosis

In Africa the most common cause of pericardial effusion is tuberculosis; and even if there is no confirmatory evidence of tuberculosis, patients must be treated with a full course of antituberculosis treatment. In countries in central and southern Africa there is a strong association between tuberculosis and HIV infection, with over 50 per cent of tuberculosis patients being HIV positive. The advent of the HIV/AIDS epidemic in Africa was associated with a large increase in the number of patients being diagnosed with tuberculosis pericardial effusion. Once in HIV-positive patients not yet on ART, a diagnosis of pericardial effusion is made, it is important to determine whether tamponade is present, with the characteristic features being syncope, tachycardia, pulsus paradoxus and hypotension. The presence of tamponade is potentially life-threatening and requires prompt pericardial aspiration. Diagnostic pericardial aspiration is usually unhelpful in the district hospital setting, because the fluid is often bloodstained and acid-fast bacilli are rarely visualized in smears of the pericardial aspirate from patients who have tuberculosis. If pericardial fluid is available for investigation, this can be examined with higher diagnostic sensitivity using the Xpert MTB/RIF assay (Cepheid, Sunnyvale, CA, USA) – a fully automated and commercially available cartridge-based nucleic acid amplification test – which allows a confirmed diagnosis of TB within 2 hours. The use of corticosteroids is recommended, especially if there is tamponade. In HIV-negative patients and HIV-positive patients on antiretroviral therapy, randomized controlled trials have shown that corticosteroids may reduce the risk of death. For HIV-positive patients not on antiretroviral drugs, corticosteroids may reduce pericardial constriction. A commonly used regimen is prednisolone administered in tapering doses during the first ten weeks of antituberculous treatment. WHO guidelines recommend that antiretroviral therapy is started within 2 to 8 weeks of the start of antituberculosis treatment. Timely antiretroviral therapy reduces mortality, is associated with excellent immunological and virological responses and reduces the risk of recurrent tuberculosis.

Further Reading

1. Thwaites G. Tuberculosis. In: Farrar J, editor. Manson's Tropical Diseases. 23rd ed. London: Elsevier; 2013 [chapter 40].
2. Mayosi BM, Wiysonge CS, Ntsekhe M, et al. Mortality in patients treated for tuberculous pericarditis in sub-Saharan Africa. S Afr Med J 2008;98:36–40.
3. George IA, Thomas B, Sadhu JS. Systematic review and meta-analysis of adjunctive corticosteroids in the treatment of tuberculous pericarditis. Int J Tuberc Lung Dis 2018;22(5):551–6.
4. Wiysonge CS, Ntsekhe M, Thabane L, et al. Interventions for treating tuberculous pericarditis. Cochrane Database Syst Rev 2017;9: CD000526.

67

A 24-Year-Old Woman from the Peruvian Andes With Fever and Abdominal Pain

FÁTIMA CONCHA VELASCO AND EDUARDO H. GOTUZZO

Clinical Presentation

History

A 24-year-old woman from the highlands of Peru is transferred to a hospital in the capital, Lima, with a 2-month history of upper abdominal pain, weight loss (5 kg), nausea and vomiting. She tried analgesics, which did not control the pain. She also reports intermittent fevers for the past 2 weeks.

Three days previously, she was seen at the emergency room of the same hospital for the above-mentioned complaints. Abdominal ultrasound revealed multiple hypoechoic lesions in her liver. She was treated with ceftriaxone and metronidazole for suspected pyogenic liver abscesses but did not show any clinical improvement.

The patient reported that about 2 to 3 months ago she started taking over-the-counter medicines to lose weight and changed her diet to vegetarian food. She also reported the consumption of energetic hot drinks made from alfalfa and watercress. Prior to her current illness, she was healthy. She is single and has no children.

Clinical Findings

The patient looks ill, with pale mucous membranes but no jaundice. Her blood pressure is 95/60 mmHg, pulse 105 bpm and temperature 38.5°C (101.3°F). On palpation of the abdomen there is right upper quadrant tenderness, and the liver is slightly enlarged with a liver span of 15 cm. The rest of the physical examination is normal.

Laboratory Results

Table 67.1 shows the patient's laboratory results, taken in the emergency room.

Imaging

A contrast-enhanced CT scan of her abdomen shows multiple hypodense, non-enhancing lesions in the liver (Fig. 67.1).

Questions

1. What are your differential diagnoses?
2. What would be the most useful investigation to establish the diagnosis?

Discussion

A young woman from the Peruvian Andes presents with a history of fever, weight loss and abdominal pain. The blood count reveals pronounced eosinophilia. The abdominal CT scan shows hypodense non-enhancing hepatic lesions.

TABLE 67.1 Laboratory Results on Admission to Emergency Room

Parameter	Patient	Reference Range
WBC ($\times 10^9$/L)	13.94	4–10
Eosinophils (%)	43	<5
Total eosinophil count	5.97	<0.5
Haemoglobin (g/dL)	12.3	12–16
AST (U/L)	34	10–40
ALT (U/L)	55	7–40
AP (U/L)	170	20–126
Amylase (U/L)	75	3–100
Lipase (U/L)	100	10–140

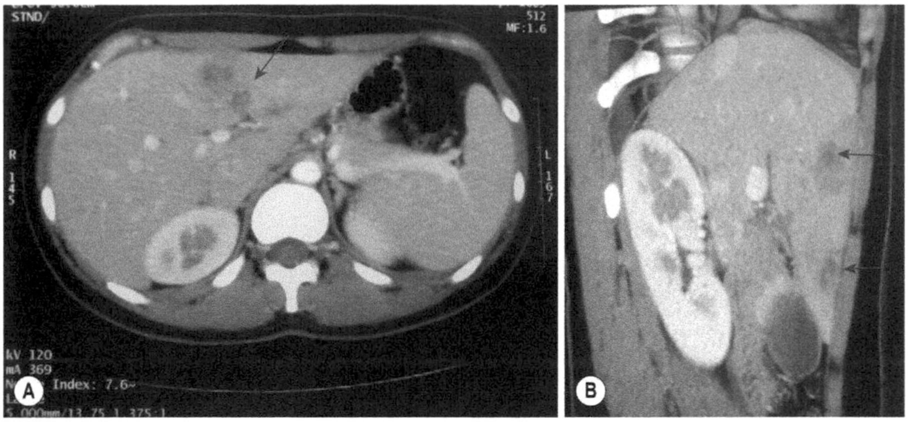

• **Fig. 67.1** A contrast-enhanced CT scan showing multiple, round, clustered, hypodense lesions in left median section of liver (A, axial cross-section; B, lateral view).

Answer to Question 1

What Are Your Differential Diagnoses?

The patient was first treated for suspected pyogenic liver abscesses based upon the presence of fever, right upper abdominal pain and hypoechoic liver lesions on ultrasound.

However, the lack of any improvement after 3 days of appropriate treatment makes this diagnosis less likely.

In a patient from the Andes with high eosinophilia and a known history of alfalfa and watercress consumption, fascioliasis is the most important diagnosis to consider. Amoebic liver abscess is also part of the differential diagnosis, but eosinophilia and the presence of multiple lesions are not typical. Also, the infection is uncommon in young women and should respond to metronidazole treatment.

Other endemic infections in Peru that could present with similar symptoms are brucellosis, visceral toxocariasis or secondary infections in the context of other infections (i.e. ascariasis and hydatid disease). *Opisthorchis,* another liver fluke, could be considered if the patient had a travel history to South-east Asia, as the condition is not present in the Americas.

Answer to Question 2

What Would Be the Most Useful Investigation to Establish the Diagnosis?

Infection with the sheep liver fluke (*Fasciola hepatica*) is top of the list of differential diagnoses in this patient with liver lesions, eosinophilia and a history of watercress consumption.

Because ova appear in the stool only later in the course of the disease, serology is the diagnostic tool of choice. The Fas2 ELISA is a serological method with good sensitivity and specificity to diagnose the acute phase of *F. hepatica* infection.

Liver biopsy is invasive and has little benefit in this context; it could be considered if tests are negative and all treatments fail.

The Case Continued...

The Fas2 ELISA titre was 0.56 (normal <0.2), supporting the suspected diagnosis of fascioliasis. The patient received one single dose of triclabendazole 10 mg/kg. Her clinical symptoms rapidly improved and her laboratory parameters went back to normal. On control tomography her liver lesions were seen to be disappearing.

SUMMARY BOX

Fascioliasis

Fascioliasis is caused by the liver flukes *Fasciola hepatica* or less frequently *F. gigantica*. Fascioliasis has the widest latitudinal, longitudinal and altitudinal distribution of any known zoonotic diseases. It is a serious public health problem, with between 2.4 and 17 million infected people worldwide and around 90 million at risk. In South America, the infection is encountered in the Andean countries, in particular in Bolivia and Peru. Egypt is another country with a very high prevalence of fascioliasis.

Ova of *Fasciola* species are shed in the faeces of herbivores. Once they reach fresh water, miracidia hatch and infect a snail which acts as an intermediate host. Additional development takes place inside the snail, then cercariae are released into the water. They develop into infective encysted metacercariae on freshwater plants. Humans acquire the disease by eating watercress (salads) or drinking water contaminated with metacercariae.

The illness includes four clinical phases: (1) incubation phase, (2) invasive or acute phase, (3) latent phase and (4) obstructive or chronic phase. The incubation phase lasts from ingestion of metacercariae to first symptoms (6–12 weeks). The invasive or acute phase begins with flukes migrating through the small intestinal wall, the peritoneal cavity, the liver capsule and the liver parenchyma.

During the acute phase, lasting 3 to 5 months, the patients typically present with intermittent fever, abdominal pain, malaise, weight loss, urticaria and respiratory symptoms (e.g. cough, dyspnoea and chest pain). Less common findings include changes in bowel habits, nausea, anorexia, hepatomegaly, splenomegaly, ascites, anaemia and jaundice. Eosinophilia is almost always present during the acute phase.

At the beginning of the subsequent latent phase the parasites have crossed the liver parenchyma to finally reach the common bile duct, where they mature and start depositing eggs. Ova appear in the stool 3 to 4 months after the ingestion of infective metacercariae. The latent phase is characterized by the progressive resolution of gastrointestinal and respiratory symptoms. An unknown percentage of patients will progress to the fourth phase of the disease characterized by biliary obstruction, cholelithiasis, ascending cholangitis, cholecystitis, or liver abscess. Haemorrhage (e.g. subcapsular haematomas), hepatic fibrosis or biliary cirrhosis might also be observed.

During the acute phase, diagnosis of human fascioliasis is based on clinical and radiological findings and immunodiagnostic assays such as the Fas2-ELISA. Eosinophilia is usually present.

During chronic infection, eosinophilia is rare but ova can be detected on stool microscopy. The yield can be improved using rapid sedimentation techniques. Microscopic detection of eggs is considered definitive diagnosis of fascioliasis. Eggs may also accidentally be discovered during surgery for biliary obstruction.

Typical lesions seen on CT scan are contrast-enhancement of the Glisson's capsule, and multiple hypodense nodular lesions.

Triclabendazole is the anthelmintic drug of choice. In acute cases a single dose of triclabendazole at 10 mg/kg is effective in almost 90% of cases and the same regimen is used in chronic disease. Triclabendazole should be taken with food to increase its bioavailability. Triclabendazole resistance seems to be an emerging problem.

Further Reading

1. Sithithaworn P, Sripa B, Kaewkes S, et al. Food-borne trematodes. In: Farrar J, editor. Manson's Tropical Diseases. 23rd ed. London: Elsevier; 2013 [chapter 53].
2. Marcos LA, Tagle M, Terashima A, et al. Natural history, clinicoradiologic correlates, and response to triclabendazole in acute massive fascioliasis. Am J Trop Med Hyg 2008;78(2):222–7.
3. Webb CM, Cabada MM. Recent developments in the epidemiology, diagnosis, and treatment of Fasciola infection. Curr Opin Infect Dis 2018;31(5):409–14.
4. Carmona C, Tort JF. Fasciolosis in South America: epidemiology and control challenges. J Helminthol 2017;91(2):99–109.
5. Kelley JM, Elliott TP, Beddoe T, et al. Current threat of triclabendazole resistance in fasciola hepatica. Trends Parasitol 2016;32(6): 458–69.

68

A 31-Year-Old Woman from Malawi With a Generalized Mucocutaneous Rash

CAMILLA ROTHE

Clinical Presentation

History

A 31-year-old woman presents to a hospital in Malawi with a generalized skin rash. The rash started 3 days before on the trunk, and then spread to the extremities and the mucosal membranes involving lips, oral mucosa, conjunctivae and genital mucosa.

There is also a productive cough with whitish sputum that started 1 day before the rash appeared, and she also reports a sore throat and dysuria for the past 2 days.

The patient had been found to be HIV positive 2 months earlier, when she was hospitalized with cryptococcal meningitis. She was treated with high-dose oral fluconazole, because amphotericin B and flucytosine were unavailable. She improved and was discharged home on a maintenance dose of fluconazole. Antiretroviral treatment with stavudine (d4T), lamivudine (3TC) and nevirapine (NVP), as well as co-trimoxazole prophylaxis, were started 1 month previously.

The rest of the medical history is unremarkable and there are no known allergies.

Clinical Findings

Her temperature is 37.7°C (99.9°F), blood pressure 120/68 mmHg, pulse 90 bpm and respiratory rate 24 breath cycles per minute. There is a generalized, non-itchy maculo-papular rash involving the skin and mucous membranes but sparing the palms and soles. There is bilateral conjunctivitis. The eyelids and lips are covered with haemorrhagic crusts (Fig. 68.1). The lips are swollen and she can hardly open her mouth; talking and eating are difficult and painful. The chest is clear.

Questions

1. What is the most likely diagnosis and what is it caused by?
2. How would you approach the patient?

Discussion

A young Malawian woman presents with a generalized rash involving her skin and mucous membranes. She also complains of a productive cough of short duration, dysuria and dysphagia.

The patient is HIV positive. Within the past month she commenced treatment with co-trimoxazole and an

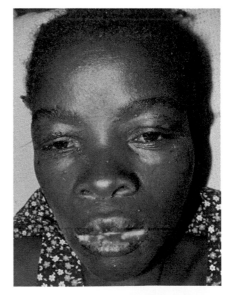

• **Fig. 68.1** The face of the patient, showing bilateral swelling of the eyes with conjunctivitis and swollen lips with haemorrhagic crusts. The maculopapular rash was non-itchy and spared the scalp.

antiretroviral triple therapy with d4T, 3TC and NVP. She has a low-grade fever, but her chest is clear.

Answer to Question 1

What is the Most Likely Diagnosis and What is It Caused By?

The most important diagnosis to consider is Stevens–Johnson syndrome (SJS)/toxic epidermal necrolysis. This potentially life-threatening mucocutaneous hypersensitivity reaction is most commonly caused by drugs. Its incidence is much higher in HIV-positive than in HIV-negative patients. If SJS involves more than 30% of the skin surface, it is called toxic epidermal necrolysis (TEN). SJS/TEN may lead to widespread epidermal detachment and erosions of the mucous membranes. Non-specific prodromal symptoms such as cough, sore throat, fever, headache and myalgias usually precede the rash by several days and may be mistaken for a bacterial or viral infection, or for malaria in a tropical setting.

Answer to Question 2

How Would You Approach the Patient?

SJS/TEN is a clinical diagnosis. Once suspected, all potentially causative drugs should be immediately withdrawn. If in doubt, all drugs need to be stopped. In general, medications initiated 2 to 4 weeks prior to the onset of symptoms are usually responsible. In this patient's case, the major culprit drugs were nevirapine and co-trimoxazole.

The patient at this stage only had a maculopapular rash. However, patients with SJS/TEN often develop large bullous skin lesions. Once they break open, this leads to considerable loss of serous fluid, similar to a burn. Therefore, patients with SJS/TEN ideally should be managed in a burns unit. Topical antiseptics will reduce skin colonization; however, wound debridement is not recommended. Steroid eye drops should be given in case of conjunctivitis, and early ophthalmological review should be sought to prevent conjunctival scarring and blindness. Patients need careful management of fluids and electrolytes and high caloric nutrition. A nasogastric (NG) tube is often helpful until the mucosal lesions have healed. Fever may be part of the clinical picture and there is no role for prophylactic antibiotics unless there are signs of sepsis. Vital signs need to be checked regularly, and blood cultures and full blood count taken repeatedly.

A urinary catheter should be inserted to prevent urethral strictures. Skin and mucosal lesions in SJS/TEN are very painful. Often, opioids are necessary to control the pain.

Upon discharge, patients should be urged to avoid the culprit drug and this should be clearly stated in the patient's documents.

The Case Continued...

Antiretroviral drugs and co-trimoxazole were stopped on admission. Because the patient was febrile, blood cultures and a rapid malaria test were taken and both came back negative. She received IV fluids and a urinary catheter. The

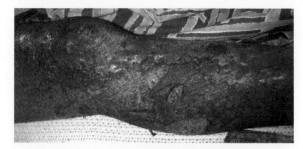

• **Fig. 68.2** The right leg of another patient with SJS/TEN showing extensive epidermal sloughing and large areas of denuded dermis.

patient and her family declined an NG tube, because they had observed that patients who had an NG tube or oxygen probes were more likely to die than patients who did not have such devices.

The patient was given 0.9% normal saline as mouthwash and dexamethasone eye ointment. Fever and cough settled spontaneously. She was discharged after 10 days in hospital.

When all lesions had completely healed, she was started on a new antiretroviral combination therapy and nevirapine was replaced by efavirenz. Co-trimoxazole was not replaced because there were no alternative drugs available. The new drug combination was tolerated well and no further rash occurred.

SUMMARY BOX

Stevens–Johnson Syndrome and Toxic Epidermal Necrolysis

SJS is a life-threatening mucocutaneous hypersensitivity reaction. It is most commonly caused by drugs. In SJS, less than 10% of the total body surface is involved. If more than 30% is affected, it is called toxic epidermal necrolysis (TEN). Between 10% and 30% it is classified as 'SJS/TEN overlap'. The extent of skin involvement is a major determinant for prognosis.

In Western industrialized countries, SJS/TEN is considered rare, with an estimated incidence of 1 to 7 per million per year. However, it is about 1000 times more common in HIV-positive individuals, and clinicians working in sub-Saharan Africa and other high-prevalence settings need to be aware of this condition.

The drugs most commonly implicated in SJS/TEN are antibiotics (in particular sulfonamides, but also other classes), the antiretroviral nevirapine, anticonvulsants and allopurinol.

Infectious agents (e.g. *Mycoplasma pneumoniae* and HSV) may also be responsible. Host genetic factors also seem to play a role.

The pathophysiology is yet to be fully elucidated. Because of an unknown mechanism there is widespread apoptosis of keratinocytes and subsequent epithelial necrosis.

SJS/TEN often starts with non-specific, flu-like symptoms. After several days a morbiliform rash sets in that becomes more and more confluent. The epidermis may slough, giving rise to flaccid bullae, leaving a characteristic denuded dermis (Fig. 68.2), which causes intense pain. Conjunctivitis is common and may lead to scarring and blindness. Involvement of the oral mucosa and haemorrhagic crusting of the lips make it difficult for the patient to eat, drink and talk. Involvement of the urogenital mucosa is very painful and may lead to urethral strictures. The oesophagus and trachea may also be affected.

Diagnosis can often be made clinically. Skin biopsies may help rule out the major differential diagnoses such as staphylococcal scalded skin syndrome, toxic shock syndrome, exfoliative dermatitis, autoimmune bullous diseases and acute paraneoplastic pemphigus.

All potentially causative drugs need to be withdrawn immediately. Treatment is supportive and there is no clear benefit of any other disease-modifying interventions. Systemic corticosteroids do not seem helpful and the use of IV immunoglobulins is disputed. However, data from large controlled clinical trials are lacking.

According to literature from the developed world, the case fatality rate of patients with SJS is up to 5%; in TEN it is 30% on average. Primary causes of death are infection and multi-organ failure.

A severity-of-illness score (SCORTEN) has been published to predict the lethality of patients with SJS/TEN. Its use in resource-constrained setting is limited, because it requires laboratory results (urea, bicarbonate, glucose) that may be difficult to obtain.

Further Reading

1. Gerull R, Nelle M, Schaible T. Toxic epidermal necrolysis and Stevens–Johnson syndrome: a review. Crit Care Med 2011;39(6): 1521–32.
2. Duong TA, Valeyrie-Allanore L, Wolkenstein P, Chosidow O. Severe cutaneous adverse reactions to drugs. Lancet 2017;390: 1996–2011.
3. Hoosen K, Mosam A, Dlova NC, Grayson W. An update on adverse cutaneous drug reactions in HIV/AIDS. Dermatopathology 2019;6:111–25.
4. Hazin R, Ibrahimi OA, Hazin MI, et al. Stevens–Johnson syndrome: pathogenesis, diagnosis, and management. Ann Med 2008; 40(2):129–38.
5. Schulze Schwering M, Kayange P, Rothe C. Ocular manifestations in patients with Stevens-Johnson syndrome in Malawi – a review of the literature illustrated by clinical cases. Graefes Arch Clin Exp Ophthalmol 2019;257(11):2343–8.

69

A 22-Year-Old Male Farmer from Rural Ethiopia With Difficulty Walking

YOHANNES W. WOLDEAMANUEL

Clinical Presentation

History

A 22-year-old male farmer from rural northern Ethiopia presents to a hospital in the capital with difficulty walking.

His problem started 10 years ago, when he woke from sleep one morning and noticed weakness in both legs. There was no history of trauma and no prodromal symptoms; he had been in excellent health before. The weakness in his legs rapidly progressed over 4 to 5 days, leading to him needing a cane for mobility. He had no back pain, sensory complaints, sphincter disturbance or upper limb symptoms.

The start of his illness coincided with a period of drought and famine, when his diet almost exclusively consisted of grass peas (*Lathyrus sativus,* local name *guaya*), which is known to be drought-resistant (Fig. 69.1). Despite the monotonous diet, he had been engaged in hard physical labour on his family farm, where he was the main breadwinner, despite his young age. He lived with his mother and three sisters, who took care of household chores; they consumed a similar diet but of overall smaller amounts of *guaya*.

During that time, several similar cases of weakness among young male farmers occurred in his village. His walking difficulty finally meant that he could not return to farm work.

At the age of 20, he moved to the capital city seeking an alternative job. He migrated along with another young male farmer from his village who had suffered a similar fate; he had weakness of both legs and arms, which he had developed during the same period of drought. There was no history of cassava exposure in the region.

Clinical Findings

An alert young man with a normal mental state. The gait is spastic ('scissor gait'), with foot-dragging and toe-scraping (Fig. 69.2). There is mild bilateral lower limb spastic weakness of pyramidal pattern, with pathological brisk deep tendon reflexes and sustained foot clonus. Extensor plantar response is elicited on the right, while equivocal on the left. Cranial nerves and upper limbs are normal. There is no sensory or bladder dysfunction.

Laboratory Results

Full blood count, liver and renal function tests, cerebrospinal fluid, nerve conduction studies and electromyography are normal. His HIV-1 serology is non-reactive. HTLV-1 and -2 serology and MRI are not available.

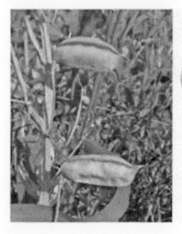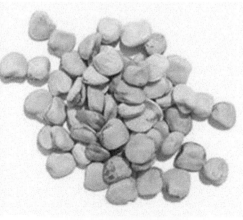

• **Fig. 69.1** *Lathyrus sativus* (local name *guaya*) grass pea plant and its leguminous seeds.

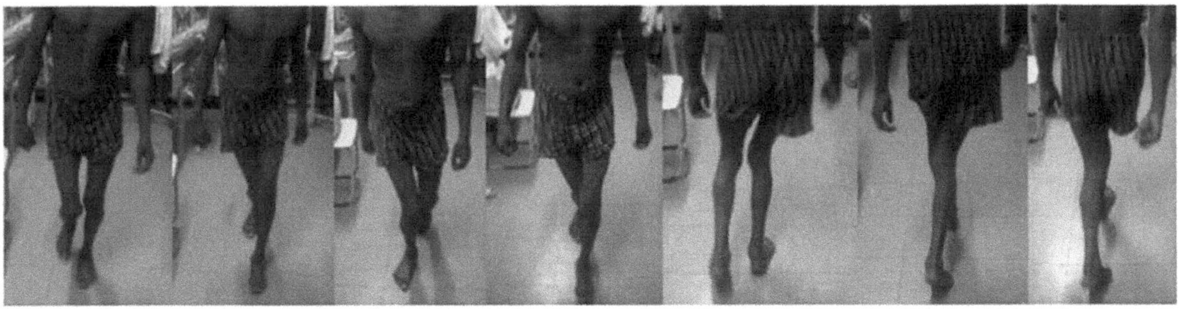

• **Fig. 69.2** Images demonstrating the patient's gait: paraplegic narrow-based 'scissor gait' with foot-dragging, and toe-scraping.

Questions

1. What clinical syndrome can you apply for a diagnostic approach and how do you narrow down your differential diagnoses?
2. What management and disease prevention plans can be used?

Discussion

A male, teenage farmer from rural northern Ethiopia develops irreversible spastic paraparesis. The onset of symptoms coincides with a period of drought when diet mainly consists of grass peas. There is no sensory deficit and no bladder dysfunction. Another young male farmer from the same village is similarly affected.

Answer to Question 1

What Clinical Syndrome Can You Apply for a Diagnostic Approach and How Do You Narrow Down Possible Differential Diagnoses?

Upper motor neuron lesion with spastic paraparesis is the clinical syndrome. Absence of radicular symptoms, sensory level, sphincter disturbance, back pain, non-progression, HIV-seronegativity and negative family history rule out most compressive, hereditary, infectious and metabolic myelopathies.

Among tropical myelopathies, HTLV-associated myelopathy (HAM) is highly unlikely. HAM has usually an insidious onset and a slowly progressive course, bladder impairment and sensory symptoms are prominent. Neurocassavism (konzo) may also present with a sudden-onset spastic paraparesis but is improbable in the absence of cassava exposure. Male gender, pre-onset physical exertion, excessive prolonged *guaya* consumption and a history of similarly affected village members favour a distinct form of toxico-nutritional disease called neurolathyrism.

Answer to Question 2

What Management and Disease Prevention Plans Can be Employed?

Neurolathyrism is a preventable neurotoxic myelopathy leading to permanent disability. Treatment is symptomatic with anti-spastic drugs and physiotherapy. Tendon and muscle release surgery can be employed to lengthen contractures of calf muscles and hip adductors. Walking canes, foot braces and wheelchairs need to be provided.

Education to avoid consumption of *L. sativus* and measures to reduce toxin burden are important public health interventions. New cases of this preventable disease continue to occur. Behaviour change communication among high-risk communities can promote positive practices to reduce toxin exposure. Such practices include the use of metallic cooking utensils rather than traditional clay pots to avoid accrued toxicity from iron-induced oxidation, addition of antioxidant seasonings, soaking seeds in lemon water and avoiding unripe seeds.

The Case Continued…

The patient received physiotherapy and muscle relaxants; however, this achieved only mild short-lasting improvement of his spasticity. A walking cane and wheelchair were provided. The patient was counselled to avoid further consumption of *L. sativus*.

SUMMARY BOX

Neurolathyrism

Neurolathyrism is a preventable toxic myelopathy caused by excessive ingestion of the *Lathyrus sativus* grass pea. Clinical presentation is an irreversible acute to subacute spastic paraparesis or quadriparesis without prominent sensory involvement. Bladder and bowel function are maintained.

L. sativus is a hardy, high-yield pest- and insect-resistant cash crop that can endure monsoon, drought or water-logging. It has been consumed in ancient Egypt, Europe, South Asia and in the northern highlands of Ethiopia. Currently more than 100 million people in drought- and monsoon-prone areas use *L. sativus* as staple crop. Being a multipurpose legume, it makes a protein-rich, filling diet. It is an 'almost perfect' crop, were it not for causing disability. *L. sativus* contains the neurotoxin β-N-oxalyl-a,b-diaminoproprionic acid (β-ODAP), a glutamate receptor agonist that results in excitotoxicity.

Toxicity is dose-dependent, and risk factors are prolonged heavy ingestion of grass peas, malnutrition, physical exertion, concurrent illness, illiteracy, male gender and young age.

Onset occurs within 3 to 6 months of monotonous excessive grass pea consumption. Weakness that develops suddenly or on waking from sleep is a classical presentation. Stage 1 neurolathyrism presents with spastic gait and independent mobility; Stage 2 is requiring a cane for mobility; Stage 3 is requiring a crutch; Stage 4 is characterized by the inability to bear weight with resultant contractures.

By virtue of affecting young breadwinners of rural families, neurolathyrism poses a high economic burden on poor communities in a setting where no social services or disability pensions are available.

Further Reading

1. Aronson JK. Plant poisons and traditional medicines. In: Farrar J, editor. Manson's Tropical Diseases. 23rd ed. London: Elsevier; 2013 [chapter 76].

2. Woldeamanuel YW, Hassan A, Zenebe G. Neurolathyrism: two Ethiopian case reports and review of the literature. J Neurol 2012;259(7):1263–8.

3. Tekle Haimanot R, Feleke A, Lambein F. Is lathyrism still endemic in northern Ethiopia? – The case of Legambo Woreda (district) in the South Wollo Zone, Amhara National Regional State. Ethiop J Health Dev 2005;19(3):230–6.

4. Bick AS, Meiner Z, Gotkine M, Levin N. Using advanced imaging methods to study neurolathyrism. Isr Med Assoc J 2016;18(6):341–5.

5. Lambein F, Travella S, Kuo YH. Grass pea (*Lathyrus sativus* L.): orphan crop, neutraceutical or just plain food? Planta 2019;250:821–38.

70

A 58-Year-Old Woman from Sri Lanka With Fever, Deafness and Confusion

RANJAN PREMARATNA

Clinical Presentation

History

A 58-year-old Sri Lankan woman who resides in a rural area presents to a local hospital with high-grade fever, chills, body aches, non-productive cough and progressive shortness of breath for 10 days. Two days previously she developed tinnitus and hearing loss. One day prior to admission she became increasingly confused.

Clinical Findings

On admission the patient is confused, with a Glasgow Coma Scale score of 13/15 (E4 V4 M5). Her hearing is severely impaired (WHO grade 3). Temperature 39.3°C (102.7°F), heart rate 120 bpm, blood pressure 90/60 mmHg. There are enlarged axillary lymph nodes on the right side. There is no rash and no neck stiffness; Kernig's and Brudzinski's signs are negative. Scattered crackles are audible on auscultation over the bases of both lungs. Her liver is enlarged to 5 cm below the right costal margin and the spleen is just palpable.

Laboratory Findings

Her basic laboratory results on admission are shown in Table 70.1; her cerebrospinal fluid results are shown in Table 70.2.

Her blood cultures grow no organisms; *Leptospira* and *Salmonella* serologies are negative. *Leptospira*-PCR is not available. A thick film for malaria parasites is negative as well.

Further Investigations

Chest radiography does not show any pathological changes. Her ECG shows sinus tachycardia. The EEG reveals widespread slowing; the CT scan of the brain is normal.

TABLE 70.1 Laboratory Results on Admission

Parameter	Patient	Reference
WBC ($\times 10^9$/L)	8.5	4–10
Haemoglobin (g/dL)	12.4	12–16
Platelets ($\times 10^9$/L)	98	150–350
AST (U/L)	74	13–33
ALT (U/L)	68	3–25
ALP (U/L)	126	40–130
Total bilirubin (µmol/L)	25.7	13.7–30.8
Blood urea nitrogen (mmol/L)	6.4	2.5–6.4
Creatinine (µmol/L)	123.8	71–106
C-reactive protein (mg/L)	48	<6

TABLE 70.2 Cerebrospinal Fluid Results on Admission

Parameter	Patient	Reference
Leukocytes (cells/µL)	35 (80% lymphocytes)	0–5/µL
Protein (g/L)	0.64	0.15–0.45
Glucose (mmol/L)	3.25*	50–75% of serum glucose

*Paired random blood glucose 7.17 mmol/L.

Questions

1. What clinical sign will you be specifically looking for?
2. What antibiotic would you include in your empirical regimen?

Discussion

A 58-year-old woman who is a rural resident of Sri Lanka presents in a septic state with confusion and hearing loss. On examination there is a regional axillary lymphadenopathy on the right side. She looks ill and is septic on admission. FBC shows a normal white cell count but slight thrombocytopenia. The liver transaminases are slightly raised, but bilirubin and AP are normal. CSF shows slight lymphocytic pleocytosis, a mildly raised protein and a slightly decreased glucose. Brain CT scan shows no abnormalities.

Answer to Question 1

What Clinical Sign Will You be Specifically Looking for?

Lymphadenopathy in the right axilla was detected on clinical examination of the patient. Her acute presentation with signs of severe sepsis make an infectious aetiology of the regional lymphadenopathy most likely. It is crucial to perform a meticulous examination in order to establish the port of entry of the microorganisms, which should be found in the skin area that drains to the enlarged regional lymph nodes.

In Asia, infection with *Orientia tsutsugamushi,* the causative pathogen of scrub typhus, is a common cause of fever, which is often associated with an eschar at the inoculation site and enlargement of the draining lymph nodes. However, the prevalence of eschar varies in different populations and its absence does not rule out the diagnosis of scrub typhus.

Answer to Question 2

What Antibiotic Would You Include in Your Empirical Regimen?

In Asia, scrub typhus must be considered in every patient presenting with an undifferentiated febrile illness, regardless of the presence or absence of an eschar.

Therefore doxycycline should be added to the empirical regimen to cover for *O. tsutsugamushi* infection. Doxycycline would also cover important differential diagnoses such as other rickettsial infections and leptospirosis.

Chloramphenicol or azithromycin is the accepted alternative treatment if tetracyclines are contraindicated, as is the case in pregnant women or patients with tetracycline hypersensitivity. Children at any age with scrub typhus can be safely treated with doxycycline.

Of note, acute hearing loss or hearing impairment in a febrile patient from Asia should always arouse strong suspicion of scrub typhus. However, no single clinical sign or laboratory test can rule in or rule out scrub typhus; therefore empirical antirickettsial treatment is given based on clinical and epidemiological evidence. A definitive laboratory diagnosis – if at all possible in the particular setting – can be established by demonstration of seroconversion in paired acute and convalescent serum samples or by PCR on pretreatment buffy coat samples of an eschar biopsy.

The Case Continued...

On day 2 after admission the patient developed coarse tremors of both upper and lower limbs associated with saccadic oscillations of her eyes in all directions with further deterioration of level of consciousness (GCS 8). At this point a careful clinical examination revealed a well-demarcated crater-like lesion in the right axilla hidden within the axillary folds. Doxycycline therapy was commenced and the patient improved over the next 48 hours. She was discharged on day 6 after admission. Her hearing had returned to normal and there were no other neurological deficits.

The patient's *O. tsutsugamushi* IFA-IgG titre came back high (>1:4096), supporting the suspected diagnosis of scrub typhus.

SUMMARY BOX

Scrub Typhus

Scrub typhus is a common cause of pyrexia in large parts of Asia and northern Australia. Its epidemiology has long been considered limited to the Asia-Pacific area but in 2016 was also first described in patients from South America.

Scrub typhus belongs to the tropical rickettsial infections and is caused by *O. tsutsugamushi*. The infection is transmitted by the bite of an infected larva (chigger) of a trombiculid mite.

Infected mite larvae are found in a wide variety of habitats, from scrubs and primary forests to gardens, beaches, bamboo fields and oil palm or rubber estates. Reservoirs of *O. tsutsugamushi* are rodents and the mites themselves, which can maintain the infection by vertical transmission. Humans are accidental hosts.

The incubation period is 6 to 10 days. A painless papule occurs at the site of the bite, which later ulcerates and transforms into a black crust or 'eschar'. Patients present with fever, severe headache and myalgia, regional or generalized lymphadenopathy and, at times, a macular or maculopapular rash. Conjunctival suffusions, vomiting and diarrhoea as well as constipation can occur.

CNS involvement is common in scrub typhus, and presentations with diffuse encephalopathy or a reversible sensorineural deafness are well documented. In contrast, focal neurological signs are rare. Cerebellar, brainstem and extrapyramidal manifestations have been reported, including opsoclonus, myoclonus and parkinsonian tremor. Further complications include myocarditis, interstitial pneumonia, ARDS and renal failure. Immunity is short-lived and strain-specific.

Diagnosis can be challenging and, in many resource-limited settings, remains clinical. The diagnostic gold standard is the documentation of a significant rise in antibody titres in paired acute and convalescent serum samples. However, these serological tests are usually unavailable in resource-poor tropical areas. Despite controversies in sensitivity and specificity, immunochromatographic rapid diagnostic tests have been developed for field use and are being used in the diagnosis of scrub typhus in several endemic countries. ELISA-based tests have a high sensitivity and specificity. PCR-based tests have been developed and are mostly employed in genotypic characterization and for research purposes or as diagnostic tools in high-resource settings. Culture of *O. tsutsugamushi* from the blood takes several weeks and requires a biosafety level 3 facility.

Scrub typhus is very responsive to antibiotic treatment, which should be given empirically once the diagnosis is suspected. Standard treatment is with doxycycline 100 mg bid for 1 week. Alternative options include tetracycline, azithromycin, rifampicin and chloramphenicol.

Further Reading

1. Paris DH, Day NPJ. Tropical rickettsial infections. In: Farrar J, editor. Manson's Tropical Diseases. 23rd ed. London: Elsevier; 2013 [chapter 22].

2. Premaratna R, Chandrasena TG, Dassayake AS, et al. Acute hearing loss due to scrub typhus: a forgotten complication of a reemerging disease. Clin Infect Dis 2006;42(1); e6–8.

3. Weitzel T, Dittrich S, López J, et al. Endemic scrub typhus in South America. N Engl J Med 2016;375(10); 954–61.

4. Saraswati K, Day NPJ, Mukaka M, Blacksell SD. Scrub typhus point-of-care testing: a systematic review and meta-analysis. PLoS Negl Trop Dis 2018;12(3); e0006330. https://doi.org/10.1371/journal.pntd.0006330.

5. Gaillard T, Briolant S, Madamet M, et al. The end of a dogma: the safety of doxycycline use in young children for malaria treatment. Malar J 2017;16:148.

71

A 71-Year-Old Man from Japan With Eosinophilia and a Nodular Lesion in the Lung

YUKIFUMI NAWA, HARUHIKO MARUYAMA AND MASAKI TOMITA

Clinical Presentation

History

A 71-year-old Japanese man is referred to a local tertiary care hospital for further work-up of a nodular lesion in his right lung. He is clinically well and does not report any complaints.

The lesion was first detected 2 years earlier during a routine health check. Initially it was of linear shape. The patient has been regularly followed up since then. At his most recent follow-up visit it was found by chest radiography (Fig. 71.1A) and CT scan (Fig. 71.1B, C) that his linear lung shadow had turned into a nodular lesion of about 2 cm in diameter.

The patient was born in Kyushu district, southern Japan, where he is still living. He has no history of travelling overseas.

Clinical Findings

The vital signs were normal. The chest was clear. The remainder of the physical examination was also normal.

Investigations

His full blood count and total IgE are shown in Table 71.1. Liver and renal function tests as well as electrolytes are normal. LDH and CRP are not raised.

Serologies

Cryptococcus Ag negative, *Aspergillus* Ag negative, β-D-glucan 6.0 pg/mL (<20 pg/mL), QuantiFERON test (QFT-2G) negative.

TABLE 71.1	Full Blood Count Results at Presentation	
Parameter	Patient	Reference
WBC ($\times 10^9$/L)	6.5	4–10
Haemoglobin (g/dL)	15.3	14–16
Platelets ($\times 10^9$/L)	190	150–300
Neutrophils (%)	46.1	30–80
Lymphocytes (%)	38.6	15–50
Monocytes (%)	6.4	1–12
Eosinophils (%)	8.3	0–6
Total eosinophil count ($\times 10^9$/L)	0.54	<0.45
Basophils (%)	0.6	0–2
IgE (U/mL)	185.7	<100

Imaging

Fluorodeoxyglucose-positron emission tomography (FDG-PET-CT) shows increased FDG-uptake into the lesion in the right upper lobe (Fig. 71.1D–F).

Questions

1. What kind of diseases should be considered in your differential diagnosis?
2. What further information should you obtain from the patient?

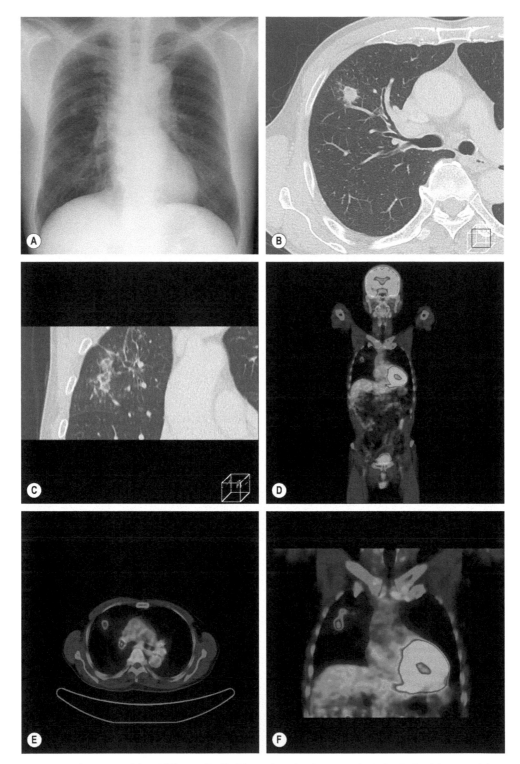

• **Fig. 71.1** Chest x-ray (A) and CT scan (B, C) of the patient showing a nodular lesion in the right upper lobe. (D–F) Fluorodeoxyglucose-positron emission tomography (FDG-PET) with increased FDG uptake into the lesion in the right upper lobe.

Discussion

A 71-year-old Japanese man who is clinically well is worked up for a nodular lesion in his right lung. Blood tests reveal a mild eosinophilia and a slightly raised IgE. On PET scan the pulmonary lesion shows an increased FDG uptake.

Answer to Question 1

What Kinds of Diseases Should be Considered in Your Differential Diagnoses?

The most important differential diagnosis for a nodular lesion with or without cavitation in the lung is either pulmonary tuberculosis or lung cancer. The PET-CT is unable to distinguish between a malignancy and an inflammatory lesion of other aetiology, e.g. an infectious process.

Systemic endemic mycoses (e.g. histoplasmosis, blastomycosis and paracoccidioidomycosis) may present with a wide variety of pulmonary lesions in otherwise asymptomatic patients; however, they are not endemic in East Asia and the patient does not have a history of travelling abroad.

In addition to abnormal findings on the chest radiograph, this patient shows eosinophilia and elevated total IgE levels. One therefore needs to consider the possibility of pulmonary helminth infections, especially of lung fluke infection (paragonimiasis).

Answer to Question 2

What Kind of Information Should You Obtain from the Patient?

When suspecting lung fluke infection, it is important to find out if the patient may at any time have been exposed to this parasite. *Paragonimus* species are endemic all over Asia, in West and Central Africa and parts of Latin America.

If the patient lives in an endemic area, or has a positive travel history, one should find out if he or she has ever eaten raw or undercooked freshwater crabs, which may harbour the infective stage (metacercariae) of *Paragonimus* species. Also, consumption of raw wild boar meat is a risk, because wild boar act as paratenic hosts, harbouring juvenile worms. Traditional medicine used in some East Asian countries may contain raw crab meat and juice and potentially act as a source of infection. However, some patients have a negative exposure history, and it has been suggested that even contaminated fingers and cooking utensils may act as a source of infection.

The Case Continued...

Bronchoscopy did not reveal any signs of malignancy. Cytology of the bronchoalveolar lavage (BAL) fluid was negative for malignant cells and acid-fast bacilli. The QuantiFERON test and a wide range of tumour markers were negative.

In view of the elevated IgE levels, the patient's eosinophilia and the fact that the patient originated from Southern Japan, paragonimiasis was strongly suspected and the patient's serum was submitted for immunodiagnosis of parasitic diseases. Multiple-dot ELISA was strongly positive for *P. westermani*.

The patient was treated with oral praziquantel 25 mg/kg tds for 3 consecutive days. The lung lesion gradually faded and eventually disappeared. His serum antibody titre also declined.

TABLE 71.2	Predominant *Paragonimus* Species by Region	
Region	Predominant *Paragonimus* spp.
East Asia	P. westermani P. skrijabini[a]
South and South-east Asia	P. heterotremus[b]
Africa	P. africanus P. uterobilateralis
North America	P. kelicottii
Central and South America	P. mexicanus

[a]syn. P. myazakii.
[b]Exception: Philippines – *P. westermani*.

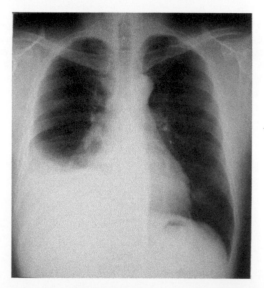

• **Fig. 71.2** Chest x-ray of a patient with acute paragonimiasis, showing right-sided pleural effusion.

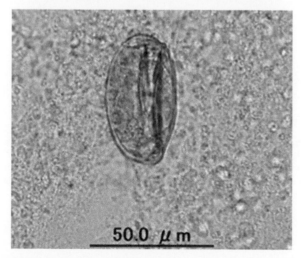

• **Fig. 71.3** Paragonimus *westermani* egg in sputum.

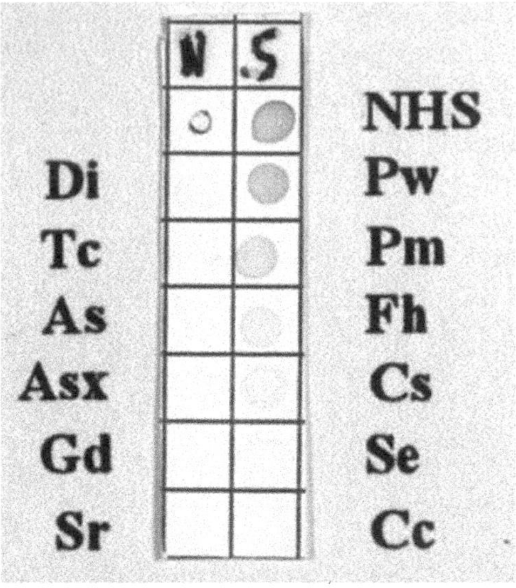

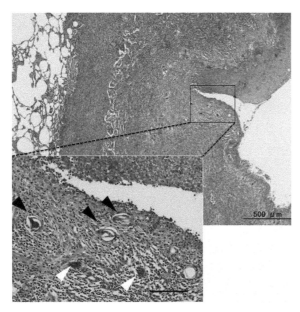

• **Fig. 71.4** Multiple-dot ELISA for helminthiases showing positive reaction against *P. westermani* antigen. NHS: normal human serum for positive control; Pw: *P. westermani*; Pm: *P. miyazakii*; Fh: *Fasciola hepatica*; Cs: *Clonorchis sinensis*; Se: *Spirometra erinacei europaei*; Cc: *Cysticercus cellulosae*; Di: *Dirofilaria immitis*; Tc: *Toxocara canis*; As: *Ascaris sum*; Asx: *Anisakis simplex*; Gd: *Gnathostoma doloresi*; Sr: *Strongyloides stercoralis*.

• **Fig. 71.5** Histopathology of the nodular lung lesion that was surgically resected after diagnosis of lung cancer based on FDG-PET imaging. Note the chronic granulomatous lesion containing numerous *Paragonimus* eggs (black arrows). Foreign body giant cells (white arrows) are also seen in the tissue.

SUMMARY BOX

Paragonimiasis

Paragonimiasis is a sub-acute to chronic lung disease caused by infection with lung flukes of the genus *Paragonimus*. *Paragonimus westermani* is the most widely distributed species in Asia, but several additional species also cause disease (Table 71.2). Apart from Asia, paragonimiasis occurs in the Americas and in sub-Saharan Africa.

Adult flukes live in the lungs of a mammalian host (felines, canines, humans). Ova are coughed up and either expectorated or swallowed and passed in the faeces. When eggs reach fresh water, miracidia hatch and infect a snail (first intermediate host). After asexual multiplication, cercariae are released and infect a crab or crayfish (second intermediate host).

Human infection occurs mainly via consumption of raw or undercooked freshwater crabs or crayfish contaminated with *Paragonimus* metacercariae. In addition, eating raw meat of wild boar, which is a paratenic host, is an important route of infection, especially in Japan. Venison (deer meet) has also been proven as the potential source of *P. westermani* infection in humans. Because the range of paratenic hosts may even be wider, eating wild animal meat in general may be a risk factor for this disease.

Metacercariae excyst in the small intestine and penetrate the intestinal wall. They pass through the liver and diaphragm, invade the pleural space and finally enter the lung parenchyma where they mature into adults and produce eggs. Juvenile worms sometimes migrate into subcutaneous soft tissue or the central nervous system to cause unexpected, potentially deleterious lesions.

Clinical features of the disease are similar to those of pulmonary TB or lung cancer. Patients may have chronic cough, haemoptysis, chest pain, fever, night sweats and abnormal findings on chest imaging. Pleural effusion (Fig. 71.2) with marked eosinophilia in the exudate and pneumothorax without apparent nodular lesion/cavitation may occur in the early stages and/or in light infections.

Extrapulmonary paragonimiasis may present as painless, mobile subcutaneous swellings. Migration into the CNS may lead to acute eosinophilic meningoencephalitis and epilepsy.

However, about 20% of patients are asymptomatic and the disease is accidentally found on routine chest radiography, when nodules, ring shadows or cavities are typically seen.

Eosinophilia is prominent during acute and sub-acute infection but may be only mild or absent in chronic disease.

The definitive diagnosis is made by detection of ova in sputum, BAL fluid or faeces (Fig. 71.3). However, sensitivity is below 50% in light infections. Instead, an immunodiagnostic screening test such as multiple-dot ELISA (Fig. 71.4) should be used in combination with the patient's history and additional laboratory results. Serological tests (e.g. ELISA) may detect early as well as chronic infections, and titres decline rapidly after cure. Praziquantel is the drug of choice. A course of 25 mg/kg tds for 3 consecutive days is usually effective against all *Paragonimus* species.

Even in paragonimiasis-endemic areas, physicians often do not pay much attention to this disease and misdiagnose it as pulmonary tuberculosis or lung cancer. Such diagnostic errors result in enormous socioeconomic loss, and create a mental and physical burden for the patient because of unnecessary hospitalization and laboratory investigations, surgical interventions and/or long-term medication. Figure 71.5 shows a typical example of such a case, in which postoperative histopathology revealed the presence of *Paragonimus* eggs in the resected nodular lesion, which had been diagnosed as a lung cancer by FDG-PET imaging.

Further Reading

1. Sithithaworn P, Sripa B, Kaewkes S, et al. Food-borne trematodes. In: Farrar J, editor. Manson's Tropical Diseases. 23rd ed. London: Elsevier; 2013 [chapter 53].

2. Kong Y, Doanh PN, Nawa Y. Paragonimus. In: Xiao L, Ryan U, Yaoyu Feng Y, editors. Biology of foodborne parasites. Boca Raton: CRC Press; 2015. p. 445–62.

3. Nawa Y, Thaenkham U, Doanh PN, Blair D. Paragonimus westermani *and* Paragonimus species. In: Motarjemi Y, Moy G, Todd E, editors. Encyclopedia of food safety: hazards and diseases. San Diego, CA, USA: Elsevier; 2014. p. 179–88.

4. Nakamura-Uchiyama F, Mukae H, Nawa Y. Paragonimiasis: a Japanese perspective. *Clin Chest Med* 2002;23(2):409–20.

5. Yoshida A, Matsuo K, Moribe J, et al. Venison, another source of *Paragonimus westermani* infection. *Parasitol Int* 2016;65: 607–12.

72

A 4-Year-Old Boy from Mozambique With Severe Oedema and Skin Lesions

CHARLOTTE ADAMCZICK

Clinical Presentation

History

An oedematous, HIV-negative 4-year-old boy from rural Mozambique is seen at the paediatric department of a central hospital in Malawi.

He was admitted 5 days earlier with the suspected diagnosis of nephrotic syndrome and was started on furosemide and prednisolone; however, his oedema did not subside.

Three weeks earlier he had been treated for pneumonia at a health centre.

Clinical Findings

The little boy is miserable, refusing to eat and apathetic with a puffy face and pitting oedema on the lower legs. His hair is brittle, sparse and fair in colour. The skin is dry and hyperpigmented; it is peeling off like 'flaky paint' (Fig. 72.1) and there are ulcerative skin lesions, most prominently in the groins (Fig. 72.2).

Laboratory Results

Albumin 2.2 g/dL (reference range 3.0–5.2 g/dL), haemoglobin 7 g/dL (12–14 g/dL).

Questions

1. What is the likely diagnosis and how can it be distinguished from nephrotic syndrome?
2. How should the child be treated and what is the prognosis?

Discussion

Three weeks after a severe bacterial infection, a 4-year old boy from rural Mozambique develops oedema. The skin is hyperpigmented and dry, peeling off and there is discoloration of his hair. Treatment with furosemide has no influence on the extent of the oedema. Clinically, the little boy

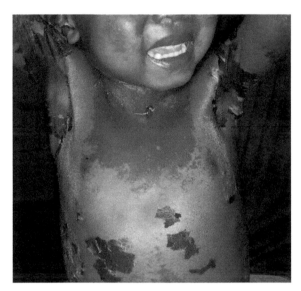

• **Fig. 72.1** A 5-year-old boy with generalized oedema. The skin is hyperpigmented and dry. It is peeling off like 'flaky paint'. Underneath, the skin is hypopigmented.

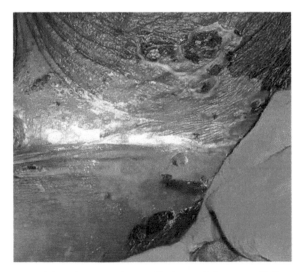

• **Fig. 72.2** Ulcerative skin lesions on the lower abdomen and in the groin (where zinc ointment and Gentian violet solution ("GV paint") has been applied).

is sick and refusing to eat or drink. He is anaemic and his serum albumin is low.

Answer to Question 1

What is the Likely Diagnosis and How Can It be Distinguished from Nephrotic Syndrome?

Generalized oedema in a child can have various causes. In nephrotic syndrome, serum albumin is low and there is heavy proteinuria. Low serum albumin is however influenced by many factors such as nutrition, liver function and intestinal resorption.

This child is displaying additional clinical features such as skin and hair changes as well as apathy. These are typical features of kwashiorkor, a form of severe acute malnutrition (see Summary Box).

A urine dipstick test should be done to check for protein. In nephrotic syndrome, proteinuria exceeds 3.5 g per day (4 + on a urine dipstick) and the urine is often macroscopically frothy. In kwashiorkor, some proteinuria may be found but rarely exceeds 1 + on a dipstick test.

Answer to Question 2

How Should the Child be Treated and What is the Prognosis?

The child needs to be admitted to the high dependency area of the nutrition ward and treated according to WHO guidelines for severe acute malnutrition with meticulously calculated amounts of feeds and close monitoring. The risks of infection, diarrhoea, anaemia, cardiac and liver failure are high. Prophylactic antibiotics, monitoring of temperature and haemoglobin as well as careful fluid replacement, are part of the treatment scheme.

The Case Continued...

The skin in the groin and armpits continued to peel off and became superinfected. The lesions could successfully be treated with Gentian violet solution.

Initially the child did not tolerate 3-hourly feeds and required feeding through a nasogastric tube. On day 5 in the nutrition rehabilitation unit he could eat by himself and the oedema started to settle. The transition to higher caloric feeds was tolerated well and he could be discharged into the community feeding program at day 15.

SUMMARY BOX

Kwashiorkor

Kwashiorkor is a form of severe, acute malnutrition characterized by hypoalbuminaemia and oedema.

Kwashiorkor mainly occurs in areas where people live on a monotonous diet and the staple food has a low protein-to-energy ratio (e.g. maize, cassava or bananas). It is uncommon in communities where diet is supplemented by animal protein. Incidence peaks during the rainy season when staple food items and vegetables are in short supply.

However, kwashiorkor is not (just) a consequence of a diet low in protein and micronutrients. Infections often precede the onset of the disease. They lead to low albumin levels in the context of acute phase reactions. Diarrhoeal diseases and capillary leakage result in further loss of protein, nutrients and fluids. An imbalance between free radicals and insufficient levels of antioxidants leads to oxidative stress and damage of cell membranes. Hypoimmunoglobulinaemia leads to severe infections, contributing to the high fatality rates associated with kwashiorkor.

The typical age at presentation is 1 to 3 years; boys and girls are equally affected.

Hepatomegaly is a common finding. The hair becomes depigmented, fair or reddish in colour and is easy to pluck. Hyperpigmented, dry, damaged and infected skin may show pale patches ('flaky paint' dermatosis) and ulcerations. Children with kwashiorkor are miserable, apathetic and often refuse to eat.

Management is challenging and involves careful feeding with slowly increasing amounts of feeds with meticulous monitoring of glucose levels, weight gain and fluid status. Prophylactic broad-spectrum antibiotics should be given to all patients, because signs of infection including fever may be absent. Diuretics are contraindicated because they further deplete the intravascular volume, causing hypotension. The oedema will settle once therapeutic feeding has been established.

Patients should also receive folic acid, anthelmintics and, once stable, measles vaccination if unvaccinated. Relapses are common and renal and liver function, as well as glucose levels, may be deranged well beyond the time of clinical recovery.

Case fatality rates from kwashiorkor are high, with a median of 20–30%. Additional infection with HIV further worsens the prognosis.

Further Reading

1. Abrams S, Brabin BJ, Coulter JBS. Nutrition-associated disease. In: Farrar J, editor. Manson's Tropical Diseases. 23rd ed. London: Elsevier; 2013 [chapter 77].

2. Bwakura-Dangarembizi M, Amadi B, Bourke CD, et al. Health Outcomes, Pathogenesis and Epidemiology of Severe Acute Malnutrition (HOPE-SAM): rationale and methods of a longitudinal observational study. BMJ Open 2019;9:e023077.

3. Coulthard MG. Oedema in kwashiorkor is caused by hypoalbuminaemia. Paediatr Int Child Health 2015;35:83–9.

4. WHO. Guideline: Updates on the management of severe acute malnutrition in infants and children. Geneva: World Health Organisation 2013. Available from: https://apps.who.int/iris/bitstream/handle/10665/95584/9789241506328_eng.pdf?ua=1

5. Heikens GT, Bunn J, Amadi B, et al. Case management of HIV-infected severely malnourished children: challenges in the area of highest prevalence. Lancet 2008;371(9620):1305–7.

73

A 21-Year-Old Male Migrant from Rural Mali With Massive Splenomegaly

CAMILLA ROTHE

Clinical Presentation

History

A 21-year-old male migrant from rural Mali is referred to the tropical medicine department of a university hospital in Germany. He has just been worked-up for splenomegaly and bicytopenia at the haematology department. However, the underlying condition could not be established.

Clinically, the patient is quite well, he only reports intermittent fever, and some "heaviness" on the left side of his abdomen for some time (the duration is difficult to specify). There are no night sweats and his weight appears to be stable.

The patient migrated from rural Mali to Germany and arrived 1 year prior. During his journey he crossed Niger and spent a few weeks at a detention centre in Libya until he made his way across the Mediterranean and through Italy to Germany. He comes from a poor family and is unable to read and write.

Clinical Findings

21-year-old young man, who appears clinically well. Temperature 36.1°C (96.98°F), BP 120/80mmHg, pulse 64 bpm. The spleen is massively enlarged (around 15 cm below the left costal margin), but there is no clinical anaemia and no lymphadenopathy. Heart sounds are clear and there are no murmurs. The rest of the examination is normal.

Abdominal Ultrasound

Spleen 21.8 cm in longitudinal diameter, the parenchyma appears homogenous. The liver is normal in size and the parenchyma looks normal. The flow of the portal and splenic veins is normal. There is no lymphadenopathy and no free fluid.

Laboratory Results

The laboratory results are shown in Table 73.1.

TABLE 73.1 Laboratory Results at First Presentation

Parameter	Patient	Reference Range
WBC ($\times 10^9$/L)	3.3	4–10
Neutrophils ($\times 10^9$/L)	2.29	1.8–7.2
Lymphocytes ($\times 10^9$/L)	1.4	1.5–4
Monocytes ($\times 10^9$/L)	0.28	0.2–0.5
Eosinophils ($\times 10^9$/L)	0.12	<0.5
Haemoglobin (g/dL)	13.8	13–15
Platelets ($\times 10^9$/L)	124	150–350
LDH (U/L)	185	<220
Total bilirubin (mg/dL)	0.5	0.2–1.2
IgM (g/l)	8.59	0.4–2.3
CRP	0.5	<0.5
ESR mm/h	9/21	<15/30
Plasmodium spp. (thick and thin film)	negative	negative
P. falciparum IFAT	1:256	<1:32

Questions

1. What are the most important differential diagnoses in this patient?
2. How would you manage him?

Discussion

A 21-year old migrant from rural Mali presents with massive splenomegaly, causing a feeling of heaviness in his abdomen and reports intermittent fever. The symptoms have been present for some time.

At presentation he appears well and is afebrile. Gross splenomegaly is the only abnormal finding confirmed by ultrasound, which otherwise yields no pathological results. Laboratory results show mild bicytopenia, normal LDH and almost 4-fold increased immunoglobulin M (IgM). The systemic inflammatory markers are not elevated. Blood films for malaria parasites are negative, but malaria serology is positive.

Answer to Question 1

What Are the Most Important Differential Diagnoses in This Patient?

Lymphoma or leukaemia is an important differential diagnosis to have in a patient with splenomegaly and fever anywhere in the world. However, in our patient it seems unlikely, because the differential count is normal, LDH, CRP and ESR are not elevated and the specialist work-up elsewhere did not yield a cause for his complaints.

Visceral leishmaniasis (VL) can present with massive hepatosplenomegaly, generalized lymphadenopathy and pancytopenia. Patients usually have a history of fever and weight loss and appear severely ill, which our patient did not.

Schistosomiasis is common in many parts of sub-Saharan Africa. Chronic *S. mansoni* infection causes liver fibrosis and secondary portal hypertension with splenomegaly and hypersplenism.

Liver fibrosis in schistosomiasis (so called "pipestem fibrosis") is usually easy to detect on ultrasound. In our patient, the liver appeared normal, and the flow of portal and splenic veins was normal as well, making portal hypertension of any cause unlikely.

Bacterial endocarditis and brucellosis may cause fever and splenomegaly; however, the spleen tends to be only moderately increased in size and there were no murmurs on cardiac examination.

EBV and CMV infections may cause ongoing fever and splenomegaly. Typical laboratory features include relative and absolute lymphocytosis, elevated LDH and liver transaminases, which our patient does not have. In Africa, most people will be exposed to both viruses already in childhood.

Our patient shows remarkably high IgM titres, positive malaria serology and a negative blood film. The most likely differential diagnosis for this patient therefore is hyperreactive malarial splenomegaly (HMS). HMS is the most common cause of massive splenomegaly in tropical areas with stable malaria transmission.

Answer to Question 2

How Would You Manage the Patient?

An HIV test should be ordered in any patient from Africa with a history of fever and/or thrombocytopenia. Serologies for schistosomiasis and visceral leishmaniasis should be done and blood cultures taken for *Brucella* species and bacterial endocarditis.

For HMS, malaria PCR should be ordered and antimalarial treatment attempted. If splenomegaly remains unexplained, a bone marrow aspirate should be done to rule out a haematological disorder and look for intracellular *Leishmania* promastigotes.

The Case Continued...

HIV serology was negative; EBV and CMV serologies indicated previous infection. Serologies for schistosomiasis and leishmaniasis were also negative, and the blood culture did not yield any pathogens. There were no ova of *S. mansoni* found in the stool.

Despite the negative blood film, PCR for *P. falciparum* came back positive, making a diagnosis of hyperreactive splenomegaly very likely.

The patient received one single course of dihydroartemisinin/piperaquine and the reported episodes of fever subsided. Malaria PCR was still positive at follow-up 2 weeks later, but has remained negative since then.

Shortly after treatment, authorities threatened to deport the patient back to Mali. A medical letter indicating that he was at high risk for splenic rupture, which at his home in rural Mali would mean certain death, was recognized and he was permitted to stay.

The patient has been monitored for a total of 2.5 years at the time of writing. IgM levels took 2 years to get back to normal. The size of the spleen slowly decreased; but at his last visit, remained slightly enlarged (14 cm in diameter).

At his last visit, the young man was well and spoke fluent German. He went to school in Germany and has learned to read and write. He planned to start vocational training to become a house painter.

SUMMARY BOX

Hyperreactive Malarial Splenomegaly (HMS)

HMS, formerly known as tropical splenomegaly syndrome (TSS), is one of the most common causes of massive splenomegaly in tropical regions with stable malaria transmission. Other important causes include lymphomas, chronic myeloid leukaemia, myelofibrosis, haemoglobinopathies, schistosomiasis and visceral leishmaniasis.

HMS is caused by an abnormal immune response to repeated infections with *Plasmodium falciparum*, *P. malariae* or *P. vivax* that results in an overproduction of polyclonal IgM. IgM forms aggregates and immune complexes, which are phagocytosed by the reticuloendothelial system, leading to massive splenomegaly and hypersplenism.

HMS is more common in women than in men and mainly affects the age group between 20 and 40 years. There seems to be a genetic background, with ethnic and familial clustering. HMS has also been described in expatriates residing in malaria-endemic regions, and more and more cases are being described in refugees and migrants from malaria-endemic areas.

Diagnostic criteria were proposed by Fakunle in 1982 and include splenomegaly extending >10cm below the left costal margin without any other cause, elevated IgM, elevated antimalarial antibodies and favourable response to antimalarial prophylaxis.

Even though commonly quoted in the literature, Fakunle's criteria are of limited practical use for clinicians practicing in resource-constrained settings, where HMS is naturally most common because malaria serology and IgM levels are usually unavailable. Under those circumstances, clinicians are often limited to presumptive treatment with antimalarials of a patient with massive splenomegaly, and HMS may be difficult to differentiate from lymphoma.

Patients most commonly present with symptoms of anaemia and abdominal heaviness or discomfort, some report episodes of low-grade fever. Full blood count usually shows anaemia, bi- or pancytopenia reflecting hypersplenism. Malaria microscopy is usually negative, because parasitaemia is kept at bay and therefore very low. However, molecular methods such as PCR may be able to detect low-level parasitaemia, as highlighted in this case.

Treatment of HMS is effective with antimalarials for the duration of exposure, i.e. in endemic settings, lifelong. In migrants living in malaria non-endemic countries, one treatment course of antimalarials is enough to eliminate parasites as shown in this case, and repeated courses are not required. However, even after clearanc of infection splenic size and increased IgM may still take a long time to get back to normal ranges.

Further Reading

1. White NJ. Malaria. In: Farrar J, editor. Manson's Tropical Diseases. 23rd ed. London: Elsevier; 2013 [chapter 43].
2. Fakunle YM. Tropical splenomegaly. Part 1: Tropical Africa. Clin Haematol 1981;10:963–75.
3. Bedu-Addo G, Bates I. Causes of massive tropical splenomegaly in Ghana. Lancet 2002;360(9331):449–54.
4. Leoni S, Buonfrate D, Angheben A, et al. The hyper-reactive malarial splenomegaly: a systematic review of the literature. Malar J 2015;14:185.
5. Bisoffi Z, Leoni S, Angheben A, et al. Chronic malaria and hyper-reactive malarial splenomegaly: a retrospective study on the largest series observed in a non-endemic country. Malar J 2016;15:320.

74

A 28-Year-Old Woman from Sierra Leone With Fever and Conjunctivitis

BENJAMIN JEFFS

Clinical Presentation

History

A 28-year-old woman presents to a small rural hospital in eastern Sierra Leone with a 6-day history of fever, weakness, sore throat and retrosternal chest pain. She has had loose stools twice a day for the past 2 days. She was seen in a local health post the day before admission and given a course of artemether with amodiaquine and amoxicillin, but she had continued to get worse on this. Her examination was unremarkable except some mild pharyngitis. On arrival in hospital she was treated with IV ceftriaxone and she completed the course of her antimalarial medications. Her malaria slide was negative. She remained on this treatment for 2 days but continued to get worse.

On the second day after admission she develops conjunctivitis. By this stage she is very unwell and is unable to walk unaided. She has developed a cough and breathlessness.

Physical Examination

Axillary temperature 38.2°C (100.8°F), blood pressure 80/55 mmHg, pulse rate 100 bpm. On chest auscultation she has bilateral fine crepitations.

Investigations

Her chest radiograph reveals diffuse bilateral infiltrates. Blood chemistry shows mild renal impairment and raised transaminases (aspartate transaminase (AST/GOT) 514 U/L (<50 U/L)).

Questions

1. What is the differential diagnosis?
2. What tests would you do and how would you manage the patient?

Discussion

A young Sierra Leonean woman has a severe febrile illness with pharyngitis, conjunctivitis and chest involvement. She deteriorates on broad-spectrum antibiotics and antimalarials.

Answer to Question 1
What is the Differential Diagnosis?

Adenovirus infections can cause conjunctivitis and pharyngitis but these are normally mild. Also, measles presents with fever, cough, coryza and a striking conjunctivitis. It may also cause pneumonitis, but at this stage you would expect to see a rash.

Mycoplasma pneumoniae can cause a pharyngitis and pneumonia but is rarely severe. Other forms of pneumonia are possible but do not normally cause conjunctivitis.

Leptospirosis can start with a non-specific febrile illness. Pulmonary involvement including haemorrhages is common and it can cause renal impairment. Patients with severe leptospirosis tend to present with conjunctival suffusions rather than with conjunctivitis.

Typhoid can present as a non-specific febrile illness. You would expect the patient to eventually improve on ceftriaxone, but prolonged clinical courses in typhoid are not uncommon. Pharyngitis and conjunctivitis are usually not part of the clinical picture.

Lassa fever is quite common in Eastern Sierra Leone, accounting for 16–20% of hospital admissions in some studies. All the signs and symptoms the patient has are consistent with Lassa fever.

Answer to Question 2
What Tests Would You do and How Would You Manage the Patient?

Lassa fever is a serious disease. It has caused nosocomial outbreaks in which many medical staff have died. Therefore all procedures should be done with caution and the possibility

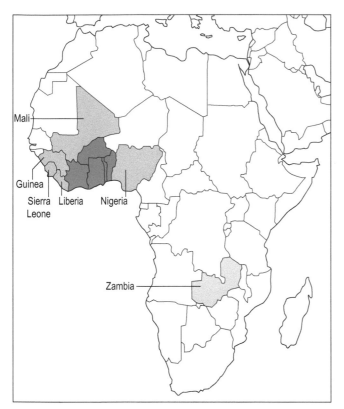

• **Fig. 74.1** Endemic areas for Old World arenaviruses. Only the two arenaviruses known to cause haemorrhagic fever, Lassa and Lujo, are shown. Countries where clinical cases of Lassa fever have been confirmed are depicted in green. Indirect evidence, such as anecdotal reports or seroprevalence data, exists for most of the other countries in West Africa, shown in red. Endemic countries for Lujo virus are shown in blue. Incidence and risk of disease may vary significantly within each country. (Adapted from Farrar, J., Hotez, P., Junghanss, T., et al., 2013. Manson's Tropical Diseases. In: Farrar, J. (Ed.) 23rd ed. Elsevier, London. Fig. 16.2. Pp. 177)

of Lassa fever should always be discussed with the laboratory. All specimens should be transported in sealed plastic containers.

Serological and PCR tests are available for the diagnosis of Lassa fever, and an antigen-based rapid point-of-care test has been licensed.

PCR tests are the most sensitive but are not available in most African countries. Antigen tests demonstrate the presence of the disease but may not detect low levels of the virus, especially if taken in the first days of illness. IgM antibody tests can show a high rate of false positive tests and may be hard to interpret.

The patient needs to be isolated until the results of the Lassa fever tests are known. Because the infection spreads through contact with blood or body fluids, the use of goggles, masks, double gloves and disposable (waterproof) surgical gowns is recommended when handling the patient until the diagnosis of a viral haemorrhagic fever has been ruled out. The patient should be isolated in a side room, which should ideally have an area outside for decontamination (i.e. removing potentially contaminated clothing). Needles and sharps

should be handled with care by experienced staff. After significant occupational exposure to the bodily fluid of a patient with Lassa fever such as a needlestick injury, post-exposure prophylaxis with oral ribavirin should be considered.

The treatment for Lassa fever is with IV ribavirin, which is expensive and not commonly available. It seems to improve survival, particularly when given during the first 6 days of symptomatic disease, but the quality of studies on this are poor.

The Case Continued...

The diagnosis of Lassa fever was confirmed with antigen testing and the patient received IV ribavirin in a specialist isolation unit. Unfortunately, the patient was already very unwell by this stage and died 2 days later. All of the patient's family, close friends and medical staff were interviewed to determine whether they had had contact with the patient. All contacts were advised to monitor their temperature and seek medical help if they became unwell within 21 days of the contact.

SUMMARY BOX

Lassa Fever

Lassa fever is a severe systemic disease caused by infection with an arenavirus. It is a zoonosis of rats of the genus *Mastomys* and infections in humans are likely to result from contact with infected rat urine. Lassa fever is common in Liberia, Sierra Leone, Ghana and Nigeria, although it probably occurs in a much larger area of sub-Saharan West Africa (Fig. 74.1). Cases have been imported to Europe from other countries such as Mali, Côte d'Ivoire and Togo. There are up to 300 000 cases estimated a year with 5000 deaths, although the confidence limits of this estimate are likely to be very broad.

Most cases are thought to be mild and patients may not even present to a health facility; but in hospitalized patients, the case fatality rate may be as high as 20%. Lassa fever is more severe in pregnant women, with a higher case fatality rate in the third trimester. It frequently results in premature labour or spontaneous abortion and about 90% of fetuses of women infected with Lassa fever die.

The incubation period is 3 to 21 days. In individuals who are not pregnant the disease normally starts insidiously with fever, body aches and weakness. Sore throat and retrosternal chest pain are common, as are vague abdominal symptoms such as pain, diarrhoea and vomiting. Cough and breathlessness may occur in some patients. Conjunctivitis is common, especially late in the disease. Frank bleeding is rare. Raised liver transaminases are markers of severity and are associated with a higher case fatality rate.

Serological and PCR tests are available for the diagnosis of Lassa fever, and antigen-based rapid point-of-care tests have been licensed, although more testing on the sensitivity for different strains is needed.

Because Lassa fever is common, it should be considered in anyone with an unexplained febrile condition who has visited an endemic area within the past 21 days and appropriate infection control precautions should be implemented. It is more common in people from rural than urban areas, but it does occur in towns. Treatment with IV ribavirin is likely to be beneficial if given early in the disease, but it should also be considered in patients who are diagnosed late.

Further Reading

1. Blumberg L, Enria D, Bausch DG. Viral haemorrhagic fevers. In: Farrar J, editor. Manson's Tropical Diseases. 23rd ed. London: Elsevier; 2013 [Chapter 16].

2. Houlihan C, Behrens R. Lassa fever. BMJ 2017;358:j2986.

3. McCormick JB, Webb PA, Krebs JW, et al. A prospective study of the epidemiology and ecology of Lassa fever. J Infect Dis 1987;155(3):437–44.

4. McCormick JB, King IJ, Webb PA, et al. Lassa fever. Effective therapy with ribavirin. N Engl J Med 1986;314(1):20–6.

5. Bonwitt J, Kelly AH, Ansumana R, et al. Rat-atouille: a mixed method study to characterize rodent hunting and consumption in the context of Lassa fever. Ecohealth 2016;13:234–47.

75

A 25-Year-Old Woman from Zambia With a New-Onset Seizure

OMAR SIDDIQI

Clinical Presentation

History

A 23-year-old HIV-positive Zambian woman is referred from a health centre to a local teaching hospital in Lusaka after suffering her first ever seizure. The seizure occurred out of sleep. Her son walked into her bedroom after hearing a noise and found his mother on the floor unresponsive and shaking all four limbs. This continued for 5 to 10 minutes.

The patient had been diagnosed with HIV infection 1 month earlier. She is not yet on antiretroviral therapy (ART) but has been taking co-trimoxazole prophylaxis for 7 days. She was successfully treated for pulmonary tuberculosis 4 years ago.

The patient is unmarried with three children. She works in the hospital cafeteria. She does not drink alcohol or use any recreational drugs.

Clinical Findings

On examination she looks well, her GCS score is 15/15, her vital signs are normal and she is afebrile. There is no meningism. The chest is clear. The neurological examination is unremarkable.

Laboratory Results

The malaria rapid diagnostic test is negative. Additional blood results are shown in Table 75.1.

A lumbar puncture is done. The opening pressure is normal. The cerebrospinal fluid (CSF) is clear. CSF results are shown in Table 75.2.

Imaging and EEG Results

Electroencephalography (EEG) demonstrates focal slowing in the right hemisphere (Fig. 75.1). A CT scan of her brain shows frontal and parietal hypodense lesions in the white matter of the right hemisphere (Fig. 75.2). No contrast enhancement is present.

TABLE 75.1 Blood Results on Admission		
Parameter	Patient	Reference Range
WBC (× 10^9/L)	5.8	4–10
Haemoglobin (g/dL)	11.0	12–14
Platelets (× 10^9/L)	215	150–350
CD4 count (cells/μL)	153	500–1200
Serum sodium (mmol/L)	135	130–145
Serum glucose (mmol/L)	4.5	3.9–5.5

TABLE 75.2 CSF Results on Admission		
Parameter	Patient	Reference Range
Leukocytes (cells/μL)	5	0–5
CSF protein (g/L)	0.78	0.25–0.55
CSF glucose (mmol/L)	2.9	2.25–2.97*
Cryptococcal antigen (CrAG)	Negative	Negative
India Ink stain	Negative	Negative
Gram stain	Negative	Negative
Ziehl–Neelsen stain	Negative	Negative

*½ to ⅔ of paired serum glucose sample.

Questions

1. How would you manage this patient?
2. What is your general approach to a patient presenting with new-onset seizures in sub-Saharan Africa?

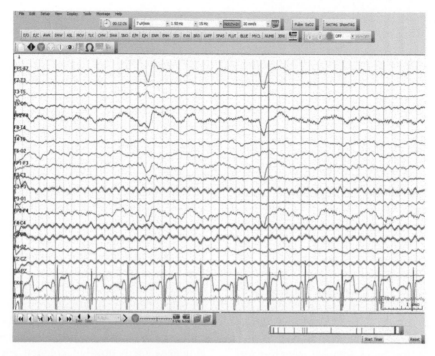

• Fig. 75.1 EEG demonstrating a slow background with superimposed delta frequency slowing of the right hemisphere.

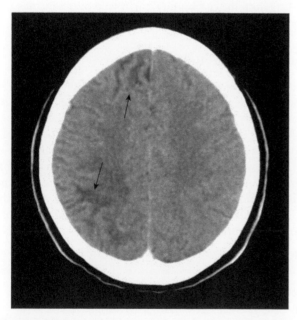

• Fig. 75.2 CT scan showing right frontal and parietal hypodensities in the subcortical white matter.

Discussion

A young Zambian woman presents with a new-onset seizure. There are no focal neurological deficits on examination. The CSF examination is normal, apart from a slightly raised protein level. Neuroimaging reveals hypodense lesions without contrast enhancement restricted to the subcortical white matter. Electroencephalography demonstrates focal slowing in the right hemisphere. The patient is HIV-positive, and her CD4 count is low. She is not yet on antiretroviral treatment.

Answer to Question 1

How Would You Manage This Patient?

The patient presents with a symptomatic seizure; there are obvious lesions in her brain and she is HIV-positive with advanced immunosuppression.

Treatment should aim at both preventing further seizures (antiepileptic treatment) and managing the underlying condition (causative treatment). The patient and her guardians should be counselled about the nature of her epileptic disorder, respecting their beliefs and attitudes. The choice for an antiepileptic drug should take into account the local availability and costs for the patient. Phenobarbitone is the most widely available and most affordable drug in sub-Saharan Africa, followed by carbamazepine. Newer drugs with fewer interactions and a better side effect profile, such as levetiracetam, are not yet routinely available. Phenytoin and valproic acid are also used but their delivery might be unreliable. Reliability of supply is an important factor to consider, because the discontinuation of the antiepileptic medication might put the patient at risk of withdrawal seizures. When starting a patient on phenobarbitone or carbamazepine, the effects of hepatic enzyme induction on antiretroviral therapy and hormonal contraception must be considered.

Syndromically, focal brain lesion is the underlying pathology in our patient. Differential diagnosis for focal brain lesions in an HIV patient with a new-onset seizure includes tuberculoma, progressive multifocal leukoencephalopathy (PML), cerebral toxoplasmosis, cryptococcoma, brain abscess and primary CNS lymphoma. Neurocysticercosis, which can occur unrelated to HIV infection, also needs to be considered.

Lesions that selectively affect the white matter without contrast enhancement and without perifocal oedema are strongly suggestive of PML. There is no causative treatment available for PML. Commencing antiretrovirals is currently the only therapeutic option.

Answer to Question 2

What is Your General Approach to a Patient Presenting With New-Onset Seizures in Sub-Saharan Africa?

The approach is influenced by (1) the high prevalence of HIV and subsequent immunosuppression; (2) the high burden of infection, including tuberculosis, bacterial meningitis and tropical diseases, e.g. cerebral malaria; and (3) the lack of resources, in particular, low availability of imaging studies and antiepileptic drugs (AEDs).

CNS infections are a prominent cause of epileptic seizures in sub-Saharan Africa. They can cause seizures during the acute illness (acute symptomatic seizures), as well as weeks or months after the acute episode, if the infection leaves an epileptogenic 'scar' in the brain (remote symptomatic seizures).

Three questions should be addressed when managing a patient with possible epileptic disorder:
1. Is it actually an epileptic seizure/epilepsy?
2. Is there an underlying cause for the seizure disorder which can be identified and treated?
3. Does the patient require antiepileptic drug treatment and for how long should it be given?

The available diagnostic and therapeutic means dictate the clinical procedure. Mimics of epileptic seizures such as syncope and psychogenic non-epileptic attacks (so-called pseudoseizures) must be considered. Here, the history taken from the patient as well as from witnesses and guardians is decisive. Feelings of lightheadedness before the loss of consciousness, pallor and brief reorientation after the fall are typical for syncope. Psychogenic non-epileptic attacks are characterized by eye closure, long duration and bizarre motor manifestations. They often occur when the patients are subjected to emotional stress, such as during spiritual rituals and church masses.

In all patients with unknown HIV status, HIV testing should be performed. In all febrile patients, a CNS infection including cerebral malaria should be ruled out. Opportunistic CNS infections should be considered in immunosuppressed patients. In areas with high prevalence of *T. solium*, neurocysticercosis should be taken into consideration. In view of the limited resources, the diagnosis will be based on clinical and epidemiological evidence; hence, the knowledge of local distribution and prevalence of possible causes is helpful.

When initiating antiepileptic treatment, the issues of availability, including reliability of supply, affordability and interactions between AEDs and the patient's medications, must be taken into consideration (particularly, antiretrovirals, antituberculous drugs and contraceptives).

Treatment of women of child-bearing age might pose some additional challenges. In all women of child-bearing age, folic acid (5 mg/day) should be added to the regimen. AEDs recommended for women of child-bearing age in resource-rich settings with low HIV prevalence, such as lamotrigine, are not available in sub-Saharan Africa and might have adverse interactions with ARVs, especially protease inhibitors. In those cases where several AEDs are available, the specific drug chosen for epilepsy treatment of a woman of child-bearing age will be a trade-off between the health of the fetus and that of the mother. Here, one should consider that leaving out a drug because of its possible fetal toxicity, such as valproic acid, and using an enzyme-inducing drug with a better record regarding foetal malformations instead, might lead to a virological failure that would jeopardize both the mother and the child.

Counselling the patients and their guardians is of paramount importance. An epileptic seizure is a dramatic event. In some African communities, epileptic disorder is still attributed to supernatural causes. Patients who have experienced epileptic seizures might become socially stigmatized. Patient-tailored, non-judgemental counselling, taking into account the patient's perception of the disease, might assist in securing the patient's cooperation. Involving local health workers from the community might help overcome misconceptions and reduce stigma.

The Case Continued...

The patient was started on carbamazepine 200 mg bid. Valproic acid was initially requested but the patient could not afford it.

JC-virus DNA was later detected in the CSF as part of a research study, further confirming the suspected diagnosis of PML. She was commenced on ART and remained on carbamazepine. After 6 months, she remained seizure-free and carbamazepine was stopped. After 1 year of ART, the patient's CD4 count reached 535 cells/μL and she had returned to work.

SUMMARY BOX

Seizure Management in HIV

HIV patients are at risk for developing seizures related to HIV-associated neurological diseases and metabolic disturbances. The decision to initiate AEDs in an HIV patient with seizures depends on their aetiology and the duration for which the patient remains at risk for seizure activity. If the cause is readily reversible, such as hypoglycemia, there is no need to initiate antiepileptic treatment. If the patient has a seizure related to a reversible process of medium duration such as an opportunistic infection (OI), it is reasonable to initiate an AED and continue it for 3 to 6 months after treatment for the OI has been completed. If a patient develops persistent seizure activity without a reversible cause, then a diagnosis of epilepsy should be given and long-term AED will be required.

Ideally, one should select an AED that avoids hepatic metabolism because of drug–drug interactions with antiretroviral therapy. However, this may not be possible in a resource-limited setting where the only available drugs are hepatically metabolized agents such as carbamazepine, phenobarbital and valproic acid. In this case valproic acid is the recommended agent, because it is a cytochrome P450 enzyme inhibitor as opposed to carbamazepine and phenobarbitone, which are cytochrome P450 enzyme inducers. When long-term treatment with carbamazepine or phenobarbital is the only option, the patient needs to be monitored closely for virological failure.

Further Reading

1. Heckmann JE, Bhigjee AI. Tropical neurology. In: Farrar J, editor. Manson's Tropical Diseases. 23rd ed. London: Elsevier; 2013 [chapter 71].

2. Siddiqi OK, Elafros MA, Bositis CM, et al. New-onset seizure in hiv-infected adult Zambians: a search for causes and consequences. Neurology 2017;88(5):477–82.

3. Radhakrishnan K. Challenges in the management of epilepsy in resource-poor countries. Nat Rev Neurol 2009;5(6):323–30.

4. Siddiqi O, Birbeck GL. Safe treatment of seizures in the setting of HIV/AIDS. Curr Treat Options Neurol 2013;15(4):529–43.

5. Bonello M, Michael BD, Solomon T. Infective causes of epilepsy. Semin Neurol 2015;35(3):235–44.

76

A 55-Year Old Woman from Turkey With Fever of Unknown Origin

ANDREAS J. MORGUET AND THOMAS SCHNEIDER

Clinical Presentation

History

A 55-year-old woman of Turkish provenance presents to a hospital in Germany with intermittent fever up to 39.5°C (103.1°F), night sweats, chest pain and fatigue. The patient had visited her relatives in Turkey several weeks before. There is a history of rheumatic fever in her childhood and mechanical mitral and aortic valve replacement at the age of 37 and 53 years, respectively (St Jude Medical prostheses).

Clinical Findings

The patient's blood pressure and heart rate are within normal limits. There are unremarkable prosthetic heart sounds and a systolic grade 1 murmur over the aortic area without radiation. Liver and spleen are not enlarged. No lymph nodes are palpable. No haemorrhages or petechiae are detectable.

Laboratory Results

There is slight anaemia (Hb 11.5 g/dL [reference >12 g/dL]). White blood cell count, lymphocyte–neutrophil ratio and platelet count are within normal limits. The C-reactive protein is 15 mg/dL (reference <0.5 mg/dL). Serum creatinine and transaminases are not elevated. Blood cultures are negative. Urinary cultures yield Enterobacteriaceae.

Additional Investigations

Chest radiography shows no infiltrates. Transthoracic echocardiography demonstrates competent prosthetic valves.

The patient is diagnosed with a urinary tract infection and treated with co-trimoxazole. Her fever settles and the patient's condition improves, but she complains of increasing dyspnoea and eventually slips into congestive heart failure.

Questions

1. What are differential diagnoses in this patient after deterioration?
2. What are the most promising next diagnostic steps?

Discussion

A 55-year old Turkish woman presents with fever of unknown origin. She has travelled to Turkey shortly before and has a history of double heart valve replacement. Treatment with co-trimoxazole results in some improvement, but then the patient develops signs of congestive heart failure.

Answer to Question 1

What Are Differential Diagnoses in This Patient After Deterioration?

Urosepsis could have been the underlying cause of the deterioration in this patient. However, urinary tract infection is usually easily managed with a short course of early antibiotic treatment. The patient's preceding stay in Turkey should raise the suspicion of another infection not detected so far, such as brucellosis, tuberculosis or Q-fever.

Answer to Question 2

What Are the Most Promising Next Diagnostic Steps?

With two prosthetic heart valves, our patient has an increased risk of infective endocarditis. Transoesophageal echocardiography is indicated to rule out cardiac involvement. Cultivation of blood cultures should be extended to up to 6 weeks in culture-negative endocarditis to reveal *Brucella* or *Coxiella* species.

The Case Continued...

After 4 weeks, the blood cultures taken initially grew *Brucella melitensis biovar 2*. Transoesophageal echocardiography revealed a large vegetation attached to the prosthetic mitral valve (Fig. 76.1). These findings led to the diagnosis of active *Brucella* endocarditis. Treatment with rifampicin, doxycycline and gentamicin was initiated. The patient improved rapidly. C-reactive protein returned to normal after 6 weeks of triple therapy. Two months later, however, an annular

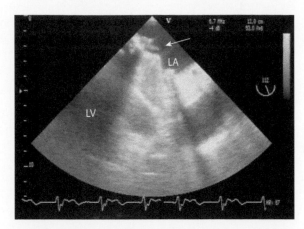

• **Fig. 76.1** Transoesophageal echocardiography showing a two-cornered vegetation (arrow) measuring about 18 mm × 7 mm attached to the posterolateral left atrial side of a St Jude Medical prosthesis in mitral position (LV, left ventricle; LA, left atrium).

abscess cavity around the aortic prosthesis was demonstrated on echocardiography; the patient at that time was on oral rifampicin and doxycycline. Finally, she gave her consent to a third thoracotomy, for prostheses exchange. After surgery she made a complete and sustained recovery.

Symptoms are non-specific, with fever, sweating, fatigue, weight loss, headache and joint pain persisting for weeks or even months. Its presentation as a non-specific febrile illness poses a differential diagnostic challenge in geographical regions where malaria and tuberculosis are highly prevalent and diagnostic resources are scarce, such as in sub-Saharan Africa. In the latter context, brucellosis is frequently missed as a major aetiology of fever, as has been shown from Tanzania.

Brucellosis may involve nearly every organ of the body. Although endocarditis is a less common manifestation of the disease, cardiac valve involvement was the most frequent cause of death from brucellosis in the past.

Definitive diagnosis requires the isolation of the bacteria from the blood, body fluids or tissues. This can be challenging as culture may take several weeks. In endemic settings, serological tests are often the only available diagnostic test and their interpretation may be challenging.

Treatment of brucellosis requires combination antibiotic therapy of several weeks' to several months' duration to prevent relapses.

The choice of the regimen and treatment duration depend upon clinical course and organ manifestation. Drugs most commonly used are doxycycline, gentamicin, rifampicin and co-trimoxazole.

In the case of cardiac valve involvement, spondylitis or neurobrucellosis, extended parenteral antimicrobial therapy is recommended. Patients with *Brucella* endocarditis will frequently require valve replacement in addition to antibiotic therapy.

SUMMARY BOX

Brucellosis

Brucellosis is one of the most common zoonotic infections worldwide. Its true incidence is unknown, because it typically affects rural communities and it is difficult to diagnose. Hot spots of the disease are Eastern Europe, the Middle East, Central and South Asia, Central and South America and Africa.

The disease is caused by intracellular bacteria of the genus *Brucella*. The *Brucella* species most importantly involved in human disease are *B. melitensis* (goats, sheep, camels), *B. abortus* (cattle), *B. suis* (pigs) and *B. canis* (dogs).

Brucellosis is most commonly acquired by eating raw or undercooked meat and offal or untreated dairy products. Also, close contact with infected livestock poses a risk. It is an important occupational hazard among herdsmen, dairy farmers, abattoir workers and laboratory technicians.

Further Reading

1. Beeching NJ, Madkour MM. Brucellosis. In: Farrar J, editor. Manson's Tropical Diseases. 23rd ed. London: Elsevier; 2013 [chapter 28].
2. Dean AS, Crump L, Greter H, et al. Global burden of human brucellosis: a systematic review of disease frequency. PLoS Negl Trop Dis 2012;6:e1865.
3. Dean AS, Crump L, Greter H, et al. Clinical manifestations of human brucellosis: a systematic review and meta-analysis. PLoS Negl Trop Dis 2012;6:e1929.
4. Crump JA, Morrissey AB, Nicholson WL, et al. Etiology of severe non-malaria febrile illness in Northern Tanzania: a prospective cohort study. PLoS Negl Trop Dis 2013;7:e2324.
5. Yagupsky P, Morata P, Colmenero JD, et al. Laboratory Diagnosis of Human Brucellosis. Clin Microbiol rev 2019;33:e00073-19.

77

A 51-Year-Old Female Traveller Returning from Central America With Conjunctivitis, Rash and Peripheral Oedema

ANDREAS NEUMAYR AND JOHANNES BLUM

Clinical Presentation

History

A 51-year-old female Swiss traveller presented to the outpatient department 6 days after returning from a 2-week holiday to Guatemala and El Salvador. Four days after her return, the patient noticed a generalized slightly pruritic maculopapular rash on the face, trunk, and extremities. There was no fever and no other accompanying symptoms. On the next day the rash worsened and a non-purulent bilateral conjunctivitis developed. The patient did not report any chronic underlying disease nor the intake of any medication.

Clinical Findings

The patient was afebrile. Upon inspection there was conjunctivitis and a generalised maculopapular rash, also involving the face. Additionally, the patient showed tender oedema of the hands, elbows, knees and feet (Fig. 77.1). There was also generalized lymphadenopathy (cervical, axillary, and inguinal).

Laboratory results

The full blood count was normal. CRP was 8 mg/L (<5) and creatinine was very mildly elevated (87 µmol/L, range 35–80 µmol/L). Liver function tests were normal.

Questions

1. What are your differential diagnoses?
2. What diagnostic tests would you perform?

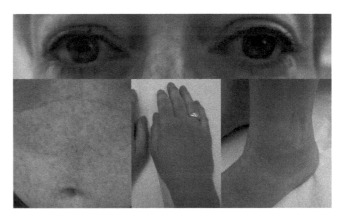

• **Fig. 77.1** Conjunctivitis, maculopapular skin rash, and peripheral oedema of the patient.

Discussion

Six days after returning from a 2-week holiday to Guatemala and El Salvador, a 51-year-old female Swiss traveller presents with a slightly pruritic disseminated maculopapular rash, conjunctivitis, peripheral painful oedema (hands, elbows, knees and feet) and a generalized lymphadenopathy.

Answer to Question 1
What Are Your Differential Diagnoses?

The clinical presentation is highly suggestive of an arboviral infection, which is also in line with the putative incubation period. The three most important arboviral infections in Central and South America are dengue, chikungunya and zika. Dengue is endemic throughout much

TABLE 77.1	**Comparative Clinical Symptom Patterns Observed in Dengue, Chikungunya and Zika Infections.**		
	Dengue	Chikungunya	Zika
Incubation period (days)	4–10	3–7	3–12
Asymptomatic infection (%)	50–80	3–28	~80
Fever	+++	+++	+
Headache	+++	++	+
Conjunctivitis	-	-	++
Arthralgias	++	+++	+
Myalgias	++	+	+
Skin rash	++	++	+++
Peripheral oedema	-	-	++
Haemorrhagic manifestations	++	(+)	-
Circulatory collapse/ shock	+	-	-
Thrombocytopenia	++	++	-
Lymphadenopathy	++	++	+

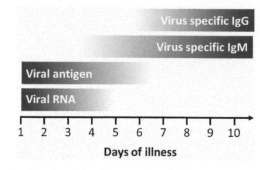

• **Fig. 77.2** Kinetics of the different arboviral test parameters.

of Central and South America, and it is the most frequent arboviral infection in travellers returning from the tropics. Chikungunya was absent in Central and South America until the virus was introduced in 2013. After its introduction, the virus spread to most tropical regions of the American continent. Zika was absent in Central and South America until 2015, when the virus was introduced to Brazil and caused a pandemic affecting most tropical regions of the American continent in the subsequent years.

Acute dengue, chikungunya, and zika infections have similar presentations and may be clinically indistinguishable. However, the presence of a skin rash, conjunctivitis and peripheral oedema in an afebrile patient is highly suggestive of a Zika virus infection (Table 77.1).

Answer to Question 2

What Diagnostic Tests Would You Perform?

When testing for arboviral infections, the kinetics of the different test parameters have to be taken into account. During the early phase of infection, viral RNA and viral antigen (e.g. dengue specific NS1) are circulating in the blood and can be detected by RT-PCR and specific antigen assays, respectively. After some days, viraemia is fading, terminated by the host's immune response, and viral RNA and antigen become undetectable in the blood samples, while now specific IgM and IgG rise and become detectable (Fig. 77.2).

The diagnosis is made by the detection of viral RNA, viral antigen or specific IgM, or by the documentation of a ≥ fourfold rise of specific IgG antibody titres in paired (acute and

convalescent) serum samples. In resource-poor countries, as well as in daily clinical practice in travel medicine, rapid diagnostic tests (RDTs) for dengue (testing for NS1-Ag, IgM, and IgG) and chikungunya (testing for IgM) are widely available and often the primarily performed diagnostic tests. RDTs to diagnose Zika virus infections are under development.

In our case, RDTs for dengue and chikungunya were negative.

The Case continued...

Because the performed RDTs for dengue and chikungunya both showed a negative result, the patient's blood samples were sent to a reference laboratory for arboviruses and our clinical suspicion of a Zika virus infection was confirmed by PCR as well as seroconversion (Table 77.2). A rise in

TABLE 77.2	**Blood Test Results**		
	First serum sample[†]	Second serum sample[‡]	Interpretation
Dengue IgM IIFT	negative	negative	negative
Dengue IgG IIFT	1:20	1:5120	*cross-reactivity*
Dengue NS1-Ag	negative	negative	negative
Chikungunya IgM ELISA	negative	ND	negative
Chikungunya IgM IIFT	ND	negative	negative
Chikungunya IgG IIFT	ND	negative	negative
Zika IgM IIFT	negative	1:640	positive
Zika IgG IIFT	1:20	1:5120	positive
Zika RT-PCR	positive	ND	positive

[†]obtained 6 days after onset of symptoms
[‡]obtained 7 days after the first serum sample
IIFT: Indirect Immunofluorescence Test; RT-PCR: real-time reverse transcription polymerase chain reaction; ELISA: Enzyme-linked Immunosorbent Assay; ND: not done.

anti-Dengue IgG was interpreted as cross-reactivity which is common among viruses of the same family.

SUMMARY BOX

Acute Arboviral Infection

Acute dengue, chikungunya, and Zika infections have similar presentations and are often clinically indistinguishable. Although the pattern of clinical symptoms can point towards the correct diagnosis, specific molecular or immunological tests are necessary to make a final diagnosis.

Interpretation of serological test results demands some caution, because cross-reactivity of antibodies directed against viruses belonging to the same family of viruses may be misleading.

Although dengue virus NS1 antigen tests are mostly specific for dengue virus infection, serological assays may show cross-reactivity with Zika virus (ZIKV) specific antibodies (as in our case). The diagnostic value of RT-PCR for detection of Zika virus RNA in the blood is limited because viraemia is usually low and limited to the first few days after disease onset. However, Zika virus RNA detection in urine provides a feasible alternative: ZIKV is detectable with higher RNA loads and for a longer period (10–20 days after onset of symptoms) in urine samples than in serum samples.

Arboviral infections are self-limiting and, in the absence of specific treatment options, clinical management is exclusively supportive. Special features of Zika virus include its sexual transmissibility, the potential to trigger post-infectious Guillan-Barré-Syndrome, and, in the case of intrauterine infection, its ability to cause severe foetopathy (primarily microcephaly).

Further Reading

1. Young PR, Ng LFP, Hall RA, et al. Arbovirus Infections. In: Farrar J, editor. Manson's Tropical Diseases. 23rd ed. London: Elsevier; 2013 [chapter 14].
2. Baud D, Gubler DJ, Schaub B, et al. An update on Zika virus infection. *Lancet* 2017;390(10107):2099–109.
3. Peters R, Stevenson M. Zika virus diagnosis: challenges and solutions. *Clin Microbiol Infect* 2019;25(2):142–6.

78

A 42-Year-Old British Man Living in Malawi With Anaphylactic Shock

ANTHONY D. HARRIES

Clinical Presentation

History

A 42-year-old British male expatriate who has lived in Malawi for 18 months presents to the local hospital emergency room with a florid itchy rash, difficulty in breathing and a feeling he is going to die. He thinks he might have been bitten on his ankle by a tick 2 days previously while out walking in the countryside. Twenty-four hours after this event he noticed a circumscribed, painless, indurated lesion on the inside of his left ankle and this was accompanied by fever and arthralgia. He went to a clinic where a blood film for malaria parasites was reported negative. He was treated with paracetamol. On the day of admission, he developed a widespread itchy rash and shortly afterwards became progressively unable to breathe and felt faint. There was a family history of allergy. He had kept bees in the United Kingdom and had frequently been stung without ill effect. However, 9 months previously he had been bitten by insects while at Lake Malawi and had developed an asthmatic attack which resolved spontaneously over 2 days.

Clinical Findings

On examination, he is clammy, in a state of collapse and has a widespread urticarial rash. There is respiratory distress and stridor. There is an indurated circumscribed swelling on the inside of his left ankle (Fig. 78.1). His vital signs are: temperature 38°C, pulse rate 130 bpm, systolic blood pressure 60 mmHg. Chest auscultation reveals expiratory wheezes.

Laboratory results

Haemoglobin 17.4 d/dL; white cell count 6.1 G/L (polymorphs 85%, lymphocytes 10%); erythrocyte sedimentation rate 5 mm/hour; blood film negative for malaria parasites; chest radiograph normal; stool and urine microscopy negative.

Questions

1. Based on the clinical history and examination and investigations done, what are the possible causes of this man's illness?
2. How should he be further managed?

Discussion

This male British expatriate presents with the clinical picture of anaphylactic shock. He relates this to a tick bite he suffered few days prior. On admission is also febrile

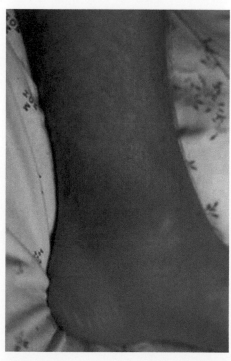

• **Fig. 78.1** Circumscribed, painless slightly erythematous swelling on the inside of the left ankle.

and besides his rash has an erythematous lesion on his ankle.

Answer to Question 1

Based on the Clinical History and Examination and Investigations Done, What Are the Possible Causes of This Man's Illness?

With a story of possible tick bite, a positive family history of allergy, a history of bee keeping, an asthmatic episode after insect bites 9 months previously in addition to the dramatic clinical presentation of urticarial rash and anaphylactic shock, the initial diagnosis was of a possible hypersensitivity reaction to a tick bite. Other differentials to include are invasive helminthiasis such as acute schistosomiasis (Katayama syndrome), acute fascioliasis and Loeffler's syndrome (the acute pulmonary stage of infection with *Ascaris lumbricoides*); rickettsial disease; and connective tissue disease. Both in allergic reactions and in invasive helminth infections though, eosinophilia would be typical which is absent in this case.

Answer to Question 2

How Should He Be Further Managed?

A firm diagnosis has not been made and he needs to remain in the hospital under observation receiving treatment as needed for his intermittent allergic manifestations.

The Case Continued…

A diagnosis of anaphylactic shock is made and 0.5ml of 1:1000 adrenaline is given by deep intramuscular injection with good effect. He is admitted to hospital and over the next 2 days he is treated with intermittent injections of intramuscular adrenaline, intravenous hydrocortisone and oral antihistaminics for intermittent episodes of widespread urticaria associated with stridor and audible wheezing.

On day 3 of his hospital admission, his condition changes. The stridor and wheezing cease, the urticarial rash is replaced by a diffuse erythematous rash (Fig. 78.2), his face becomes

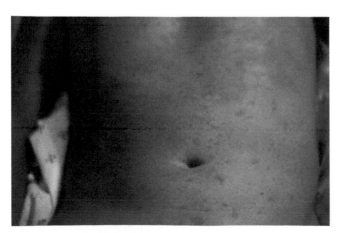

• **Fig. 78.2** Abdominal rash.

slightly puffy, he has a bad headache and a sustained fever of 38 to 39°C. On direct enquiry, he says he visited a national game park 2 weeks before this current illness where he has suffered numerous painful bites by tsetse flies. The fever, headache, puffy face and erythematous rash suggest trypanosomiasis and the circumscribed swelling on the ankle is now recognized to be a "trypanosomal chancre". A thick blood film reveals 5 to 10 trypanosomes per high power field and the diagnosis of trypanosomiasis is confirmed. He is given a test dose of suramin 0.25 g with no ill effect, 0.5 g 2 days later, 1.0 g another 2 days later and this is followed by weekly doses of 1.0 g to a total of 5.75g suramin without ill effect. 24 hours after the first dose of suramin, his cerebrospinal fluid (CSF) is examined by lumbar puncture to assess whether there has been central nervous system invasion – his CSF is normal. His urine is monitored weekly during the suramin treatment; towards the end of treatment his urine shows protein, casts and white cells, but these all disappear a few weeks after treatment has finished.

TABLE 78.1	Standard Treatment for Human African Trypanosomiasis by Species and Stage	
	West African trypanosomiasis (*T. brucei gambiense*)	East African trypanosomiasis (*T. brucei rhodesiense*)
First stage	Pentamidine IM or IV OD × 7 days or Fexinidazole PO OD × 10 days	Suramin IV, 6 injections, e.g. days 0,1,3,7,14, 21. Or Pentamidine IM or IV OD × 7 days
Second stage	Nifurtimox-Eflornithine combination therapy (NECT) (Nifurtimox PO TDS × 10 days + Eflornithine IV BD × 7 days) or Fexinidazole PO OD × 10 days	Melarsoprol IV OD × 10 days

IM = intramuscularly, IV = intravenously, PO = orally, OD = once daily, BD = twice daily, TDS = three times a day
After Büscher, P., et al. 2017. Lancet.

SUMMARY BOX

Human African Trypanosomiasis (HAT)

The patient was diagnosed with HAT. East African trypanosomiasis (*Trypanosoma brucei rhodesiense*) appears epidemiologically and clinically likely. It is primarily a zoonosis, and animal reservoir hosts include domestic and game animals; its clinical course therefore tends to be rapid with a high case fatality rate if untreated. In contrast, West African trypanosomiasis is considered an anthroponotic disease. The parasite, *T. brucei gambiense,* is adapted to the human host, causing chronic symptoms and leading to the classic picture of "sleeping sickness", i.e. a chronic encephalopathy.

The reasons for the dramatic presentation of trypanosomiasis with anaphylaxis as with the case of this patient can only be speculative, but his "allergic" preponderance may have made him hypersensitive to the invasive trypanosomes as they migrated from the subcutaneous tissues of the chancre to the blood. Gold standard of diagnosis is the demonstration of trypanosomes in blood smears by microscopy. Why trypanosomes were not identified in the first blood smear 24 hours after his illness started is not clear – they may not have been present in sufficient numbers in the blood at that stage or they may have been missed by the laboratory technician who was focused on searching for malaria parasites. Suramin is the treatment of choice for early stage East African trypanosomiasis (Table 78.1). It needs to be administered carefully with an initial test dose in case of hypersensitivity reactions. It is potentially nephrotoxic, hence the need for urine monitoring.

In all cases of trypanosomiasis, it is essential to check the CSF for stage determination. It is best to perform the lumbar puncture 24 hours after the first dose of suramin to avoid introducing trypanosomes from the blood into the CSF during lumbar puncture. If there are >5 cells/µl in the CSF or trypanosomes are found, this is considered stage 2 (neurological involvement). Treatment in case of second stage East African trypanosomiasis is with melarsoprol, a trivalent arsenical drug with severe potential toxic effects (Table 78.1).

Further Reading

1. Burri C, Chappus F, Brun R. Human African Trypanosomiasis. pages 606-621. In: Farrar J, Hotez P, Junghanss T, Kang G, Lalloo D, White NJ, editors. Manson's Tropical Diseases. 23rd ed. London: Elsevier Saunders; 2013 [Chapter 45].
2. Thwaites GE, Day NPJ. Approach to fever in the returning traveler. N Engl J Med 2017;376:548–60. https://doi.org/10.1056/NEJMra1508435.
3. Büscher P, Cecchi G, Jamonneau V, et al. Human African Trypanosomiasis. Lancet 2017;390:2397–2409. https://doi.org/10.1016/S0140-6736(17)31510-6.
4. World Health Organization. Human African Trypanosomiasis. Available from: http://www.who.int/trypanosomiasis_african/en/.
5. Neuberger A, Meltzer E, Leshem E, et al. The changing epidemiology of Human African Trypanosomiasis among patients from Nonendemic countries – 1902-2012. PLoS One 2014;9(2): e88647. https://doi.org/10.1371/journal.pone.0088647.

79

A 34-Year-Old Male Immigrant from Peru With Chronic Diarrhoea and Severe Weight Loss

THOMAS WEITZEL AND CRISTINA GOENS

Clinical Presentation

History

A 34-year-old man presents to a hospital in Chile with a 6-month history of severe chronic diarrhoea associated with colicky abdominal pain and weight loss of approximately 20 kg. For more than 12 years he has suffered from recurrent episodes of diarrhoea and abdominal cramps; the frequency of these episodes appears to have increased in the past 2 years.

The patient originates from northern Peru but has been living in Chile for the past 9 years. He reports that his Peruvian wife and children are healthy, but that his mother and one brother suffered from chronic abdominal symptoms of unknown origin, leading to wasting and subsequent death at the age of 45 and 28 years, respectively.

Clinical Findings

The patient is cachectic with a severe loss of muscle mass and a body weight of 44 kg (BMI 17). Apart from slight pain on abdominal palpation, the physical examination is normal: He is afebrile, liver and spleen are not enlarged, there is no palpable lymphadenopathy and no peripheral oedema.

Laboratory results

His laboratory results on admission are shown in Table 79.1.

Other Investigations

Abdominal CT scan and abdominal MRI are without any pathological findings. Oesophagogastroduodenoscopy appeared macroscopically normal. Histology of a duodenal biopsy is shown in Fig. 79.1.

TABLE 79.1 Laboratory Results		
Parameter	Patient	Reference
WBC ($\times 10^9$/L)	11.7	4.5–11.0
Platelets ($\times 10^9$/L)	644	150–450
Haemoglobin (g/dL)	12.4	13.5–17.5
Protein (g/dL)	4.9	6.0–8.0
Albumin (g/dL)	2.2	3.5–5.0
ESR (mm/h)	26	1–14
HIV test	negative	-

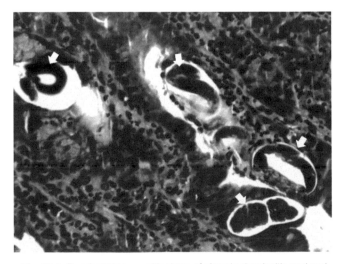

• **Fig. 79.1** Duodenal biopsy with signs of chronic duodenitis and multiple elongated structures (arrows) compatible with a helminth infection (H&E stain, magnification ×400).

Questions

1. Which helminth infections can cause such clinical manifestations and which parasitological examination(s) should urgently be performed to clarify the histopathology report?
2. Would you order any additional investigations?

Discussion

A migrant of Peruvian origin living in Chile presents with chronic diarrhoea and abdominal pain, leading to severe weight loss and cachexia. Laboratory values show signs of malabsorption and inflammation. The physical examination, abdominal imaging and upper GI endoscopy are unremarkable, but the pathologist reports structures compatible with helminth infection in duodenal biopsies.

Answer to Question 1

Which Helminth Infections Can Cause Such Clinical Manifestations and Which Parasitological Examination(s) Should Urgently Be Performed to Clarify the Histopathology Report?

Chronic diarrhoea, malabsorption and wasting are usually not associated with intestinal helminth infections. Therefore diagnosis and treatment are often delayed. The two main helminth species capable of causing chronic diarrhoea and wasting are *Strongyloides stercoralis* and *Capillaria philippinensis* (see Case 58). In immunocompromised patients, intestinal protozoa such as *Cryptosporidium* species or *Cystoisospora belli* might cause similar manifestations. Our patient originated from northern Peru, a tropical region highly endemic for *S. stercoralis*. Routine ova and parasite stool tests might be ordered; but most importantly, specific tests to detect larvae of *S. stercoralis* such as an agar plate method or the Baermann technique should be performed. The latter has the advantage of being technically simple and providing results within a few hours. If stool samples are positive, respiratory samples and urine should also be examined for *S. strongyloides* larvae.

Answer to Question 2

Would You Order Any Additional Investigations?

Because *S. stercoralis* is the most probable cause of this severe disease, serology for HTLV-1 should be ordered. HTLV-1 is an important risk factor for *S. stercoralis* hyperinfection syndrome, and Peru is endemic for this retrovirus. The family history of the patient also hints at this virus that is commonly transmitted by breastfeeding.

The Case Continued…

The patient was hospitalized and stabilized under symptomatic treatment and parenteral nutrition. After the histopathology report was received, a fresh stool sample was sent to the parasitology laboratory for Baermann testing, which demonstrated a high load of rhabditiform larvae of *S. stercoralis* (Fig. 79.2A). Numerous larvae were also present in respiratory secretions (Fig. 79.2B), but not in urine. Oral treatment with ivermectin (200 µg/kg per day × 7 days) was initiated and repeated after 2 weeks. HTLV-1 co-infection was confirmed by serology. The patient recovered from diarrhoea and other abdominal symptoms within weeks. Parasitological follow-up examination after 3 months was negative. At that point, the patient had gained 13 kg and was without postprandial abdominal cramps for the first time in more than 10 years. Baermann testing of the family and other household members revealed asymptomatic *S. stercoralis* infection of his wife and one of the two children. His wife tested HTLV-1 positive, but both children were negative.

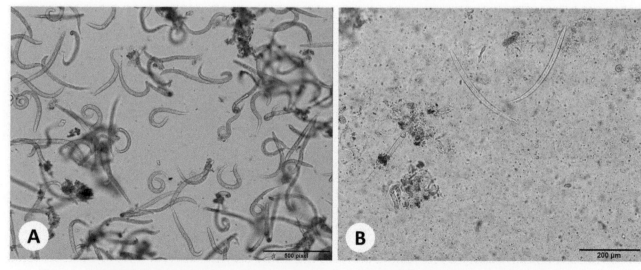

• **Fig. 79.2** (A) Baermann technique showing high load of motile rhabditiform larvae of *S. stercoralis* in a stool sample. (B) Rhabditiform larvae are also present in a wet mount preparation of respiratory secretion.

SUMMARY BOX

HTLV-1-Associated *Strongyloides stercoralis* Hyperinfection Syndrome

S. stercoralis is a soil-transmitted nematode, capable of maintaining chronic intestinal infection through a cycle of auto-infection. It is a poverty-associated neglected disease, endemic in most tropical and subtropical regions worldwide. Strongyloidiasis is not unusual in returning travellers, who typically present with non-specific gastrointestinal complaints and/or eosinophilia (see Case 20). In immunocompromised patients, the parasite may multiply massively, resulting in severe and potentially fatal complications, commonly called "hyperinfection syndrome". Corticosteroids play a major role as a risk factor for strongyloides hyperinfection syndrome. In addition, HTLV-1 infection is an important predisposing condition.

HTLV-1 is a neglected retrovirus, which is primarily transmitted by breastfeeding, but also by sexual contact and blood products. It causes a Th1-predominant T-cell proliferation and a marked shift towards type 1 cytokines. This immunological imbalance affects the Th2-mediated control of *S. stercoralis,* with the risk of accelerated auto-infection leading to increased loads of *Strongyloides* adults and larvae.

In HIV/AIDS, T-cell response is shifted towards Th2 cytokines; therefore HIV infection is not usually associated with strongyloides hyperinfection syndrome, even though some cases have been described, e.g. in the context of immune reconstitution inflammatory syndrome (IRIS).

HTLV-1-associated *S. stercoralis* hyperinfection syndrome mostly presents as severe chronic diarrhoea, malabsorption, and wasting. Disseminated forms, which are characterized by invasion of extraintestinal tissues (apart from the lung passage of larvae), a more rapid progress and a high lethality, are more typically found in patients under corticosteroid therapy. Because patients with hyperinfection lack common hallmarks of strongyloidiasis, such as eosinophilia and elevated IgE levels, diagnosis is often delayed or missed.

The drug of choice for patients with strongyloides hyperinfection syndrome is ivermectin given over prolonged periods of time (e.g. 7 days for two or more cycles). Patients with signs of dissemination (e.g. larvae in urine) should be treated with ivermectin and albendazole in combination with broad-spectrum antibiotics to prevent Gram-negative infections (e.g. sepsis or meningitis) commonly associated with larval dissemination.

Management can be challenging in severely ill patients incapable of resorbing ivermectin from the gastrointestinal tract, e.g. in paralytic ileus, because no parenteral anthelminthic drugs are licensed for use in humans. However, parenteral ivermectin is commonly administered in veterinary medicine and some case reports describe successful subcutaneous treatment with a veterinary formulation of the drug. Because treatment failures might occur, patients require close follow-up. Family members should be screened for both *S. stercoralis* and HTLV-1 infection. Patients originating from endemic countries should be screened for *Strongyloides* infection before initiation of any immunosuppressive therapy.

Further Reading

1. Brooker SJ, Bundy DAP. Soil-transmitted Helminths (Geohelminths). In: Farrar J, editor. Manson's Tropical Diseases. 23rd ed. London: Elsevier; 2013 [chapter 55].
2. Solomon T. Virus Infections of the Nervous System. In: Farrar J, editor. Manson's Tropical Diseases. 23rd ed. London: Elsevier; 2013 [chapter 21].
3. Keiser PB, Nutman TB. Strongyloides stercoralis in the immunocompromised population. Clin Microbiol Rev 2004;17:208–17.
4. Carvalho EM, Da Fonseca Porto A. Epidemiological and clinical interaction between HTLV-1 and Strongyloides stercoralis. Parasite Immunol 2004;26:487–97.
5. Toledo R, Muñoz-Antoli C, Esteban JG. Strongyloidiasis with emphasis on human infections and its different clinical forms. Adv Parasitol 2015;88:165–241.

80

A 62-Year-Old Man from Thailand With a Liver Mass

PRAKASIT SA-NGAIMWIBOOL AND YUKIFUMI NAWA

Clinical Presentation

History

A 62-year-old male Thai police sergeant major from Kalasin Province in northeast Thailand presents at an urban hospital for his annual physical check-up. On abdominal ultrasonography, a solitary mass is found in the liver. He denies any clinical symptoms, there is no weight loss, no jaundice and no other gastrointestinal symptoms.

He is referred to a hospital in Khon Kaen for further investigations and treatment.

Clinical Findings

He appears in good health and vital signs are normal. Physical examination shows no jaundice. Liver and spleen are not palpable. No liver stigmata are found nor is any lymphadenopathy detected.

Laboratory results

His laboratory results are shown in Table 80.1.

Imaging

Abdominal MRI reveals a single solid liver mass in the right liver lobe (segments VI/VII), Fig. 80.1.

Questions

1. What is your differential diagnosis?
2. What additional information should you obtain from the patient?

Discussion

A 62-year-old asymptomatic Thai man undergoes his annual physical check-up. Ultrasound incidentally detects a solitary liver mass. Liver function tests are normal, and Hepatitis B

TABLE 80.1	Laboratory Results of the Thai Patient With a Liver Mass	
Parameter	Patient	Reference
AST (U/L)	26	4–36
ALT (U/L)	32	12–32
ALP (U/L)	84	42–121
Total bilirubin (mg/dL)	0.6	0.3–1.5
Direct bilirubin (mg/dL)	0.2	0.0–0.5
HBsAg (MEIA)	Negative	Negative
Anti-HBs (ELISA, IU/L)	24.13	0.0–10.0
HBeAg (ELISA)	Negative	Negative
Anti-HBc (ELISA)	Positive	Negative
Anti-HCV	Negative	Negative
AFP (U/mL)	2.8	0.0–10.0
CEA (µg/L)	18.96	0.0–2.5
CA19-9 (U/mL)	342.80	0.0–37.0

serology suggests previous infection. The CA19-9 level is markedly elevated.

Answer to Question 1

What is Your Differential Diagnosis?

The most important differential diagnoses in this Thai man in his sixties are hepatocellular carcinoma, cholangiocarcinoma (CCA), a metastatic tumour and some infections, including tuberculosis.

In an otherwise asymptomatic patient with a high serum CA19-9 level without a history and signs of chronic viral hepatitis, CCA is the most likely diagnosis. Metastatic cancer should be considered and thorough investigation is required to detect the primary site of the tumour.

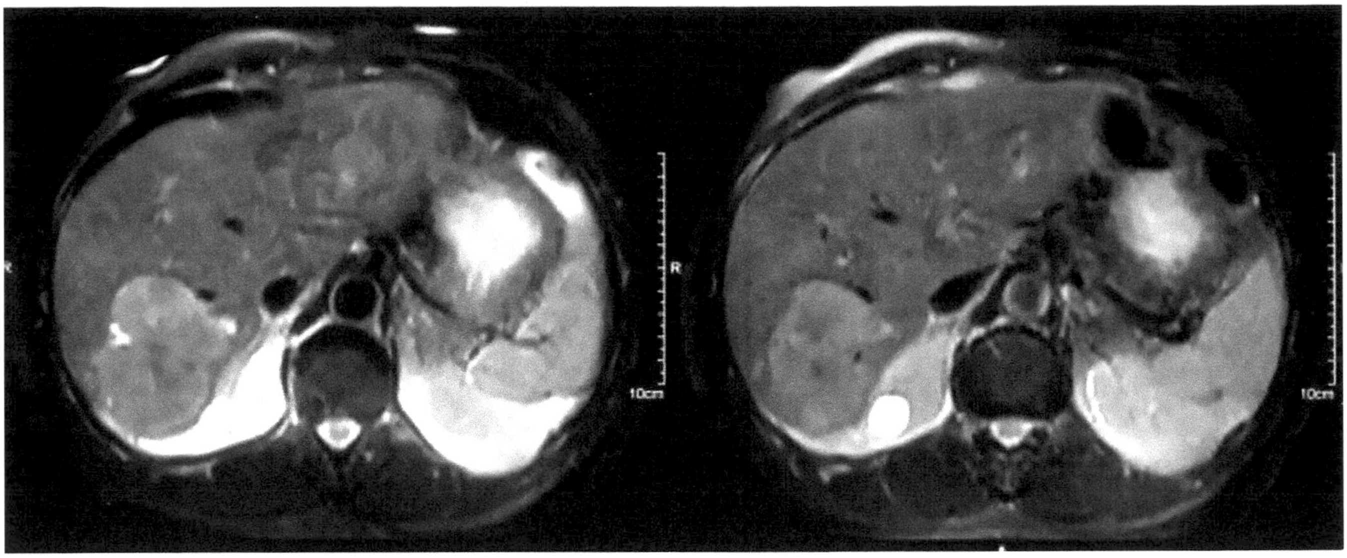

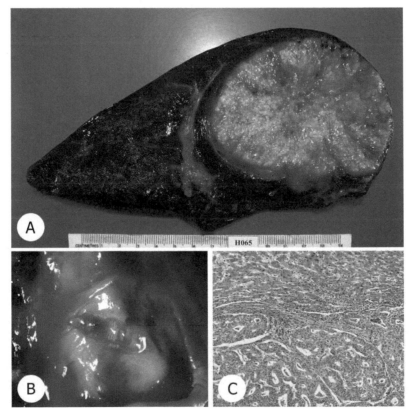

• **Fig. 80.1** Abdominal MRI revealing a single solid liver mass lesion at the segment VI/VII. No marked bile duct dilatation is seen.

• **Fig. 80.2** (A) A single heterogenous whitish-yellow mass, size 9 × 9 cm in diameter at the segment VII and VIII. The dilated bile duct with a small parasite (arrow). The liver parenchyma appears non-cirrhotic; (B) The adjacent dilated bile duct contains a few liver flukes *(O. viverrini);* and (C) The histology of the tumour shows infiltrative compact glandular structures, lined by dysplastic columnar cells with necrosis.

Answer to Question 2

What Additional Information Should You Obtain from the Patient?

Kalasin, where the patient comes from, is a province in northeast Thailand. Given his region of origin it is important to ask for a history of eating raw or undercooked freshwater fish, which frequently contains metacercariae of the liver fluke, *Opisthorchis viverrini*.

Traditional food containing undercooked freshwater fish is usually eaten among the villagers in the region including their children. Exposure to the fluke early in life is an important risk factor for the development of CCA. Liver fluke infection is easily treated with praziquantel; however, re-infection is common in an area where traditional food is regularly consumed.

The Case Continued...

The patient was admitted to the hospital and underwent hemihepatectomy. A large tumour (9 × 9 cm) of whitish-yellowish colour was found in the right liver lobe. In addition, liver flukes were detected in the adjacent bile duct (Fig. 80.2A and B). The liver parenchyma itself appeared non-cirrhotic.

Histology confirmed intrahepatic CCA (Fig. 80.2C) and the patient was started on postoperative chemotherapy. Additional past medical history taken after surgery revealed that he had a history of liver fluke infection and praziquantel treatment in the past 10 years at the local primary care unit.

SUMMARY BOX

Cholangiocarcinoma

CCA is strongly associated with chronic liver fluke infection. *O. viverrini* and *Clonorchis sinensis* are therefore classified by WHO as biological carcinogens.

The Greater Mekong subregion has the highest reported incidence of liver fluke-associated CCA in the world. It is also endemic in East Asia (southern China, Korea, northern Vietnam) because of *C. sinensis* infection, and in Kazakhstan, Siberia, other parts of Russia and various European countries, where *O. felineus* is the major parasite.

The infection is acquired by eating raw freshwater fish and uncooked fermented fish containing metacercariae of the parasites. Adult worms live in the small intrahepatic bile ducts of their definitive host, which includes humans, cats, dogs and other mammals. They can live in the bile duct for over 20 years and re-infection may occur. Prevalence and intensity of infection increase with age.

Chronic infection may lead to periductal fibrosis, cholecystitis and gallstones. Mutagenesis is thought to be triggered by chronic mechanical and chemical irritation as well as immunological factors. Besides the infection itself, cultural and lifestyle factors have recently been found to be relevant risk factors for CCA; among others, a combination of alcohol use and smoking.

The complex interaction of risk factors besides fluke infection may explain why despite the widespread availability of praziquantel and massive control efforts, CCA remains a major health problem in endemic regions in Asia.

CCA may long be asymptomatic, as shown in this case. Screening and early detection of CCA is crucial but challenging.

In Thailand, a comprehensive approach to prevention and control of liver fluke infection has been implemented under the "Cholangiocarcinoma Screening and Care Program" (CASCAP). Also, EcoHealth-based integrated control programmes such as the "Lawa model" have been successfully propagated at the community level. The "Lawa model" (referring to the fluke-endemic Lawa lake region in Thailand) is a programme which includes treatment with anthelmintic drugs, intensive health education methods, ecosystem monitoring and active community participation.

Further Reading

1. Sithithaworn P, Sripa B, Kaewkes S, et al. Food-borne trematodes. In: Farrar J, editor. Manson's Tropical Infectious Diseases. 23rd ed. London: Elsevier; 2013 [chapter 53].

2. Sithithaworn P, Andrews RH, De NV, et al. The current status of opisthorchiasis and clonorchiasis in the Mekong Basin. Parasitol Int 2012;61(1):10–6.

3. Sripa B, Tangkawattana S, Sangnikul T. The lawa model: a sustainable, integrated opisthorchiasis control program using the Eco-Health approach in the lawa lake region of Thailand. Parasitol Int 2017;66(4):346–54.

4. Khuntikeo N, Titapun A, Loilome W, et al. Current perspectives on opisthorchiasis control and cholangiocarcinoma detection in Southeast Asia. Front Med (Lausanne) 2018;5:117.

5. Steele JA, Richter CH, Echaubard P, et al. Thinking beyond *Opisthorchis viverrini* for risk of cholangiocarcinoma in the lower Mekong region: a systematic review and meta-analysis. Infect Dis Poverty 2018;7:44.

81

A 33-Year-Old Refugee from Afghanistan With Recurrent Fever and Back Pain

PETER SOTHMANN AND CASSANDRA ALDRICH

Clinical Presentation

History

A 33-year-old male refugee from Afghanistan presents to a German clinic with a 6-month history of recurrent fever, night sweats and progressive back pain. After leaving Afghanistan with his wife and two children, the family first lived in a refugee camp in Iran. There, the patient started feeling ill about 6 months ago and was treated with tablets for several weeks. Initially he also received intragluteal injections. His symptoms subsided whilst on medication but recurred after the treatment ended. After crossing Turkey and Eastern Europe, the family reached Germany 4 months ago. All medical documents were lost during the journey.

Clinical Findings

The patient is afebrile and in fair general condition. Vital signs are normal. On examination, there is marked spinal tenderness in the lumbar region. The remaining examination is unremarkable.

Laboratory Results and Imaging

Differential blood count, liver and renal function tests as well as LDH are normal. C-reactive protein and erythrocyte sedimentation rate are slightly raised at 26 mg/L (<5 mg/L) and 40 mm/hour (<20 mm/hour), respectively. Urinalysis is unremarkable.

MRI of the spine reveals signal enhancement of the L3 and L4 vertebral bodies, the corresponding vertebral disc and the right psoas muscle, as well as disc space narrowing and irregularities of both adjacent vertebral endplates (Fig. 81.1A and B). A chest x-ray shows no abnormalities.

Questions

1. What are the most likely differential diagnoses in this patient?
2. Which investigations are useful to determine the causative agent?

Discussion

A male Afghan refugee presents with a 6-month history of recurrent fever, night sweats and progressive back pain. Physical examination reveals localized lumbar spinal tenderness. CRP and ESR are slightly raised and an MRI of the spine shows spondylodiscitis of L3/L4 with involvement of the psoas muscle.

Answer to Question 1

What are the Most Likely Differential Diagnoses in This Patient?

Spondylitis in a febrile young adult is likely to be infectious. Globally, tuberculosis is the main cause of infectious spondylitis. Spinal brucellosis may be equally common or even predominant in highly endemic countries, such as Afghanistan.

Other infectious causes of spondylitis mirror those of osteomyelitis and usually follow haematogenous spread from a distant site of infection. The spectrum of pathogens includes *Staphylococcus aureus*, pyogenic and non-pyogenic streptococci and Gram-negative bacteria such as *Salmonella* species. In addition, histoplasmosis, actinomycosis and melioidosis may be relevant causes depending on local epidemiology.

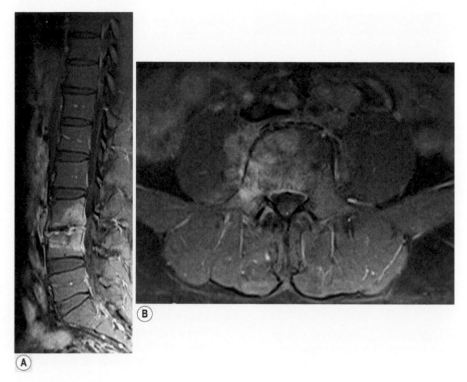

• **Fig. 81.1A and B** MRI of the spine reveals signal enhancement of the L3 and L4 vertebral bodies, the correspond-ing vertebral disc and the right psoas muscle, as well as disc space narrowing and irregularities of both adjacent vertebral endplates.

Answer to Question 2

Which Investigations are Useful to Determine the Causative Agent?

It is not possible to reliably distinguish spinal tuberculosis from brucellosis by x-ray or CT/MRI imaging; microbiolog-ical testing is required. In patients from highly endemic countries, serological testing and interferon gamma release assays (IGRA) are of limited diagnostic value, because they are not able to distinguish between active and latent/past infection. Definitive diagnosis requires isolation of the caus-ative agent from blood or tissue samples.

Spinal tuberculosis is rarely accompanied by pulmonary involvement, and sputum samples often remain negative. In brucellosis, the sensitivity of blood culture is generally high in acute disease and decreases over time. Bone marrow cultures have a better yield at all stages of disease.

CT-guided percutaneous vertebral biopsy and subsequent tissue culture and molecular analysis is the diagnostic gold standard in infectious spondylitis. Histopathology should be performed simultaneously to rule out malignancy and to confirm granulomatous inflammation, which is a feature of both tuberculosis (caseous) and brucellosis (non-caseous).

It is important to notify laboratory staff that brucellosis is suspected: *Brucella* cultures are highly infectious and require biosafety level 3 handling; they may also have a prolonged

time to positivity (although this is less of an issue with mod-ern automated blood culture systems).

The Case Continued…

Several blood cultures are taken but remain negative. Spu-tum samples are negative for acid-fast bacilli. A CT-guided biopsy of the lesion is performed without complications. Culture of the tissue sample reveals *Brucella melitensis* as the causative agent. No additional sites of infection are iden-tified on imaging. Importantly, there is no sign of endocar-ditis on echocardiography.

The presentation is classified as "complicated brucellosis" with spondylitis and para-vertebral abscess formation accord-ing to WHO criteria, which requires a prolonged course of antimicrobial combination therapy. The patient is treated with doxycycline 100 mg twice daily and rifampicin 900mg daily for 16 weeks. Additionally, intramuscular strep-tomycin (1 g daily) is given for the first 3 weeks of treatment.

The fever subsides after several days and inflammation parameters return to normal several weeks after initiation of antimicrobial therapy. A second MRI at the end of treat-ment shows full resolution of the paravertebral abscess. One year post treatment completion, the patient shows no signs of relapse.

SUMMARY BOX

Brucellosis

Brucellosis is a common zoonotic bacterial infection and an important differential diagnosis in prolonged febrile illness. Currently, around 500 000 cases of brucellosis are reported to the WHO each year, with global incidence rates increasing. *B. melitensis* is the most common cause of brucellosis worldwide and mainly infects camels, sheep and goats. Frequent routes of animal-to-human transmission include consumption of unpasteurized dairy products as well as exposure to bodily fluids and aerosols during animal birth or slaughter. The possibility of airborne transmission requires special safety precautions while handling *Brucella* cultures in the laboratory (biosafety level 3).

In the early stages, brucellosis usually presents as a non-focal febrile illness. Clinical signs and symptoms are non-specific and may include night sweats, fatigue, lymphadenopathy and hepatosplenomegaly. Localized infection develops frequently during the course of disease and may affect the musculoskeletal, genitourinary, central nervous or cardiovascular system. Osteoarticular involvement is particularly common (up to 40% of cases) and often presents as peripheral arthritis, sacroiliitis or spondylitis.

Serological diagnostic tests are widely available but fail to distinguish current from past infection in areas of high endemicity. Blood culture has a high sensitivity in acute disease and tissue culture is considered the gold standard in localized infection.

Brucellosis therapy generally requires a combination of antimicrobials with activity in the acidic intracellular environment, as well as a prolonged course of treatment to avoid treatment failure and relapse. Preferred drug combinations of brucellosis are doxycylin plus an aminoglycoside (streptomycin or gentamicin) or plus rifampicin. In neurobrucellosis, ceftriaxone is combined with doxycyclin and rifampicin. If contraindications occur, ciprofloxacin and cotrimoxazole may be used. Treatment duration is between six weeks and several months depending upon organ manifestation and severity.

Although most osteoarticular complications can be treated with a standard course of 6 weeks' duration, brucella spondylitis requires prolonged treatment for at least 12 weeks to avoid relapse. Furthermore, surgical intervention may be required in cases of vertebral instability or epidural and paravertebral abscess formation.

Further Reading

1. Beeching NJ, Monir Makdour M. Brucellosis. In: Farrar J, editor. Manson's Tropical Diseases 23rd ed. London: Elsevier; 2014 (chapter 28).

2. Gouliouris T, Aliyu SH, Brown NM. Spondylodiscitis: Update on diagnosis and management. J Antimicrob Chemother 2010;65 (Suppl. 3):11–24. https://doi.org/10.1093/jac/dkq303.

3. Pappas G, Akritidis N, Bosilkovski M, et al. Brucellosis. N Engl J Med 2005;352(22):2325–36. https://doi.org/10.1056/NEJMra050570.

4. Corbel MJ. Brucellosis in humans and animals. WHO; 2006. p. 1–102.

5. Yousefi-Nooraie R, Mortaz-Hejri S, Mehrani M, et al. Antibiotics for treating human brucellosis. Cochrane database Syst Rev 2012;10(10):CD007179. https://doi.org/10.1002/14651858. CD007179.pub2.

82

A 31-Year-Old Man from Guatemala With Acute Weakness and Numbness of the Leg

CESAR G. BERTO AND CHRISTINA M. COYLE

Clinical presentation

History

A 31-year-old Guatemalan man with no past medical history presents to a hospital in New York City with several minutes of weakness and numbness of the leg. His symptoms resolved just before his arrival at the hospital. Two weeks previously, he also had two episodes of facial twitching that subsided without intervention after 10 seconds.

He was born and lived in a rural area of Guatemala before immigrating to New York 5 years ago. In Guatemala, his family owned uncorralled pigs and his house did not have sanitation services.

Clinical Findings

His vitals were normal. Cranial nerves were intact. Motor and sensory examinations were normal. Deep tendon reflexes and gait was normal. The rest of the exam was unremarkable.

Laboratory Results

Cell blood count and serum chemistry were within normal limits.

Imaging

The computed tomography (CT) and magnetic resonance imaging (MRI) on admission are shown in Figures 82.1 and 82.2. A CT angiography showed patent cerebral arteries.

Questions

1. What is the most likely diagnosis and what is the pathophysiology of this disease?
2. What is the approach to diagnosis and treatment?

Discussion

A young, previously healthy man from Guatemala presents with transitory ischemic attack. Imaging reveals parenchymal calcified lesions, complex cystic structures in the subarachnoid space and an old lacunar infarct proximal to a cyst with a normal CT angiography.

Answer to Question 1

What is the Most Likely Diagnosis and What is the Pathophysiology of This Disease?

These findings and the epidemiological risk factors are highly suggestive of subarachnoid neurocysticercosis.

The clinical expression of neurocysticercosis is pleomorphic and depends on the location, burden of disease and host

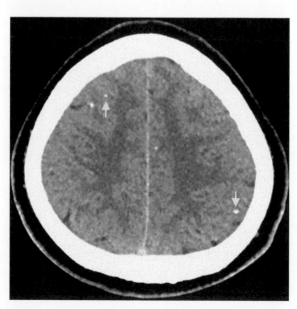

• **Fig. 82.1** CT of the head demonstrates multiple calcifications in the brain parenchyma (yellow arrows).

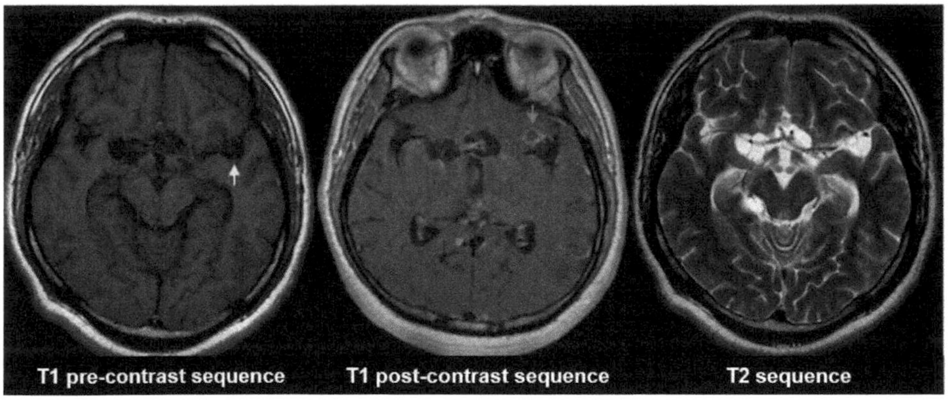

T1 pre-contrast sequence   **T1 post-contrast sequence**   **T2 sequence**

• **Fig. 82.2** MRI of the head on T1 sequence reveals dilation of the suprasellar and Sylvian cistern (yellow arrow). Peripheral enhancement (orange arrow) is evidenced after the administration of gadolinium. Corresponding fluid filled septated cystic lesions (blue arrow) are seen surrounding the proximal middle cerebral arteries on T2 sequence. An old lacunar infarct in the right frontal white matter proximal to an interhemispheric cyst was also found (not shown).

inflammatory response. Disease in the parenchyma behaves differently from neurocysticercosis involving the extra-parenchymal space. Therefore clinical presentation and therapeutic interventions for each location are different. Sub-arachnoid neurocysticercosis (SANCC) is probably the most severe form of neurocysticercosis. In the subarachnoid space, the parasite can undergo an aberrant continued growth and reach large sizes, especially when it is located in the Sylvian fissure. SANCC also has a high frequency of concomitant asymptomatic spinal involvement. Therefore an MRI of the spine should always be included.

The pathogenesis of the subarachnoid form is largely mediated by the host's inflammatory response. Clinically, it can manifest as meningitis, communicating hydrocepha-lus, focal neurological symptoms and cerebrovascular disease. Increased intracranial pressure because of hydrocephalus is the most common presentation. Vascular involvement is a common, but frequently unrecognized manifestation of SANCC. The inflammation of the vessel can result in occlu-sive endarteritis, aneurysm formation and thrombosis. Small perforating vessels are most affected, resulting in lacunar infarcts proximal to cysts as seen in this patient. In many instances, the CT angiography will be negative.

Answer to Question 2

What is the Approach to Diagnosis and Treatment?

Imaging is the cornerstone in the diagnosis of SANCC. CT is sensitive at detecting parenchymal calcifications, but MRI is superior in delineating cysts in the subarachnoid space and assessing the amount of inflammation. The serological gold standard, the immunoblot, has a sensitivity of 98% and spec-ificity close to 100% in patients with two or more lesions; the sensitivity decreases in cases with a single or calcified lesion. The immunoblot is always positive in SANCC because of the high burden of disease. Circulating parasite antigen pro-vides additional information on the presence of viable cysts, and can be used to monitor efficacy of therapy.

Principles of treatment for parenchymal neurocysticerco-sis cannot be extrapolated to those patients with SANCC. Antiparasitics are always indicated in the treatment of SANCC and many experts recommend dual therapy with albendazole and praziquantel.

The duration of treatment is still controversial, but cur-rent guidelines recommend treating until resolution on neuroimaging.

Corticosteroids are also critical to reduce the inflamma-tion secondary to antiparasitic treatment. A careful taper of steroids should be employed to avoid complications, such as hydrocephalus, meningitis, and vasculitis. Patients may need a long course of treatment with neuroimaging every 3 months to assess the clinical response.

The Case Continued...

A serum immunoblot for cysticercosis run at the Centers for Disease Control and Prevention (CDC) was positive. The serum cysticercosis antigen was positive at the beginning of therapy. A spine MRI did not show evidence of spinal involvement. The patient was begun on a high dose of pred-nisone followed by a taper, and dual therapy with albenda-zole and praziquantel. After 9 months of treatment, his serum antigen was negative and his lesions resolved on imag-ing. He has been followed closely with no recurrence.

SUMMARY BOX

Subarachnoid Neurocysticercosis

Neurocysticercosis is caused by the larval form of *Taenia solium* in the central nervous system. It is endemic in Latin America, Asia and Africa, where its transmission is favoured by poor sanitary conditions. The mechanism of transmission is faecal-oral and person to person, but requires the presence of free-roaming pigs to perpetuate the life cycle.

Subarachnoid neurocysticercosis is the most severe form because of the large dimension of the cysts, exuberant inflam-matory response leading to complications and slow response to therapy. Neuroimaging and serology are complementary for diagnosis. MRI is superior for the detection of subarachnoid cysts than CT, and the serological gold standard is the immunoblot. Compared with the parenchymal form, SANCC needs a longer duration and usually double the antiparasitic treatment along with corticosteroids. Neuroimaging and serum antigen should be repeated periodically to assess for clinical response and decision to stop treatment.

Further Reading

1. Baily G, Garcia HH. Other cestode infections: intestinal cestodes, cysticercosis, other larval cestode infections. In: Farrar J, editor. Manson's Tropical Diseases. 23rd ed. London: Elsevier; 2013 [chapter 57].

2. Coyle CM. Neurocysticerosis: an individualized approach. Infect Dis Clin North Am 2019;33(1):153–68. https://doi.org/10.1016/j.idc.2018.10.007.

3. Garcia HH, Nash TE, Del Brutto OH. Clinical symptoms, diagnosis, and treatment of neurocysticercosis. Lancet Neurol 2014;13(12):1202–15. https://doi.org/10.1016/s1474-4422(14)70094-8.

4. White AC Jr., Coyle CM, Rajshekhar V, et al. Diagnosis and Treatment of Neurocysticercosis: 2017 Clinical Practice Guidelines by the Infectious Diseases Society of America (IDSA) and the American Society of Tropical Medicine and Hygiene (ASTMH). Clin Infect Dis 2018;66(8):1159–63.

5. Fleury A, Carrillo-Mezo R, Flisser A, et al. Subarachnoid basal neurocysticercosis: a focus on the most severe form of the disease. Expert Rev Anti Infect Ther 2011;9(1):123–33. https://doi.org/10.1586/eri.10.150.

83

An 18-Year-Old Man from India With a Pale Patch on His Right Upper Limb

STEPHEN L. WALKER AND SABA M. LAMBERT

Clinical Presentation

History

An 18-year-old man from India has noticed a pale patch on his right arm and forearm for 3 months. It is not itchy or painful, but he reports reduced sensation in the affected area. He also complains of mild numbness of the little finger of the right hand but no weakness (he is right-handed). Otherwise he is well. There is no family history of skin problems.

Clinical Findings

There is a 20 cm by 10 cm hypopigmented macule on the outer aspect of the right arm extending on to the forearm (Fig. 83.1). The affected skin is dry. The sensation within the hypopigmented area is reduced compared with the normally pigmented skin. The rest of the skin examination is normal. Both ulnar nerves are palpable, however the right ulnar nerve is thickened. There is reduced sensation on the tip and ulnar border of the right little finger. There are no other neurological abnormalities.

Questions

1. What common skin conditions cause hypopigmentation?
2. What further investigations are required?

Discussion

An 18-year-old man from India presents with a hypopigmented macular lesion on the right arm with reduced sensation.

A hypopigmented anaesthetic patch is a cardinal sign of leprosy. The combination of a skin problem and signs of a neuropathy should always raise the suspicion of leprosy.

Answer to Question 1

What Common Skin Conditions Cause Hypopigmentation?

Hypopigmented skin lesions are very common. Hypopigmentation may be a non-specific sequela of any inflammatory or traumatic process such as dermatitis or a burn.

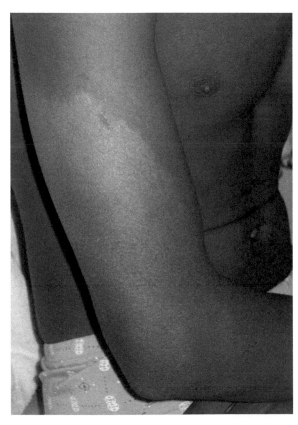

• **Fig. 83.1** A hypopigmented macular skin lesion with reduced sensation on the right arm of an 18-year-old Indian male.

Common causes of hypopigmentation include pityriasis alba, pityriasis versicolor and seborrheic dermatitis. Vitiligo causes depigmentation rather than hypopigmentation. In leprosy-endemic countries any skin problem causing reduced pigmentation may cause an individual to seek advice because of concern about leprosy. Leprosy awareness campaigns often advise people to get pale patches checked.

Answer to Question 2
What Additional Investigations are Required?

No additional investigations are required because the patient has the two clinical cardinal signs of leprosy – a hypopigmented skin lesion with reduced sensation and a thickened nerve. However, where available, clinicians may elect to perform a skin biopsy and slit-skin smears. In this case a skin biopsy is likely to show granulomatous dermatitis with destruction of cutaneous nerves and a slit-skin smear is likely to be negative.

The Case Continued…

The patient was diagnosed with paucibacillary leprosy and commenced on rifampicin and dapsone which he took for 6 months. The sensory neuropathy was treated with oral prednisolone 30 mg daily which was reduced by 5 mg each month. The patient was counselled extensively about the cause of leprosy and that he was not an infection risk to his family or friends, who were examined and had no signs of leprosy. He was advised how to care for his hands and avoid trauma. He made a full recovery.

TABLE 83.1	WHO Classification of Leprosy and Recommended Duration of Treatment	
Classification	Number of Patches	Duration of Treatment
Paucibacillary	≤5	6 months

TABLE 83.2	WHO Treatment of Leprosy (2018)	
	Once Monthly	All Other Days Daily
Rifampicin	600 mg	-
Clofazimine	300 mg	50 mg
Dapsone	100 mg	100 mg

SUMMARY BOX

Leprosy

Leprosy is a disease predominantly of the skin and peripheral nerves caused by *Mycobacterium leprae* (and *Mycobacterium lepromatosis*). The organisms cannot be grown in culture. The vast majority of individuals exposed to the infection do not develop clinical disease, but those who do develop a variety of clinical signs determined by their immunological response to the bacteria.

Individuals with high cell-mediated immunity develop tuberculoid leprosy or borderline tuberculoid leprosy with one or a few hypopigmented anaesthetic skin patches and thickened peripheral nerves. Bacteria are usually not seen in the skin biopsies or slit-skin smears of these individuals. Individuals who do not mount a cell-mediated response to *M. leprae* develop lepromatous leprosy with infiltration of the skin and many skin lesions. These individuals have lots of bacteria in their skin and nasal secretions.

The World Health Organization categorises leprosy according to the number of skin lesions for the purpose of treatment with multi-drug therapy. Individuals with paucibacillary leprosy (five skin lesions or fewer) are treated for 6 months and those with multibacillary leprosy (six or more) for 12 months (Table 83.1). In 2018, the WHO recommended that all leprosy patients receive treatment with three drugs. The WHO regime is rifampicin 600 mg, clofazimine 300 mg, dapsone 100 mg once per month and dapsone 100 mg and clofazimine 50 mg daily on the other days (Table 83.2). Prior to this, patients with paucibacillary leprosy received two drugs (dapsone and rifampicin) for 6 months. Multi-drug therapy is provided free of charge to patients.

Individuals with recent onset of sensory or motor loss (defined as within the last 6 months) are treated with oral corticosteroids, in addition to multi-drug therapy, to improve nerve function. In rare circumstances leprosy may manifest without skin changes – pure neural leprosy – which makes the diagnosis challenging.

The diagnosis of leprosy remains largely clinical as there is no diagnostic or screening test for all cases. Presentations and clinical forms are very varied. The majority of individuals with leprosy do not have identifiable bacteria in slit-skin smears or skin biopsies.

Further Reading

1. Walker SL, Withington SJ, Lockwood DNG. Leprosy. In: Farrar J, editor. Manson's Tropical Diseases. 23rd ed. London: Elsevier; 2013 [chapter 41].
2. The World Health Organization. Guidelines for the Diagnosis, Treatment and Prevention of Leprosy. New Delhi: WHO, Regional Office for South-East Asia; 2018. Available at:http://nlep.nic.in/pdf/WHO%20Guidelines%20for%20leprosy.pdf (accessed 11 October 2019).
3. Lockwood DNJ, Lambert S, Srikantam A, et al. Three drugs are unnecessary for treating paucibacillary leprosy-A critique of the WHO guidelines. PLoS Negl Trop Dis 2019;13(10):e0007671. https://doi.org/10.1371/journal.pntd.0007671.
4. Saleem MD, Oussedik E, Picardo M, et al. Acquired disorders with hypopigmentation: a clinical approach to diagnosis and treatment. J Am Acad Dermatol 2019;80(5):1233–50.

84

A 64-Year-Old Japanese Man With Generalized Tonic-Clonic Seizures

MASAHIDE YOSHIKAWA, FUMIHIKO NISHIMURA, YUKITERU OUJI AND HIROYUKI NAKASE

Clinical Presentation

History

A 64-year-old Japanese man is admitted to a local hospital in Japan because of generalized tonic-clonic seizures followed by weakness of the right lower extremity.

He has a medical history of hypertension and right cerebellar infarction; however, recent simple partial seizures were well controlled by administration of an antiepileptic agent.

Clinical Findings

On admission, the patient is afebrile, GCS is 15/15 and the neurological examination does not reveal any abnormality.

Laboratory Results

Laboratory results show no abnormalities, including no eosinophilia or leukocytosis.

Imaging

Head CT reveals a small high-density nodule with an enhanced perifocal low-density area in the left occipital lobe.

MRI shows a ring-enhancing, tunnel-shaped lesion in the left occipital lobe (Fig. 84.1).

Angiography findings are normal, except for right vertebral artery occlusion, reflecting the history of right cerebellar infarction.

Further Investigations

Open surgery with craniotomy targeting the lesion is performed. With manipulation of the aspirator and forceps, a white tape-like body at the centre of the targeted lesion is exposed, and complete removal of a live worm-like structure is carefully performed (Fig. 84.2A-C). A presumed diagnosis of sparganosis is made.

Questions

1. What is the cause of sparganosis?
2. What is the treatment of choice for cerebral sparganosis?

Discussion

A 64-year old Japanese man presents with a generalized tonic-clonic seizure. Imaging reveals an elongated structure in the right occipital lobe. During neurosurgery, a live worm-like structure is removed from the brain, identified as a sparganum.

Answer to Question 1

What is the Cause of Sparganosis?

Spargana are the larvae of zoonotic tapeworms of the genus *Spirometra*. Adult worms inhabit the intestines of cats and dogs, and produce eggs that are discharged in faeces. In fresh water, coracidia hatch from the eggs to be ingested by copepods and develop into first stage (procercoid) larvae.

When copepods are ingested by the second intermediate host (e.g. frogs, fish, snakes, birds), the procercoid larvae mature into plerocercoid sparganum larvae and migrate to the muscle and subcutaneous tissue. The cycle is completed when a carnivorous mammal eats the second intermediate host.

Humans can become infected by ingesting the first or second intermediate host, i.e. by drinking water containing infected copepods, eating undercooked meat from infected snakes, frogs, or birds, or by the use of poultices produced from infested frog or snake flesh or skin on open wounds or eyes.

In the human body, the sparganum commonly migrates into subcutaneous tissue or muscle, and sometimes into the eye, the spinal cord or brain, the latter resulting in cerebral sparganosis. The infection route in the present case was probably through consumption of raw chicken meat, which the patient ate approximately once a month before the generalized seizure.

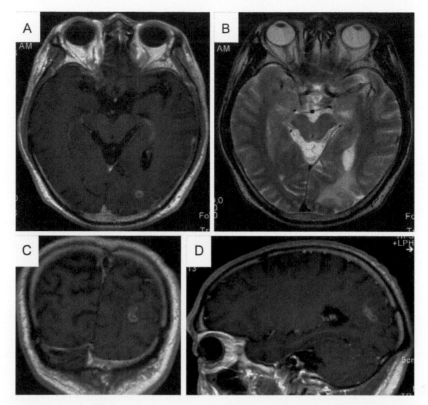

• **Fig. 84.1** MRI A. T1-weighted MRI showing a ring-shaped nodule with gadolinium enhancement in the left occipital lobe. B. T2-weighted image showing an area of hyperintensity associated with an adjacent ventricular dilation. C, D. Post-contrast coronal and sagittal T1-weighted images demonstrating a tunnel-shaped enhancement, so-called tunnel sign.

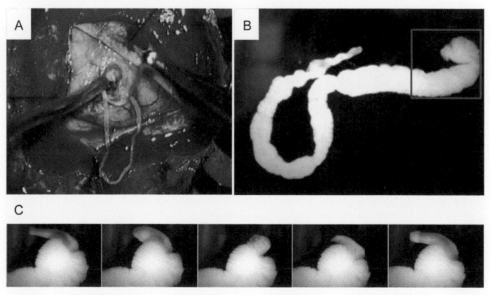

• **Fig. 84.2** Images of the Sparganum A. Intraoperative photograph showing a live sparganum during removal from the cortex. B. Whole body of extracted sparganum with anterior end enclosed by red square. The sparganum was wrinkled and whitish, and measured 1 to 3 mm in width and up to 12.5 cm in length at maximum extension. C. Five successive images from video recording. The anterior end showed active repeated movements of extension and constriction.

Cerebral sparganosis is a rare disease, but should be considered in patients from endemic areas presenting with symptoms suggestive of a space-occupying lesion. Cases have been mainly reported from Asian countries, especially China, South Korea, Thailand and Japan, and the most commonly observed clinical manifestation is epileptic seizures. Diagnosis is based upon dependable history taking and serological investigations. Neuroimaging, especially MRI, is helpful for the diagnosis of cerebral sparganosis. The most characteristic finding is the "tunnel sign" in post-contrast MRI, which appears as hypointensity in T1-weighted and hyperintensity in T2-weighted images.

Answer to Question 2

What is the Treatment of Choice for Cerebral Sparganosis?

The treatment of choice is the removal of the sparganum from the brain. However, in a small-sample non-randomized retrospective study, high-dose praziquantel had an efficacy similar to that of surgical removal with respect to the primary outcome (complete disappearance of active lesions in cerebral MRI findings).

The Case Continued...

After surgical removal of the worm, the patient was well without seizures at the most recent examination. Enzyme-linked immunosorbent assay (ELISA) results of serum and cerebrospinal fluid revealed strong positivity for Spirometra mansoni.

SUMMARY BOX

Cerebral Sparganosis

Cerebral sparganosis is the infestation of the human brain by larvae of a zoonotic cestode of carnivorous mammals. It is a food-borne zoonosis acquired by drinking untreated freshwater or eating undercooked meat of snakes and frogs or by application of infested flesh on open wounds or the eyes during medical procedures. The incubation period is 6 to 11 days but may be longer. The larvae can survive in the human host for up to 20 years.

Most cases occur in Asia, but sporadic cases have been reported from many other parts of the world.

Cerebral infestation may manifest like any space-occupying lesion with headache, confusion, seizures, paraesthesias or palsies. Spinal sparganosis may lead to paraplegia, as well as urinary and bowel incontinence.

Diagnosis of cerebral sparganosis is made on the basis of a combination of clinical history, laboratory tests (eosinophilia, positive serology), CT and MRI, and histopathology findings including the identification of the larva itself, if available. Recent advances in imaging technology, especially MRI, are key for diagnosis.

Differential diagnoses include brain tumours or metastases, neurocysticercosis, cerebral schistosomiasis and paragonimiasis.

An HIV test should be done in any person with unclear CNS lesions. In immunocompromised patients, cerebral toxoplasmosis has to be considered, as well as cerebral cryptococcomas and tuberculomas.

Further Reading

1. Baily G, Garcia HH. Other cestode infections: intestinal cestodes, cysticercosis, other larval cestode infections. In: Farrar J, editor. Manson's Tropical Diseases. 23rd ed. London: Elsevier; 2013 [chapter 57].
2. Liu Q, Li MW, Wang ZD, et al. Human sparganosis, a neglected food borne zoonosis. Lancet Infect Dis 2015;15(10):1226–35.
3. Song T, Wang WS, Zhou BR, et al. CT and MR characteristics of cerebral sparganosis. Am J Neuroradiol 2007;28(9):1700–5.
4. Li YX, Ramsahye H, Yin B, et al. Migration: A Notable Feature of Cerebral Sparganosis on Follow-Up MR Imaging. Am J Neuroradiol 2013;34(2):327–33.
5. Hong D, Xie H, Wan H, et al. Efficacy comparison between long-term high-dose praziquantel and surgical therapy for cerebral sparganosis: a multicenter retrospective cohort study. PLoS Negl Trop Dis 2018;12(10):e0006918.

85

A 55-Year-Old Female Pig Farmer from Vietnam With Fever and Impaired Consciousness

THI THUY NGAN NGUYEN AND JEREMY DAY

Clinical Presentation

History

A 55-year-old woman presents to a hospital in rural Vietnam with a 1-day history of fever, headache and vomiting. Her blood film is negative for malaria and she is treated with fluids and paracetamol.

On the second day of illness she develops confusion and is referred to a hospital in Ho Chi Minh City for further investigation.

The patient has a history of type 2 diabetes and hypertension, she has been on treatment for 4 years. She raises pigs on her smallholding and works as a butcher in a local market selling pork and chicken.

Clinical Findings

On admission, she is confused with a Glasgow Coma Score of 12/15 (E3 M5 V4), there is fever (38.5°C or 101.3°F), tachycardia (124 bpm), hypotension (85/60 mmHg), tachypnoea (32 breaths per minute), and hypoxia (O$_2$ saturation 86% on ambient air). She has neck stiffness and photophobia. There are no focal neurological signs. She has a diffuse petechial rash over her trunk (Fig. 85.1) and marked purpuric non-blanching lesions on her left leg (Fig. 85.2). The rest of her examination is unremarkable.

Laboratory Results

Her laboratory results on admission are shown in Table 85.1.

Further Investigations

Non-contrast-enhanced CT scan of the brain is unremarkable. Electrocardiogram shows sinus tachycardia and is otherwise normal. Chest x-ray is unremarkable.

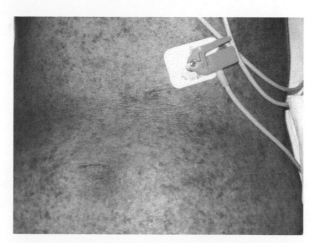

• **Fig. 85.1** Petechial rash on the trunk of the patient.

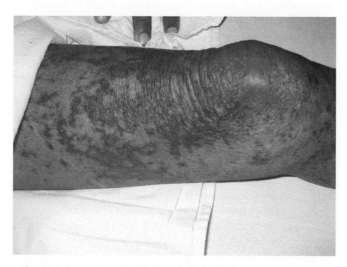

• **Fig. 85.2** Purpuric, non-blanching rash on the leg.

TABLE 85.1	Laboratory Results on Admission	
Parameter	Patient	Reference
WBC ($\times 10^9$/L)	10.25	4–10
% Neutrophils	86.5	45–75
Haemoglobin (g/dL)	11.8	12–17
Platelets ($\times 10^9$/L)	56	200–400
Creatinine (mg/dL)	0.86	0.7–1.5
Blood urea nitrogen (mg/dL)	7	7–20
Na+ (mmol/l)	137	135–150
K+ (mmol/l)	3.2	3.5–5.5
Random blood glucose (mmol/L)	15.4	3.9–7.8
HbA1c (%)	8.5	4–7
Lactate (mmol/L)	11.2	0.5–2.2

Questions

1. What is the differential diagnosis and what empirical treatment would you give?
2. What additional investigations are needed?

Discussion

This middle-aged Vietnamese woman from a rural area presents with a syndrome consistent with meningitis complicated by shock. She has a widespread non-blanching purpuric rash.

Answer to Question 1

What is the Differential Diagnosis and What Empirical Treatment Would You Give?

The patient presented at the rural district hospital with fever and malaise and developed confusion. There is malaria in rural Vietnam and both *P. falciparum* and *P. vivax* are endemic; therefore severe malaria must be excluded. Enteric fever, an important disease in low-income tropical countries, can cause confusion and should be considered, but the rate of disease progression in this case is uncharacteristic. Dengue fever is endemic in South-east Asia and should also be considered. Skin changes in dengue usually present with transient flushing erythema of the face followed by a diffuse erythematous, blanching rash on days 3 to 6. A small proportion of patients develop severe disease during a second, immune-mediated phase (usually on day 4–6). This phase may be complicated by capillary leak, shock, mucocutaneous bleeding and organ involvement. Dengue may also present as encephalitis.

In this case the rapid deterioration with signs of meningitis and shock is not typical for dengue.

Melioidosis is another differential diagnosis to consider. In some areas of South-east Asia, it is the commonest cause

of community-acquired sepsis, and diabetes is known to be a risk factor for the disease. Melioidosis may also cause brain abscess and encephalitis. However, melioidosis is comparatively rare in Vietnam, where the true burden of disease remains to be elucidated.

The most likely diagnosis though seems to be acute bacterial meningitis complicated by septic shock. Globally, the common causes of acute bacterial meningitis are *Streptococcus pneumoniae*, *Neisseria meningitidis*, and *Haemophilus influenzae*. Both *S. pneumoniae* and *N. meningitidis* infections can be complicated by development of a purpuric rash; this is more common with *N. meningitidis* septicemia.

In Vietnam, however, the commonest identified cause of acute bacterial meningitis in adults is *Streptococcus suis*. Like its counterparts, *S. suis* infection can cause both meningitis and septic shock; the syndromes overlap. A florid purpuric rash is common (6%–31% of patient cases).

Other forms of meningitis seen in Asia and the tropics include tuberculous and cryptococcal meningitis. Although each of these tends to have a more insidious onset, the duration of symptoms before presentation can be as short as 4 to 5 days; these diagnoses therefore should always be considered. However, they are not associated with shock or purpuric rash.

Meningitis is a medical emergency requiring prompt treatment. Lumbar puncture is the investigation of choice but should not delay administration of broad-spectrum intravenous antibiotics. A typical choice is ceftriaxone; where resistance is suspected or common epidemiologically, vancomycin is also administered. The value of adjunctive corticosteroids in acute bacterial meningitis is difficult to generalize. Large studies in Africa found no benefit; this contrasts with Western Europe, where steroids reduced the risk of death, and Vietnam, where in microbiologically confirmed disease they reduced the risk of complications.

Answer to Question 2

What Additional Investigations are Needed?

The patient requires a lumbar puncture and blood cultures. CSF should be sent for microscopy, Gram stain, cell count, protein, glucose and culture. A simultaneous blood glucose measurement should be performed. If resources are limited, then CSF glucose with simultaneous blood glucose is the most important test informing clinical management, because a normal ratio (i.e. a CSF/serum glucose ratio of 0.6) excludes acute bacterial meningitis and TB. In both bacterial and Tb meningitis, the CSF/serum glucose ratio is expected to be markedly diminished. Rapid diagnostic tests such as pneumococcal antigen can be performed on CSF, blood or urine, and meningococcal polymerase chain reaction on blood or CSF if available. Because the patient is from a malaria-endemic area, the blood film should be repeated.

The Case Continued...

The patient received empirical treatment with intravenous ceftriaxone and vancomycin, and supportive treatment including intravenous fluids. Lumbar puncture revealed turbid cerebrospinal fluid with 2870 cells/µL (<5), 92% neutrophils, protein 541.16 mg/dL (15–45) and CSF glucose 2.44 mmol/l (2.5–4.4). Blood glucose was 19 mmol/L (3.9–6.1), CSF/serum glucose ratio 0.12 (normal 0.6).

Gram stain showed a Gram-positive coccus in short chains, and negative India ink, mycobacterial GeneXpert and Herpes simplex virus PCR. Repeat malaria film and malaria rapid diagnostic tests were negative. Five days later, both blood and CSF cultures grew *S. suis*, sensitive to penicillin and ceftriaxone.

The patient received 12 days of antibiotic therapy. Dexamethasone was administered for the first 4 days of treatment. She responded to treatment but had residual bilateral hearing impairment.

SUMMARY BOX

Streptococcus suis meningitis

S. suis is the most frequently confirmed cause of acute bacterial meningitis in adults in Vietnam. Globally, it is an economically important zoonotic pathogen of pigs causing septicaemia, joint and genitourinary tract infections. Human disease is almost exclusively caused by serotype 2. It is reported globally but seems particularly frequent in East and South-east Asia.

Outbreaks of severe sepsis have been reported from China. The prevalence of disease in Asia is probably driven by farming and food practices; disease is more common in those in contact with pigs and raw pork. Infection is rare in children because culturally they are protected from contact with pigs. Antibiotic resistance is rarely reported in human isolates. First-line treatment is ceftriaxone; adjunctive treatment with steroids reduces the risk for deafness in adults, which occurs in up to 70%.

Further Reading

1. Mai NT, Hoa NT, Nga TV, et al. Streptococcus suis meningitis in adults in Vietnam. Clin Infect Dis 2008;46(5):659–67.
2. Nghia HD, Tu Le TP, Wolbers M, et al. Risk factors of Streptococcus suis infection in Vietnam. A case-control study. PLoS One 2011;6(3):e17604.
3. Yu H, Jing H, Chen Z, et al. Human Streptococcus suis outbreak, Sichuan. China Emerg Infect Dis 2006;12(6):914–20.
4. Nguyen TH, Tran TH, Thwaites G, et al. Dexamethasone in Vietnamese adolescents and adults with bacterial meningitis. N Engl J Med 2007;357(24):2431–40.
5. de Gans J, van de Beek D. European Dexamethasone in Adulthood Bacterial Meningitis Study. Dexamethasone in adults with bacterial meningitis. N Engl J Med 2002;347(20):1549–56.

86

A 14-Year-Old Girl in the Solomon Islands With a Non-Healing Leg Ulcer

MICHAEL MARKS AND ORIOL MITIÀ

Clinical Presentation

History

A 14-year-old girl was seen in the Solomon Islands. She reported a painless, non-healing large ulcer of her left leg that began 1 month earlier.

Clinical Findings

On examination there was a large lesion (approximately 3 cm diameter) on the left lower leg covered by a layer of crust (Fig. 86.1). Lower down the leg a smaller, similar lesion

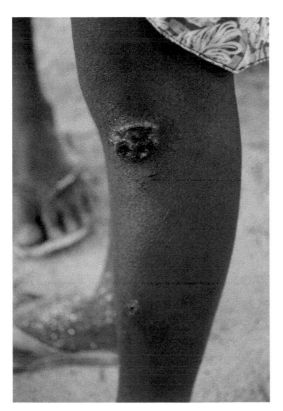

• **Fig. 86.1** Leg ulcer in a 14-year-old girl from the Solomon Islands.

was noted. There was no regional lymphadenopathy or evidence of any other skin or bone lesions.

Laboratory results

A rapid plasma reagin (RPR) test was positive at a titre of 1:64 (Normal – Negative).

Questions

1. What is the most likely diagnosis when the patient first presents and how should she be treated?
2. How would you manage her? How should she be followed up?

Discussion

A 14-year-old girl from the Solomon Islands presenting with a chronic leg ulcer.

Answer to Question 1

What is the Most Likely Diagnosis When the Patient First Presents and How Should She Be Treated?

The patient has a clinical lesion suspicious for yaws, which is still a common problem in the West Pacific. The satellite lesion on the leg is also very typical of early yaws lesions. The patient has a high-titre positive RPR test which is consistent with the diagnosis. A number of other bacteria, in particular *Haemophilus ducreyi,* can cause skin lesions that clinically appear similar to those of early yaws. Other relevant differential diagnoses are pyoderma, tropical ulcer, cutaneous diphtheria, and *Aeromonas hydrophila* infection.

Answer to Question 2

How Would You Manage Her? How Should She Be Followed Up?

A single oral dose of azithromycin (30 mg/kg single dose; maximum dose 2 g) or a single intramuscular (IM) dose of benzathine benzylpenicillin (<10 years of age: 0.6 million units single dose; $\geq$10 years of age: 1.2 million units single dose) is the treatment of choice. A four-fold fall in titre at 6 months indicates cure.

The Case Continued...

She was treated with a single IM dose of benzathine benzylpenicillin and the skin lesion resolved over the next 10 days. The patient was seen again at the hospital 12 months later with a similar ulcer on the right leg.

The RPR test was repeated and was positive at a titre of 1:8. Given a greater than four-fold fall in the RPR titre this was considered cure after the recent treatment. The other leg ulcer was therefore interpreted to be of a different aetiology.

SUMMARY BOX

Yaws

Yaws is a chronic infectious disease caused by *Treponema pallidum* subspecies *pertenue,* which is spread by skin-to-skin contact in warm, humid environments. In the Pacific region, yaws remains highly endemic in the Solomon Islands, Papua New Guinea and Vanuatu, as well as in Indonesia and Timor-Leste. There is also evidence for a re-emergence of yaws in the Philippines were the disease was considered eradicated since the 1970s. The disease is also still endemic in parts of West and Central Africa. Yaws is normally seen in young children; it is associated with overcrowding and poor hygiene. The disease consists of primary, secondary and tertiary phases. The primary lesion usually starts as a localized papule 2 to 10 weeks after inoculation. Common sites are the lower legs and the face. The papule may develop into a large nodule 2 to 5 cm in diameter that ulcerates. Secondary lesions appear from a few weeks to 2 years after the primary lesion and may include a variety of skin lesions. Arthralgias and malaise are the most common additional symptoms and may be accompanied by early osteoperiostitis of the proximal phalanges of the fingers (dactylitis) or long bones (forearm, tibia, or fibula). Late-stage disease is characterized by destructive lesions of soft tissues and bones. Diagnosis is predominantly based on serology and relies on both treponemal tests (such as the *Treponema pallidum* particle agglutination assay, TPPA) and non-treponemal tests (such as RPR test). Benzathine benzylpenicillin and azithromycin are the treatments of choice, with the latter the preferred drug to use in mass treatment campaigns. A four-fold fall in the RPR titre over 6 months (for example from 1:64 to 1:16) is considered to indicate cure. Similar lesions to those of early yaws may be caused by other bacteria, in particular *H. ducreyi,* but PCR is required to make this diagnosis.

Further Reading

1. Salazar JC, Bennett NJ. Endemic treponematosis including yaws and other spirochaetes. In: farrar j, editor. Manson's tropical diseases. 23rd ed. London: Elsevier; 2013 [chapter 36].
2. Mitjà O, Asiedu K. Mabey D. Yaws Lancet 2013;381:763–73.
3. Mitjà O, Houinei W, Moses P, et al. Mass treatment with single-dose azithromycin for yaws. N Engl J Med 2015;372:703–10.
4. Marks M, Chi K-H, Vahi V, et al. Haemophilus ducreyi associated with skin ulcers among children, Solomon Islands. Emerg Infect Dis 2014;20:1705–7.
5. Mitjà O, Godornes C, Houinei W, et al. Re-emergence of yaws after single mass azithromycin treatment followed by targeted treatment: a longitudinal study. Lancet 2018;391:1599–607.

87

A 27-Year-Old Male Traveller Returning from the Peruvian Amazon With Persisting Polyarthralgias

ANDREAS NEUMAYR

Clinical Presentation

History

A 27-year-old male Swiss tourist spent 3.5 weeks travelling in the rainforests of the Amazon Basin in northern Peru. During the second week of his stay he developed an acute febrile illness with chills, malaise, frontal headache, generalized myalgia and a transient, non-pruritic maculopapular rash.

The rash started on the forearms about 1 week after the onset of fever and spread to the trunk, neck and face before fading after 3 days. In addition, there were slowly progressive debilitating polyarthralgias affecting the peripheral joints accompanied by transient joint swelling. He also noticed painful cervical and inguinal lymphadenopathy, which was self-limiting, lasting for about 1 week.

The traveller presented at the local hospital, where physicians made a clinical diagnosis of dengue fever, and he received symptomatic treatment with paracetamol. Although the fever and the other symptoms subsided within 1 week, the polyarthralgias did not improve, showing a symmetrical pattern mainly affecting the small joints of the hands and feet as well as the wrists, ankles, and knees.

Upon return home to Switzerland a few weeks later, the patient consulted his general practitioner because of persisting, incapacitating polyarthralgias. The patient reported stiffness of the affected joints, mainly in the morning and after immobility. Physical examination of the affected joints did not reveal any clinical signs of inflammation (swelling, redness, effusion). Laboratory tests were performed including serological testing for dengue virus, chikungunya virus, parvovirus B19, Epstein-Barr virus, *Borrelia burgdorferi*, *Chlamydia trachomatis*, *Salmonella Typhi*, and S. Paratyphi but none revealed a cause for the symptoms. For two more months, the joint pains did not improve; thus the patient was referred to a rheumatologist and subsequently to a tropical medicine clinic for evaluation of a putative travel-related cause of his polyarthralgias.

Clinical Findings

The physical examination was completely unremarkable. The affected joints did not reveal any clinical signs of inflammation (no swelling, no redness, no effusion).

Laboratory results

Full blood count was normal. C-reactive protein was mildly elevated at 9 mg/L ($<$5), liver function tests were normal.

Questions

1. What are your differential diagnoses?
2. What diagnostic test would you perform?

Discussion

A 27-year-old male Swiss tourist presents with persisting and incapacitating symmetrical polyarthralgias primarily affecting the small peripheral joints after returning from a trip to the Amazon Basin of northern Peru. The patient reports an acute self-limiting febrile illness accompanied by a rash before the onset of the polyarthralgias, which had clinically been diagnosed as dengue infection at a local hospital in Peru.

Answer to Question 1
What Are Your Differential Diagnoses?

Two main differential diagnoses should be considered in patients presenting with persisting or prolonged arthritis/arthralgias and a history of a preceding infection:

Reactive arthritis (Reiter's syndrome):

Reactive arthritis is a rheumatoid factor (RF)-seronegative, HLA-B27-linked arthritis often preceded by an infection. The most common triggers are gastrointestinal infections (caused by *Salmonella*, *Shigella* or *Campylobacter*) and sexually transmitted infections *(Chlamydia trachomatis)*. Reactive arthritis may manifest as monoarthritis (often affecting the knee or sacroiliac joint) or as oligoarthritis (usually of the lower extremities). The course may be additive (i.e. more joints becoming inflamed in addition to the primarily affected one) or migratory (new joints becoming inflamed after the initially inflamed joint has already improved). It usually develops within 2 to 4 weeks of the preceding infection. Reactive arthritis may also manifest with the classical triad of symptoms termed "Reiter's syndrome": (i) inflammatory arthritis of large joints, (ii) inflammation of the eyes manifesting as conjunctivitis or uveitis and (iii) urethritis in men or cervicitis in women. Other musculoskeletal manifestations include enthesitis (often involving the Achilles tendon) and dactylitis. In some cases, mucocutaneous lesions *(circinate balanitis)* or psoriasis-like skin lesions *(keratoderma blennorrhagicum)* may be present. Clinical manifestation may vary widely and patients may be oligosymptomatic. In the majority of cases the complaints are self-limiting and subside under symptomatic treatment with non-steroidal drugs over weeks to months.

Viral arthritis:

Although self-limiting polyarthralgias are present during the acute phase of many viral infections, prolonged polyarthritis/polyarthralgias are characteristic for certain viral infections. Worldwide, parvovirus B19, hepatitis B and C, HIV, rubella and the alphaviruses are the most common infections to consider in the differential diagnosis. Although rubella has become rare because of vaccination, the vector-borne, alphaviral infections are becoming increasingly relevant in endemic regions and in returning travellers (see Table 87.1). Unlike reactive arthritis, viral arthritis primarily presents as symmetrical polyarthritis of peripheral small joints.

TABLE 87.1 **Characteristics of Human Pathogenic Alphaviruses**

Virus	Epidemiology and Endemic Regions	Occurrence and Number of Reported Cases	Frequency of Main Symptoms (%)
Chikungunya	Tropical and subtropical regions of Asia, Africa and Latin America	Large sporadic epidemics	Fever: 90 Rash: 40–50 Myalgia: 90 Arthralgia/arthritis: >95
Sindbis Virus Group	Eurasia, Africa, Australia, Oceania; primarily reported from West Russia ("Karelian fever"), Finland ("Pogosta disease"), and Sweden ("Ockelbo disease")	Geographically most widely distributed alphavirus (lack of data on human cases) Karelian fever: rare (no data) Pogosta disease: ~140 cases (range 1–1282)/year Ockelbo disease: ~30 cases/year	Fever: 15–40 Rash: 90 Myalgia: 50 Arthralgia/arthritis: 95
Ross River	Australia, Papua New Guinea, West Papua	~5000 cases per year in Australia; in 1979–1980 an epidemic with >60000 cases hit some pacific islands (New Caledonia, Fiji, Samoa, Cook Islands)	Fever: 20–60 Rash: 40–60 Myalgia: 40–80 Arthralgia/arthritis: 80–100
Barmah Forest	Australia	~2000 cases/year	Fever: 50 Rash: 40–60 Myalgia: 50–80 Arthralgia or arthritis: 70–95
O'Nyong Nyong	East Africa	Rare epidemics; >2 million cases in 1959–1961	Fever: 80–100 Rash: 70–90 Myalgia: 70 Arthralgia/arthritis: 60–100
Mayaro	South America, primarily the Amazonian rainforest, Caribbean	Sporadic single cases and small outbreaks (involving ~10–100 cases)	Fever: 100 Rash: 30–50 Myalgia: 75 Arthralgia/arthritis: 50–90

Adapted from Suhrbier, A., Jaffar-Bandjee, M.C., Gasque, P., 2012. Arthritogenic alphaviruses - an overview. Nat Rev Rheumatol, 8(7):420–9.

TABLE 87.2   Results of the Serological Testing for Alphavirus Infections Performed in Our Case

Virus	Blood Sample Taken on 29 August			Blood Sample Taken on 12 September			Interpretation of test result
	IgM-IFA	IgG-IFA	PRNT	IgM-IFA	IgG-IFA	PRNT	
Mayaro	1280	2560	40	40	2560	160	positive
Sindbis	<20	160	<20	<20	160	<20	negative
Chikungunya	<20	160	n.d.	<20	160	n.d.	negative
Ross River	<20	160	n.d.	<20	160	n.d.	negative
Barmah Forest	<20	20	n.d.	<20	20	n.d.	negative

IFA: indirect immunofluorescence assay (screening assay)
PRNT: plaque reduction neutralization test (confirmatory assay)
n.d.: not done (screening assay negative [and epidemiologically not supported])

Answer to Question 2

What Diagnostic Test Would You Perform?

The diagnostic principles for most alphaviruses are the same: During the first days of the acute infection, detection of viral RNA in the blood by PCR may confirm the diagnosis. Beyond the acute phase, the diagnosis is based upon serological detection of specific IgM and IgG antibodies against the respective virus. Cross-reactivity within the same virus family is common. Reference laboratories therefore usually perform parallel testing for potentially cross-reacting viruses (see Table 87.2) and apply a two-step approach, using highly sensitive screening assays followed by highly specific confirmatory assays.

The Case Continued...

Given the patient's travel history, the course of the illness and the clinical signs and symptoms experienced during the journey, Mayaro virus (MAYV) infection was strongly suspected. (Chikungunya was not yet endemic in the Americas at the time this patient was seen).

The serological results (Tab. 87.2) confirmed the suspected diagnosis of Mayaro infection. The patient received symptomatic treatment with ibuprofen, and the polyarthralgias subsided slowly over the following weeks and months before finally disappearing completely.

SUMMARY BOX

Mayaro-Fever

Mayaro-virus is an alphavirus. Alphaviruses are arthropod-borne viruses (arboviruses) that circulate among a wide variety of wild animals in relative mosquito vector-specific and host-specific enzootic cycles; infection of humans (dead-end hosts) is exclusively incidental. The Mayaro virus (MAYV) circulates in an enzootic, sylvatic cycle (similar to that for yellow fever) involving forest-dwelling *Haemagogus* species mosquitoes as vectors and non-human primates as natural hosts. Infections in humans mostly occur sporadically, are strongly associated with occupational or recreational exposure in rainforest environments and represent spillover from the enzootic cycle. MAYV has so far been only reported from South America and the Caribbean.

Mayaro infection presents as a dengue-like, febrile illness lasting 3 to 7 days. It typically manifests with chills, headache, retro-orbital and epigastric pain, myalgia, arthralgia, nausea, vomiting, diarrhoea and a maculopapular rash (sometimes followed by desquamation). Haemorrhagic manifestations have been described but are rare. Like other alphaviruses, Mayaro may cause debilitating and long-lasting polyarthralgias, which are suspected to arise from the inflammatory immune response stimulated by the prolonged virus persistence in joint tissues. Treatment is exclusively symptomatic with non-steroidal drugs. Symptoms subside slowly over weeks to months. Permanent damage of the affected joints is not reported.

Further Reading

1. Young PR, Ng LFP, Hall RA, et al. Arbovirus Infections. In: Farrar J, editor. Manson's Tropical Diseases. 23rd ed. London: Elsevier; 2013 [chapter 14].
2. Schmitt SK. Reactive Arthritis. Infect Dis Clin North Am 2017; 31(2):265–77.
3. Suhrbier A, Jaffar-Bandjee MC, Gasque P. Arthritogenic alphaviruses-an overview. Nat Rev Rheumatol 2012;8(7):420–9.
4. Acosta-Ampudia Y, Monsalve DM, Rodríguez Y, et al. Mayaro: an emerging viral threat? Emerg Microbes Infect 2018;7(1):163.
5. Blohm G, Elbadry MA, Mavian C et al. Mayaro as a Caribbean traveler: Evidence for multiple introductions and transmission of the virus into Haiti. Int J Infect Dis 2019;87:151–3.

88

A 74-Year-Old Man from Japan With Fever, Nausea and Drowsiness

KOHSUKE MATSUI, KENSUKE TAKAHASHI, KOYA ARIYOSHI AND CHRIS SMITH

Clinical Presentation

History

74-year-old Japanese man is brought to a hospital with a history of fever, joint pain, headache, and nausea over the past 5 days. He has a history of cerebral infarction without neurological sequelae, hypertension and ulcerative colitis. He is taking antiplatelet, and antihypertensive medicine and subcutaneous injection of the TNF-alpha Blocker adalimumab once every 2 weeks.

He lives in a suburb of a city in Kyushu district, southwestern Japan and has opportunities to encounter wild animals such as boars and deer. He is retired and does grape farming once in a while.

He does not have any recent history of overseas travel.

Clinical findings

On examination the patient looks unwell and drowsy. His body temperature is 37°C (98.6°F), pulse rate 101 bpm, blood pressure 120/70 mmHg, SpO$_2$ 96% with 7l oxygen, and respiratory rate 32 breaths per minute. Chest examination is normal. The Glasgow Coma Scale on arrival is 13/15 (E3V4M6). There is livedo reticularis bilaterally on his lower extremities but otherwise no rash is seen. His left inguinal lymph node is enlarged.

Laboratory results

His laboratory results on admission are shown in Table 88.1.

Questions

1. What are your differential diagnosis and diagnostic approach?
2. How would you manage this patient?

Discussion

A 74-year-old man living in south-western Japan presents with fever, arthralgia, impaired consciousness and respiratory distress. Laboratory results show elevated AST/ALT, LDH, CK and low platelets.

Answer to Question 1
What Are Your Differential Diagnosis and Diagnostic Approach?

Acute fever with respiratory distress and impaired consciousness are signs of sepsis. Pneumonia, meningitis or infective endocarditis need to be investigated as soon as possible. In addition, considering the patient's lifestyle and habitat, tick- and mite-borne infectious diseases should be included in the differential diagnosis. There are two rickettsial infections and one viral infection that are transmitted by mites or ticks, respectively, in Japan: Japanese spotted fever (caused by *Rickettsia japonica*), scrub typhus (caused by *Orientia tsutsugamushi*) and severe fever with thrombocytopenia syndrome (SFTS).

SFTS should be suspected when a patient at risk of tick bite develops acute fever with thrombocytopenia or pancytopenia, abnormal liver function tests, and an elevated serum creatinine kinase. SFTS and rickettsioses are sometimes difficult to

TABLE 88.1 Laboratory Results on Admission

Parameter	Patient	Reference Range
WBC (× 10^9/L)	5.3	3.3–8.6
Haemoglobin (g/dL)	17.7	13.7–16.8
Platelets (× 10^9/L)	90	158–348
AST (U/L)	413	13–30
ALT (U/L)	95	10–42
LDH (U/L)	1025	124–222
CK (U/L)	7442	59–248
CK-MB (U/L)	41	0–15
CRP (mg/dL)	0.1	0.00–0.14

differentiate from each other because both show similar clinical manifestations and laboratory results. In this case, however, a negative CRP is suggestive of SFTS rather than rickettsiosis.

Diagnosis of SFTS is confirmed by detecting SFTS virus in blood serum by PCR. It is reported that real-time RT-PCR of serum is 98.6% sensitive and 99.1% specific.

Answer to Question 2

How Would You Manage This Patient?

Symptomatic and supportive treatment such as adequate fluid administration and respiratory support play an essential role in management. Vasopressors should be started if the patient develops hypotension. Laboratory results have to be monitored closely because there are risks of worsening thrombocytopenia, disseminated intravascular coagulation, multi-organ failure and haemophagocytic syndrome. Antibiotics should be administered until the PCR result is available and other infectious diseases have been ruled out.

Medical staff should be aware that there is a chance of human-to-human transmission through blood or body fluids. Contact precaution is needed until the SFTS viral load becomes undetectable.

The Case Continued...

The patient was intubated and admitted to the intensive care unit immediately. Meropenem and vancomycin were initiated for possible bacterial sepsis. His blood sample was sent to the reference laboratory, and SFTS virus PCR came back positive. Antibiotics were subsequently discontinued because no bacterial infection was identified.

Despite adequate fluid administration and other supportive therapies, the patient experienced worsening of his respiratory condition and protracted hypotension for a week. Noradrenaline was initiated, and then hydrocortisone 200 mg/day was added for non-responsive septic shock before he started showing gradual improvement. His platelet count decreased to 65×10^9/L on day 4 of admission but subsequently recovered to the normal level. His CK was highest on admission and decreased to the normal level on day 7.

He was extubated on day 12 and discharged on day 35 without any sequelae.

SUMMARY BOX

Severe Fever With Thrombocytopenia Syndrome (SFTS)

SFTS is an emerging infectious disease caused by infection with the SFTS virus and transmitted by tick bites. The first case was reported in China in 2009; and since then, cases have been reported in both Japan and Korea. As of 2019, 491 cases had been reported in Japan from when the first case was reported in 2012.

The SFTS virus belongs to the family Bunyaviridae, which also includes the Crimean Congo haemorrhagic fever virus and hantavirus. Its incubation period is 6 to 14 days. Despite being a tick-borne disease, it is reported that an eschar is rarely seen. Clinical manifestations of SFTS include fever, nausea, diarrhoea, arthralgia, myalgia and neurological symptoms. Laboratory results typically show leukopenia, thrombocytopenia and elevated serum AST, ALT, LDH and CK levels. Patients sometimes develop multi-organ failure and hemophagocytic syndrome, which results in a high case-fatality rate.

Supportive treatment is the main treatment strategy. There is no effective antiviral agent against SFTS. Patients require close monitoring of their respiratory condition and blood pressure. Adequate fluid administration, close monitoring and management of thrombocytopenia, haemophagocytic syndrome and secondary bacterial infection are important.

The case-fatality rate has been reported to range from 6.3% to 30% in China and be 23.2% in Japan. Older age, impaired consciousness and high serum LDH and CK levels are associated with high lethality.

Further Reading

1. Sun Y, Liang M, Qu J, et al. Early diagnosis of novel SFTS bunyavirus infection by quantitative real-time RT-PCR assay. J Clin Virol 2012;53:48–53.
2. Kim WY, Choi W, Park SW, et al. Nosocomial transmission of severe fever with thrombocytopenia syndrome in Korea. Clin Infect Dis 2015;60:1681–3.
3. Kida K, Matsuoka Y, Shimoda T, et al. A Case report of cat-to-human transmission of severe fever with Thrombocytopenia syndrome. Jpn J Infect Dis 2019;72:356–8. https://doi.org/10.7883/yoken.JJID.2018.526.
4. Yasukawa M. Diagnosis and treatment of SFTS (In Japanese). Jpn J Chemother 2017;65:558–63.
5. Liu Q, He B, Huang SY, et al. Severe fever with thrombocytopenia syndrome, an emerging tick-borne zoonosis. Lancet Infect Dis 2014;14:763–72.

89

A 30-Year-Old Woman from Bolivia With Exertional Dyspnoea

ISRAEL MOLINA

Clinical Presentation

History

A 30-year-old woman presents to the outpatient clinic of a hospital in Spain. She was born in Santa Cruz (Bolivia) and arrived in Europe 4 months prior. She has been living in an urban environment for the past 20 years but grew up in a rural area during her childhood.

She reports a 2-year history of progressive dyspnoea at moderate exertion (New York Heart Association grade II) along with self-limiting palpitations. She has no other relevant medical history and does not take any medication. She expresses the wish to become pregnant.

Clinical Findings

On examination, the blood pressure is 110/65 mmHg. The pulse is regular at 40 bpm. SpO_2 is 99% on ambient air. On auscultation, cardiac sounds are clear and there are no murmurs. The chest is clear. There is no peripheral oedema and the jugular venous pressure is not raised.

Laboratory Results

Full blood count and basic blood chemistry tests are normal. Her ECG is shown in Figure 89.1. Her chest radiograph is shown in Figure 89.1B.

Questions

1. In a recent migrant from Bolivia, which different pathologies should be screened for?
2. If a patient was diagnosed with Chagas disease, how would you proceed to assess organ involvement? Which are the indications for treatment of Chagas disease?

Discussion

A Bolivian woman of childbearing age presents to an outpatient clinic for the first time. She complains of progressive dyspnoea and palpitations. She has no clinical signs of heart failure. However, CXR shows moderate cardiomegaly and there is sinus bradycardia with right bundle branch block on her ECG.

Answer to Question 1

In a Recent Migrant from Bolivia, Which Different Pathologies Should Be Screened For?

Following the guidelines of the European Centre for Disease Prevention and Control (ECDC), newly arrived migrants from highly endemic countries should be offered a screening panel including screening for active and latent tuberculosis, HIV, hepatitis B, hepatitis C and strongyloidiasis. In migrants from Latin America, especially from Bolivia, this screening panel should include Chagas disease, because prevalence rates are high and Chagas may be asymptomatic.

If a chronic phase of Chagas disease is suspected, screening is usually performed with serological testing through detection of IgG antibodies against *Trypanosoma cruzi* using two different serological testing methods.

Answer to Question 2

If a Patient Was Diagnosed With Chagas Disease, How Would You Proceed to Assess Organ Involvement? Which Are the Indications for Treatment of Chagas Disease?

The heart is the most frequently affected organ. Alterations most commonly seen include conduction disorders such as bundle branch blocks and sinus node dysfunction (Fig. 89.1). Myocardial involvement can progress to dilated cardiomyopathy (Fig. 89.1B). Gastrointestinal involvement is less common and manifestations comprise motility disorders or megaviscera.

As a general approach it is therefore reasonable to start with an ECG, chest x-ray and barium enema. In addition, referral to a cardiologist for echocardiography and 24-hour Holter ECG would be recommended.

There are two trypanocidal treatments: benznidazole and nifurtimox. Treatment is always recommended for acute and congenital Chagas disease as well as for patients younger than

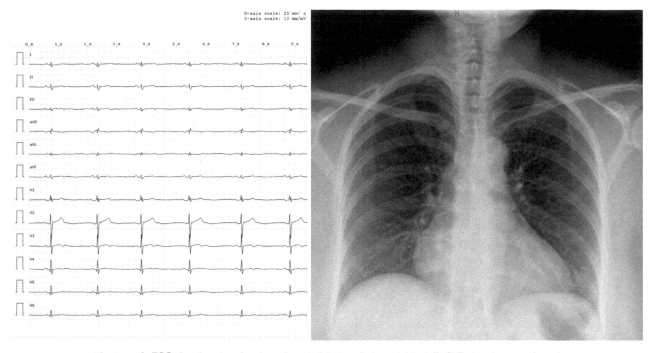

• **Fig. 89.1** **A:** ECG showing sinus bradycardia with right bundle branch block **B:** CXR showing a moderately enlarged cardiac silhouette.

18 years in the chronic phase. In older patients with chronic disease, treatment is controversial. Trypanocidal treatment is usually offered to patients in the indeterminate phase with mild-to-moderate organ involvement. In order to avoid vertical transmission, guidelines usually recommend treatment of women of childbearing age.

The Case Continued...

Both serological tests for Chagas disease came back positive. The patient was classified as having chagasic cardiomyopathy; and as she intended to become pregnant, antitrypanosomal therapy was offered. She started treatment with benznidazole 5 mg/kg per day for 60 days at the outpatient clinic.

Fifteen days into treatment, she presented with a pruritic maculopapular rash (Fig. 89.2) and mild eosinophilia. Benznidazole treatment was discontinued and the patient received corticosteroids and antihistamines for 5 days which lead to complete resolution of the skin rash. Re-introduction of benznidazole was tolerated well and she was able to complete the entire 60-day course without any additional problems.

Complete cardiological evaluation revealed sinus dysfunction without symptomatic bradycardia or syncope. Echocardiography showed a hypertrophic left ventricle without obstruction. Follow-up was ensured, and 5 years after, cardiac function was stable and she gave birth to a healthy child.

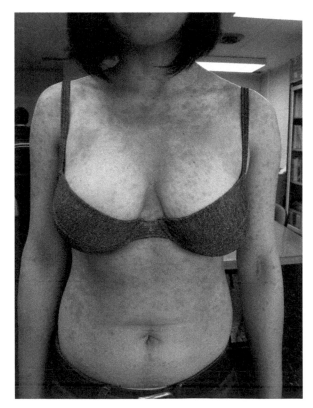

• **Fig. 89.2** Maculopoapular rash with pruritus after 15 days on benznidazole.

SUMMARY BOX

Chagas Disease

Chagas disease is an anthropozoonosis caused by the protozoan *T. cruzi*. It is a neglected tropical disease endemic in 21 Latin American countries with prevalence rates as high as 6.1% in Bolivia. In endemic areas, it is mainly transmitted by triatomine bugs. However, in non-endemic countries mother-to-child transmission, blood transfusions or transplants play a major role. Rarely, Chagas can be orally acquired by ingestion of food items and drinks contaminated with bug faeces.

Diagnosis in the acute phase is usually made by direct microscopic visualization of trypomastigotes on blood films. In the chronic phase when parasitaemia is low and intermittent, diagnosis relies on serological testing through detection of IgG antibodies against *T. cruzi* using two different tests. PCR is also used with varying sensitivities.

Chagas disease has two different clinical phases. The acute phase is usually asymptomatic but can present as inflammation at the inoculation point and fever. It is followed by a chronic phase that is usually asymptomatic (indifferent phase). About 30% to 40% of patients with chronic Chagas disease will go on to develop organ involvement 10 to 20 years after initial infection. The heart is the most frequent organ involvement, predominantly affecting conduction system and myocardium. Alterations most frequently seen include bundle branch blocks and segmental ventricular wall motion abnormalities that can progress to sinus node dysfunction, ventricular arrhythmias and dilated cardiomyopathy. Gastrointestinal involvement is less common and manifestations comprise of motility disorders or megaviscera (megaoesophagus and megacolon).

There are two approved drugs for Chagas disease: benznidazole and nifurtimox. Although benznidazole is the preferred drug for Chagas disease, about 50% of patients receiving this treatment will present with adverse events. Hypersensitivity reactions with skin involvement are the most frequently observed side effects followed by gastrointestinal disturbances, bone marrow depression and peripheral neuropathy. Mild-to-moderate reactions can be solved with symptomatic treatment with or without temporal withdrawal of trypanocidal treatment. However, in about 10% of cases treatment discontinuation is definite.

Prevention relies on vector control, improving living conditions in endemic countries, screening of blood and organs for donation and screening of women of childbearing age to avoid mother-to-child transmission.

Further Reading

1. Franco-Parades C. American Trypanosomiasis: Chagas Disease. In: Farrar J, editor. Manson's Tropical Diseases. 23rd ed London: Elsevier; 2013 [chapter 46].
2. European Centre for Disease Prevention and Control. Public health guidance on screening and vaccination for infectious diseases in newly arrived migrants within the EU/EEA. Stockholm: ECDC; 2018.
3. Pérez-Molina JA, Molina I. Chagas disease. Lancet 2018;391 (10115):82–94.
4. Norman FF, López-Vélez R. Chagas Disease: comments on the 2018 PAHO guidelines for diagnosis and management. J Trav Med 2019;26(7):1–7.
5. Lattes R, Lasala MB. Chagas disease in the immunosuppressed patient. Clin Microbiol Infect 2014;20:200–9.

90

A 55-Year-Old Couple Both Returning from Chile and Argentina With Acute Respiratory Distress Syndrome

CORNELIA STAEHELIN

Clinical Presentation

History

A 55-year-old Swiss couple, both fitness instructors, travelled for 3 months from Ecuador to Chile. The last month of their trip they spent hiking, camping and taking occasional mud baths in the Chile-Argentinian border region. On their flight back to Switzerland, the husband developed a fever (39°C, 102.2°F), myalgias and generalized weakness that did not respond to symptomatic treatment. At presentation at the hospital in Switzerland 4 days later, he continued to be febrile and felt too weak to walk to the toilet unassisted or even hold up a newspaper. He developed shortness of breath with oxygen desaturation and bilateral interstitial infiltrates were seen on chest x-ray (Fig. 90.1).

The respiratory pathogen panel from a nasopharyngeal swab (including influenza A/B, parainfluenza, RSV, adenovirus, rhinovirus, bocavirus, coronavirus and human metapneumovirus) as well as an HIV test came back negative. The following day he was transferred to the intensive care unit for non-invasive ventilator support.

Three weeks later, his wife presented with similar complaints and was admitted to the same hospital. She deteriorated rapidly over the 24 hours after admission, developed cardiorespiratory failure and fulfilled fast-entry criteria for extracorporeal membrane oxygenation (ECMO). Furthermore, she experienced multi-organ failure requiring hemodialysis, and she developed profuse bleeding from puncture sites in the context of disseminated intravascular coagulation. During the following days, she required mass transfusions of blood products.

Clinical Findings

Husband: BP 90/55 mmHg, pulse 120 beats per minute, oxygen saturation 94% on ambient air, and temperature 39°C (102.2°F). No abnormal findings on cardiopulmonary auscultation.

Wife on admission (3 weeks after her husband's admission): normal blood pressure, heart rate and oxygen saturation, temperature 38.6°C (101.5°F). No abnormal findings on auscultation.

Laboratory Results

Husband, on admission: WCC 7.3 G/L (reference: 3.0–10.5), 35% band neutrophils; platelets 48 G/L (reference: 150–450); CRP 68 mg/L (reference: <5); glomerular

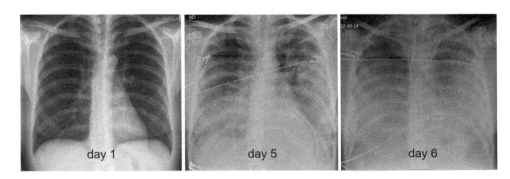

• **Fig. 90.1** Chest x-ray findings of the female patient on day 1, day 5 and day 6 of admission.

filtration rate >90 mL/min (reference: >90 mL/min); transaminases normal.

Wife, on admission: WCC 1.88 G/L; platelets 98 G/L; CRP 7 mg/L; glomerular filtration rate >90 mL/min; transaminases normal.

Chest radiography at presentation was normal in both patients; however, during the course of the disease both developed extensive bilateral infiltrates with pleural effusions.

Questions

1. What is your differential diagnosis for this couple?
2. How would you manage these patients clinically? Is there any need to consider particular hospital hygiene precautions?

Discussion

A previously healthy Swiss couple in their mid-50s present with varying degrees of cardiorespiratory failure of 2 and 21 days, respectively, after their return from a 3-month trip down the western coast of South America. They spent the last month travelling along the Chile-Argentinian border. The cardiorespiratory collapse in the female patient occurs precipitously and requires ECMO treatment.

Answer to Question 1

What Is Your Differential Diagnosis for This Couple?

Conditions that may present with acute respiratory distress syndrome (ARDS) and possible multi-organ failure after travel to South America include influenza and other respiratory viruses. Of the viral infections, New World hantaviruses cause cardiopulmonary disease; their incubation period is comparatively long and human-to-human transmission has been described, which could explain why husband and wife presented 3 weeks apart.

Pneumococcal pneumonia should also be in the differential diagnosis as a common cause of community-acquired pneumonia worldwide. Rickettsial diseases have to be considered: of the spotted-fever group, in particular *Rickettsia rickettsiae*, which notoriously causes severe disease should be on the list of differentials; and scrub typhus, which was long thought to be limited to Asia, has recently been described from Chile. Pulmonary plague is also focally endemic in South America. Fungal infections (Histoplasmosis, Cryptococcosis) also have to be considered. Severe malaria may cause ARDS and is a possibility, too.

Given the bleeding tendency seen in the wife, most viral haemorrhagic fevers can be excluded based on the incubation time alone, which is well below 21 days for most endemic viral haemorrhagic fevers (yellow fever, dengue and the New World arenaviruses, e.g. Junín virus and Machupo virus). There is only one exception to this rule, which is hantavirus infections: their incubation time may be up to 35 days.

Answer to Question 2

How Would You Manage These Patients Clinically? Is There Any Need to Consider Particular Hospital Hygiene Precautions?

Both patients should be referred to a tertiary care setting, which is equipped to handle ARDS and haemorrhagic fevers. Clinically, securing cardiorespiratory function is the main priority. Broad-spectrum antibiotics are indicated as empirical treatment until further results are back.

Although the aetiology is still unclear, a patient with respiratory symptoms must be treated under standard hygiene and droplet precautions (at least) to prevent potential nosocomial transmission. Depending on local hospital hygiene requirements, airborne precautions may be required.

The Case Continued...

Both patients were confirmed by PCR and serology to be infected with Andesvirus (ANDV), a New World species of the family *Hantaviridae*, belonging to the order of *Bunyavirales*. The New World hantaviruses are the causative agent of the Hantavirus Cardiopulmonary Syndrome (HCPS).

The husband was treated with non-invasive ventilation for 5 days. He made a full recovery after a month of rehabilitation. His wife experienced a dramatic course with nearly a full month on ECMO treatment. Multi-organ failure requiring renal replacement therapy and haemorrhagic complications with mass transfusions of blood products ensued. As a result of bleeding complications at the inguinal ECMO insertion sites (compartment syndrome and leg ischemia) ECMO was replaced centrally (Fig. 90.2). After additional bleeding complications at inguinal and thoracic insertion sites, she underwent several surgical interventions. Nosocomial infections followed, and she remained in intensive care for 5 months and an additional 12 months in rehabilitation. The mode of transmission remained unclear; both human-to-human-transmission and acquisition from a common source were possible.

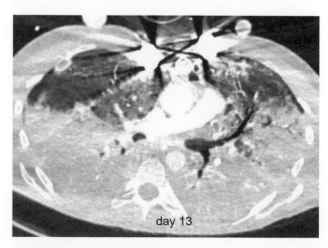

• **Fig. 90.2** Computed tomography of the chest (lung window) of the female patient on day 13 showing extensive and dense dorsal infiltrations and the centrally placed ECMO cannulae.

SUMMARY BOX

Hantavirus Cardiopulmonary Syndrome (HCPS)

HCPS is caused by ANDV. This New World hantavirus is endemic in the border region between Chile and Argentina. The vast majority of infections occur through inhalation of excreta from the long-tailed pygmy rice rat *(Oligoryzomys longicaudatus),* the reservoir host. Accordingly, outdoor activities are the major risk factor for acquiring ANDV infection.

The incubation period is typically 2 to 3 weeks (range 7–39 days) in case of common exposure.

After non-specific prodromal symptoms over 2 to 8 days, the clinical course varies from a mild disease to its most severe form, HCPS, which is characterized by microvascular leakage and is mainly attributed to host immune response. It presents with rapidly progressing respiratory failure and precipitous haemodynamic instability because of cardiogenic shock and consecutive pulmonary oedema. Capillary leak leads to hypovolemia, which may further impair cardiac and renal function. A haemorrhagic course may occur, although uncommon.

Diagnosis is confirmed by RT-PCR from whole blood or by serology, either with presence of specific IgM antibodies or at least a 4-fold increase in IgG titres in paired samples.

There is no specific treatment or vaccine against ANDV. The use of ribavirin and corticosteroids in ANDV infection still remains to be elucidated. Organ supportive therapy is therefore the mainstay of treatment. Patients should be transferred to a tertiary intensive care unit immediately upon suspicion of ANDV infection, because ECMO support might be required. Case fatality rate in patients with HCPS attributable to ANDV is 20% to 40%.

ANDV is the only hantavirus for which person-to-person transmission has been described, though this occurs very rarely. Nosocomial outbreaks were first reported in 1995. The incubation period in such a scenario is usually around 20 days. Person-to-person transmission is much less common than infection by inhalation of rodent excreta and occurs through close interpersonal contacts in the hospital setting (caring for a person with respiratory or haemorrhagic symptoms) or at home (such as sexual contacts, deep kissing or sharing the same bed).

In the nosocomial setting, standard hygiene and droplet precautions should be adopted, and it is recommended to treat the patients in a single room. During aerosol-generating procedures, however, healthcare workers are advised to wear high-efficiency respirator masks and ocular protection.

Further Reading

1. Blumberg L, Enria D, Bausch DG. Viral haemorrhagic fevers. In: Farrar J, editor. Manson's Tropical Diseases. 23rd ed London: Elsevier; 2013 [chapter 16].

2. Figueiredo LT, Souza WM, Ferrés M, Enria DA. Hantaviruses and cardiopulmonary syndrome in South America. Virus Res 2014;187:43–54.

3. Wells RM, Sosa Estani S, Yadon ZE, et al. An unusual Hantavirus outbreak in southern Argentina: person-to-person transmission? Hantavirus Pulmonary Syndrome Study Group for Patagonia. Emerg Infect Dis 1997;3:171–4.

4. Martinez-Valdebenito C, Calvo M, Vial C, et al. Person-to-person household and nosocomial transmission of Andes hantavirus, southern Chile, *2011.* Emerg Infect Dis 2014;20:1629–36.

5. Riquelme R, Rioseco ML, Bastidas L, et al. Hantavirus pulmonary syndrome, southern Chile, *1995–2012.* Emerg Infect Dis 2015;21:562–8.

91

A 20-Year-Old Male from India With Fever and Quadriparesis

REETA S. MANI

Clinical presentation

History

A previously healthy 20-year-old man from southern India is admitted to a local hospital with fever and quadriparesis.

He has had fever for 4 days, followed by tingling and weakness initially in his left leg, subsequently involving all four limbs over the next 2 days. He gives a history of a stray dog bite (WHO category III) on his left lower limb 1 month before onset of symptoms, for which he received five doses of anti-rabies vaccine (purified chick embryo cell vaccine), but no rabies immunoglobulin (RIG).

Clinical Findings

On admission, he is conscious and his mental functions are normal (GCS 15/15). His blood pressure is 110/70 mmHg, pulse 90 beats per minute, respiratory rate 26 breaths per minute and temperature 38.5°C (101.3°F). Neurological examination reveals a flaccid, areflexic quadriparesis.

Laboratory Results

His blood investigations including serum electrolytes, renal and liver function test are normal. Cerebrospinal fluid (CSF) shows 52 mg/dL protein (reference: 15–50mg/dL), 60 mg/dL glucose (reference: 50–75mg, provided a normal serum glucose) and 340 cells/mm^3 (60% polymorphs and 40% lymphocytes; normal $\leq$5 cells/mm^3).

Questions

1. You are suspecting rabies. How could you secure the diagnosis? What are the differentials?
2. How could rabies have been prevented in this case?

Discussion

A 20-year-old male Indian with a history of dog-bite presents with fever and rapidly progressive quadriparesis a month after the incident. He has received a full course of five active anti-rabies vaccinations, but no anti-rabies immunoglobulin.

Answer to Question 1

How Could You Secure the Diagnosis? What Are the Differentials?

A young male with a history of dog bite in a rabies-endemic country, presenting with fever and rapidly progressive ascending paresis a month later should elicit a high clinical suspicion of paralytic rabies. Laboratory confirmation must be done wherever feasible to rule out clinical mimics (Table 91.1) amenable to treatment and to institute prompt infection control measures. Testing at least three saliva samples at 3- to 6-hour intervals (owing to intermittent shedding of the virus in saliva), along with a nuchal skin biopsy for viral RNA by RT-PCR, can secure the diagnosis in most cases of the encephalitic form of rabies. Though serological diagnosis has a limited role in

TABLE 91.1	Clinical Mimics of Rabies
Syndrome or Disease
Guillain Barré Syndrome
Post-vaccination encephalomyelitis
NMDAR antibody-mediated/Autoimmune encephalitis
Campylobacter-associated summer paralysis syndrome
Cerebral malaria
Herpes simplex encephalitis
Arthropod-borne encephalitides (e.g. Japanese encephalitis, West Nile Virus encephalitis, etc.)
Poliomyelitis
B-virus (Cercopithecine herpesvirus 1) encephalomyelitis
Tetanus
Snake- or Scorpion-envenomation
Organophosphate poisoning
Illicit drug use, CNS intoxicants
Psychiatric disorders

the first week of illness, detection of rabies-specific antibodies in serum (of an unvaccinated individual) or CSF can aid in diagnosis, especially in cases where survival is prolonged beyond a week. If laboratory confirmation cannot be done ante-mortem, antigen detection by direct fluorescent antibody (dFA) test or RT-PCR on brain tissue obtained post-mortem can confirm or rule out a diagnosis of rabies (Table 91.2).

Answer to Question 2

How Could Rabies Have Been Prevented in This Case?

Prompt and appropriate post-exposure prophylaxis (PEP) after an exposure from a suspect rabid animal can prevent rabies in almost 100% of cases. True PEP failures are extremely rare and may occur because of short incubation periods resulting from multiple exposures on highly innervated areas of the body like the face, neck, hands etc. or because of direct inoculation of the virus into nerves.

In severe exposures (WHO category III) PEP consists of thorough wound washing, active vaccination with anti-rabies vaccines and passive vaccination with anti-rabies immunoglobulin (RIG). While it may take about 5 to 7 days for vaccine-induced antibodies to be produced, RIG, which is locally infiltrated into and around the wounds neutralizes the virus deposited at the site of the bite and prevents its entry into the nerves. Even though the patient received adequate doses of active vaccine, he did not receive RIG, which is life-saving in individuals

with severe exposures. Administration of human or equine RIG (or recently available monoclonal antibodies) could have possibly prevented rabies in this case.

The Case Continued…

After admission, the patient developed autonomic instability evidenced by increased perspiration and significant variability in heart rate and blood pressure. He developed dysphagia and respiratory distress requiring mechanical ventilation on the third day after hospitalization. His saliva sample collected at admission was positive for rabies viral RNA by RT-PCR; a CSF sample was negative. The patient died because of a sudden cardiac arrest on the fifth day of hospitalization (9 days post-onset of symptoms).

SUMMARY BOX

Rabies

Rabies is a progressive, fatal encephalomyelitis caused by viruses of the *Lyssavirus* genus (Order *Mononegavirales*, Family *Rhabdoviridae*). Rabies lyssavirus (RABV), the prototype virus of the *Lyssavirus* genus, is the most common causative agent of rabies, usually transmitted through the bite of infected mammals, mostly dogs. About 61 000 human global deaths occur because of rabies annually, mostly in Asia and Africa.

The incubation period is usually 20 to 90 days, but may vary. Two distinct clinical forms of rabies are recognized: Encephalitic ("furious") and paralytic ("dumb"). The encephalitic form rarely poses diagnostic difficulties because of the classical clinical features like hydrophobia, aerophobia, agitation and

---

TABLE 91.2 Tests for Laboratory Diagnosis of Rabies

	Sample(s)	Test(s)	Detection	Sensitivity	Remarks
Ante-mortem Diagnosis*	Saliva	RT-PCR	Viral nucleic acid	Moderate to high sensitivity	Testing serial/pooled samples recommended to increase sensitivity
	Nuchal skin biopsy	RT-PCR	Viral nucleic acid	Moderate to high sensitivity	Full thickness biopsy and adequate hair follicles required
	CSF, Urine	RT-PCR	Viral nucleic acid	Low sensitivity	
	CSF, Serum	RFFIT, FAVN, ELISA	Neutralizing Antibodies (RFFIT, FAVN); Antibodies against viral glycoprotein (ELISA)	Low sensitivity in first week of illness; rises with increased duration of survival (>90% by 2 weeks)	Presence of antibodies in CSF (irrespective of prior vaccination status) and serum (in previously unvaccinated cases) diagnostic of rabies
Post-mortem Diagnosis**	Brain tissue	dFA, RT-PCR	Viral antigen	High sensitivity (nearly 100%)	Gold standard for laboratory confirmation (dFA)

RT-PCR: Reverse transcriptase polymerase chain reaction; RFFIT: Rapid fluorescent focus inhibition test; FAVN: Fluorescent antibody virus neutralization; dFA: Direct fluorescent antibody
*A positive test confirms rabies; negative test results cannot rule out a diagnosis of rabies completely
**A positive test on brain tissue confirms rabies; negative test rules out rabies

autonomic dysfunction; however, paralytic rabies may clinically mimic Guillain Barré syndrome (GBS), post-vaccination encephalomyelitis and other conditions (Table 91.1) posing a challenge in diagnosis and management. Fever at onset, paraesthesia in the bitten limb, rapid progression, quadriparesis with predominant involvement of proximal muscles, bowel and bladder involvement, percussion myoedema, presence of hydrophobia/aerophobia and CSF pleocytosis seen in paralytic rabies can help differentiate it from GBS. Post-vaccination complications historically observed with nerve tissue vaccines used in the past are rarely seen with the currently used rabies vaccines derived from tissue culture or embryonated eggs. High titres of neutralizing antibodies in CSF and serum and predominant involvement of grey matter in brain and spinal cord on neuroimaging in paralytic rabies can help distinguish it from post-vaccination neurological complications.

Nerve conduction studies (an axonal neuropathy supports rabies), neuroimaging and laboratory tests (Table 91.2) can aid in the diagnosis.

Currently, there is no specific antiviral therapy of proven efficacy for rabies. Management consists of symptomatic treatment and supportive care. Prognosis is dismal in both forms of rabies, resulting in death within one to 2 weeks of symptom onset. Survival from rabies is extremely rare, though critical care can reportedly prolong survival by a few weeks or months in some cases.

This fatal disease can be prevented in most cases with appropriate PEP after exposure. Pre-exposure prophylaxis is recommended in individuals at high risk, including travellers to rabies-endemic countries.

Further Reading

1. Warell MJ. *Rabies*. In: Farrar J, editor. Manson's Tropical Diseases. 23rd ed. London: Elsevier; 2013 [chapter 52].
2. Willoughby RE. Jr. Rabies: rare human infection - common questions. Infect Dis Clin North Am 2015;29(4):637–50.
3. Rupprecht CE, Fooks AR, Abela-Ridder B, editors. An overview of antemortem and postmortem tests for diagnosis of human rabies. In: Laboratory Techniques in Rabies. 5th ed vol. 1. Geneva: World Health Organization; 2018 [chapter 5].
4. World Health Organization. WHO Expert Consultation on Rabies: Third report. World Health Organization Technical Report Series 1012. Geneva: WHO; 2018.
5. Fooks AR, Cliquet F, Finke S, et al. Rabies. Nat Rev Dis Primers 2017;3:17091.

92

A 42-Year-Old Traveller Returning from Thailand With Fever and Thrombocytopenia

CAMILLA ROTHE, MARIA S. MACKROTH AND E. TANNICH

Clinical Presentation

History

A 42-year-old German man presents to a hospital in Germany. For the past 6 days he has had a fever of up to 40°C (104°F), arthralgias and retro-orbital pain.

The day before presentation, he returned from a 10-week trip to Thailand, where he had spent 2 months on Little Koh Chang, an island in the Andaman Sea. After that, he spent 5 days in Hua Hin at the Gulf of Thailand and another 5 days in Bangkok. He has not taken any antimalarial chemoprophylaxis, which is in line with the national recommendations in his home country for this trip.

His past medical is unremarkable.

Clinical Findings

On examination, GCS is 15/15, Temperature 39.1°C (102.4°F), BP 156/80 mmHg, pulse 106 beats per minute, respiratory rate 16 breath cycles per minute, SpO$_2$ 95% on ambient air. There is no skin rash and no lymphadenopathy. Upon auscultation, his chest is clear. Abdominal examination does not show any intercostal tenderness, no tenderness on palpation and no organomegaly.

Laboratory results

FBC shows thrombocytopenia of 81×10^9/L (reference: 150–300) and is otherwise normal, CRP 55 mg/L (reference: <5), AST 62 U/L (reference: 10–50 U/L), ALT 106 U/L (reference: 10–50).

Dengue NS1 antigen test is negative, the rapid diagnostic test for malaria (which detects *Plasmodium falciparum*-specific histidine-rich protein II and the panmalarial aldolase) is negative.

Questions

1. What is your differential diagnosis?
2. How do you proceed?

Discussion

A 42-year old German man presents with a fever for 6 days, retro-orbital pain and arthralgias after extensive travel in southern Thailand. He is febrile, but otherwise physical examination is unremarkable. Full blood count reveals thrombocytopenia, CRP and liver function tests are slightly elevated. Rapid diagnostic tests for dengue and malaria are negative.

Answer to Question 1
What Is Your Differential Diagnosis?

Given the clinical syndrome of fever, retro-orbital pain, arthralgias and thrombocytopenia after a visit to Thailand, the most likely differential diagnosis to suspect is dengue fever. Dengue is the most common febrile tropical disease seen in returning travellers from South and South-east Asia. The duration of fever, however, is borderline long for dengue. The dengue NS1 antigen test reflecting dengue viraemia may already be negative at day 6 and does not reliably rule out the infection. Chikungunya and Zika are additional important arboviral infections to suspect.

Influenza is another important differential diagnosis to have in this patient. Fever and associated symptoms are usually of shorter duration but may last as long as 8 days. Acute HIV infection may present with persistent fever and thrombocytopenia, and possible exposures should definitely be inquired. Enteric fever presents with persistent febrile temperatures and otherwise non-specific symptoms. Because food hygiene in Thailand is overall very good, typhoid and paratyphoid fever are nowadays rarely seen imported from this country. Malaria has to be ruled out in any febrile traveller returning from a possibly endemic area, thrombocytopenia also being a hallmark feature. Malaria is nowadays rarely seen in travellers returning from Thailand; however, overlooking it could be lethal. A negative rapid diagnostic test (RDT) does not rule out malaria because RDTs are of unsatisfactory sensitivity for diagnosis of non-falciparum malaria. Also, in falciparum malaria high parasitaemia may cause a prozone phenomenon with a false negative RDT.

Answer to Question 2

How Do You Proceed?

To reliably rule out dengue and indeed any of the arboviral infections, serology at this point is the diagnostic test of choice, because viraemia is short and IgM should be positive by day 6 of fever. Convalescent samples taken 10 to 14 days later should show a further rise in titres.

For diagnosis of influenza a deep nasopharyngeal swab should be obtained, and care must be taken to apply the correct technique. For acute HIV infection fourth-generation diagnostic tests which include p24 antigen, should be able to diagnose acute infection. Western Blot may still be negative at this stage, but in case of doubt, HIV PCR would help establish the diagnosis. Blood cultures would be the appropriate test to rule out enteric fever.

For malaria, microscopy (thick and thin films) remains the diagnostic gold standard. Three negative films taken on consecutive days are considered to safely rule out malaria.

If malaria parasites are detected but the species remains unclear even at a referral laboratory, species-specific polymerase chain reaction (PCR) may be useful.

The Case Continued...

A thick blood film showed *Plasmodium* species trophozoites at a density of 920/µL. On thin film however, the microscopist on duty was unable to determine the *Plasmodium* species. Based on the negative result of the rapid diagnostic test, non-falciparum malaria was suspected. The patient was admitted to the infectious diseases ward. Treatment was started with atovaquone/proguanil 250/100mg, 4 tablets once daily for 3 days. The patient rapidly recovered and was discharged on the fourth day. For further parasite differentiation, malaria microscopy was repeated by the head parasitologist. After intense reading of the Giemsa-stained thin blood film, 2 parasite-infected erythrocytes were identified with morphological characteristics compatible with *Plasmodium malariae* or *P. knowlesi* infection (Figs. 92.1 and 92.2). Subsequently, species-specific PCR confirmed the presence of a mono-infection with *P. knowlesi*.

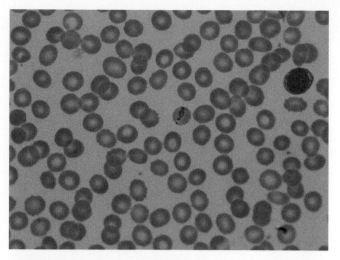

• **Fig. 92.1** Young trophozoite (ring form) of *P. knowlesi* (Giemsa-stained thin film).

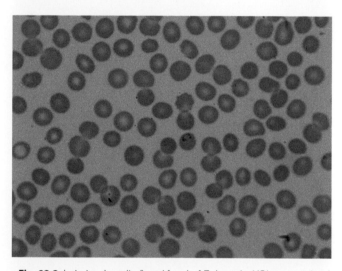

• **Fig. 92.2** Late trophozoite (band form) of *P. knowlesi* (Giemsa-stained thin film).

SUMMARY BOX

Knowlesi Malaria

P. knowlesi is primarily a zoonotic parasite reported increasingly in humans across South-east Asia. Its reservoir is in various species of macaques.

Knowlesi malaria is now recognized as the most common form of malaria in Malaysia and parts of western Indonesia and it is increasingly reported from other parts of South-east Asia.

Its prevalence may have long been underestimated because of the inability to reliably distinguish *P. knowlesi* from other *Plasmodium species*, in particular *P. malariae*. PCR-based methods have been a major breakthrough in recognizing the importance of *P. knowlesi*. Rapid diagnostic tests lack sensitivity and specificity for this parasite, and physicians practising in the region or seeing returned travellers from South-east Asia need to be aware of these pitfalls.

P. knowlesi has a 24-hour erythrocytic cycle and therefore causes a quotidian (daily) fever pattern with relatively high parasitaemias seen in some patients. It may cause severe disease, similar to falciparum malaria. Treatment is the same as for acute falciparum malaria.

Further Reading

1. White NJ. Malaria. In: Farrar J, editor. Manson's Tropical Diseases. 23rd ed. London: Elsevier; 2013 [chapter 43].

2. Antinori S, Galimberti L, Milazzo L, et al. *Plasmodium knowlesi:* the emerging zoonotic malaria parasite. Acta Trop 2013;125:191–201.

3. Singh B, Daneshvar C. Human Infections and Detection of *Plasmodium knowlesi*. Clin Microbiol Rev 2013;26(2):165–84.

4. Zaw MT, Lin Z. Human *Plasmodium knowlesi* infections in South-East Asian countries. J Microbiol Immunol Infect 2019;S1684–1182:30078. https://doi.org/10.1016/j.jmii.2019.05.012.

5. Froeschl G, Nothdurft HD, von Sonnenburg F, et al. Retrospective clinical case series study in 2017 indentifies *Plasmodium knowlesi* as most frequent Plasmodium species in returning travellers from Thailand to Germany. Euro Surveill 2018;23(29).

93

A 35-Year-Old Male Logger from Peru With Fever, Jaundice and Bleeding

PEDRO LEGUA

Clinical Presentation

History

A 35-year-old Peruvian man is referred to a hospital in Lima. Eight days prior, he developed fever and retro-orbital headache. Two days into the illness he was admitted to a local hospital in the jungle after he had developed jaundice, coffee-ground vomiting, gross haematuria and increasing mental obtundation. During the transfer to the referral hospital in Lima the patient had a generalized seizure. His past medical history included hepatitis of unknown aetiology 20 years before.

The patient was born in Lima, but for the past 5 years has been working as a logging supervisor in a remote jungle area near Pucallpa on the shores of the Ucayali River (which joins the Marañón to form the Amazon river). He has not taken any malaria prophylaxis and has not received any vaccinations since his early childhood.

Clinical Findings

Temperature 38.8°C (101.8°F), blood pressure 110/70 mmHg, heart rate 110 beats per minute, respiratory rate 24 breaths per minute. He is agitated, unresponsive to verbal commands and intermittently stuporous. There is marked flapping of hands, no focal neurological signs and no meningeal signs. He is jaundiced, and there is spontaneous bleeding of his oral mucosa and at venipuncture and IV sites. There are multiple large ecchymoses on the face, the trunk and all limbs (Fig. 93.1). On auscultation of the lungs there are crepitant rales in both bases. The heart sounds are normal. The liver is felt 3 cm below the right costal margin; the spleen is not palpable and there is no lymphadenopathy.

Laboratory Results

His routine laboratory results on admission are shown in Table 93.1. His malaria thick film is three times negative. Blood cultures are negative. Brucella serology is negative. Hepatitis B IgM anti-Hbc are negative.

TABLE 93.1	Laboratory Results on Admission
Parameter	**Result (Reference Range)**
Haematocrit	30% (41–53)
White cell count	8700/µL (4500–11000)
	Bands: 4% (0–10)
	Neutrophils: 62% (40–70)
	Eosinophils: 0% (0–8)
	Basophils: 0% (0–3)
	Monocytes: 6% (4–11)
	Lymphocytes: 28% (22–44)
Platelets	110000/µL (150000–450000)
AST (GOT)	2890 U/L (0–35)
ALT (GPT)	2676 U/L (0–35)
AP	496 U/L (38–126)
Total Bilirubin	11.6 mg/dL (0.3–1.2)
Direct Bilirubin	9.2 mg/dL (0–0.4)
Urea	89 mg/dL (17–49)
Creatinine	1.2 mg/dL (0.6–1.2)
Glucose	80 mg/dL (70–110)
Serum Protein	4.2 g/L (5.5–8.0)
Albumin	2.8 g/L (3.5–5.5)
Prothrombin Time	17 s (11.1–13.1)
INR	2.6 (0.9–1.3)
aPTT	80 s (22.1–35.1)
Fibrinogen	250 mg/dL (150–400)
CK	6200 U/L (52–336)
Urine	Proteins 3+, RBC: 50–60/f, WBC: 4–6/f

Questions

1. What is your differential diagnosis?
2. What tests will you do to confirm the diagnosis?

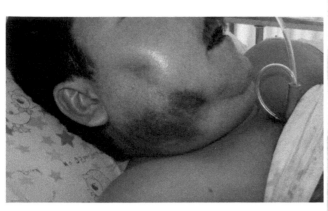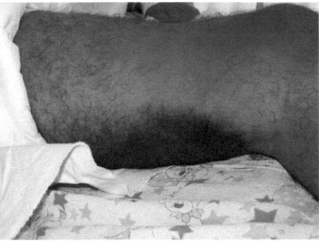

• **Fig. 93.1** Extended ecchymoses in a febrile Peruvian logger with fever and jaundice

Discussion

A young male Peruvian logger working in the South American jungle presents with fever, jaundice, bleeding, encephalopathy and seizures. Laboratory results indicate liver failure.

Answer to Question 1

What is your differential diagnosis?

This patient presents with an acute febrile illness that produces liver failure. Severe malaria is a possibility, although transaminases are usually not so high. The differential diagnosis includes viral hepatitis (A, B, C, D, and E) and toxin-mediated hepatitis.

Leptospirosis seems possible, but the transaminases in leptospirosis are usually only mildly elevated (less than 200 U/L) and jaundice is caused by cholestasis rather than hepatocellular damage. Typhoid fever and brucellosis are other bacterial infections to be taken into account.

Severe dengue has to be considered, although 8 days of fever appears long for dengue and usually jaundice is not so prominent. Also, haematocrit would be increased rather than low, as in this case.

Other viral haemorrhagic fevers (VHFs) with jaundice are possible, particularly given his occupation as a logger in the Peruvian jungle with possible contact to sylvatic mosquitoes and animals. The most prominent VHF in Peru is yellow fever and he does not appear to be vaccinated against this disease.

Answer to Question 2

What Tests Will You Do to Confirm the Diagnosis?

Serial thick blood smears for malaria should be ordered.

Dengue NS1 and dengue IgM should be performed (because NS1 might have turned negative after more than 1 week of illness).

Blood cultures should be done to look for *Brucella* species, as well as *S.* Typhi and *S.* Paratyphi. If brucellosis is suspected, microbiologists must be informed because specimens have to be handled under special biosafety precautions to prevent laboratory infections.

If available, PCR of urine and blood should be done to look for leptospirosis; microscopic agglutination test is an alternative if PCR is not available.

Laboratory tests should include IgM antibodies for the different viral hepatitis viruses (except for acute hepatitis D because of delayed antibody production).

IgM antibodies against the yellow fever virus persist for several weeks and can be detected by various methods, e.g. IgM capture ELISA. Detection of viral RNA by RT-PCR could also be attempted.

The Case Continued…

The patient received presumptive treatment for malaria, broad-spectrum antibiotics, and supportive care. Over the next 3 days, he developed increasing hepatic encephalopathy, renal failure, coma, and DIC with increasing spontaneous bleeding. The chest x-ray showed bilateral pulmonary infiltrates compatible with ARDS (Fig. 93.2). Repeat laboratory results on day 3 showed deterioration of his kidney function (creatinine 6.5 mg/dL, urea 120 mg/dL) and a sudden drop in his liver transaminases (AST 100 U/L, ALT 200 U/L), most likely indicating acute hepatic disintegration. Sadly, the patient passed away 1 day later.

IgM capture ELISA for yellow fever came back highly positive at 1:10000. Anti-dengue IgM was negative. Direct viral isolation in culture was negative on a blood specimen drawn on admission (8 days into the illness), which is not surprising because viraemia in yellow fever is short (4–5 days). Permission for autopsy was refused, therefore liver histology was not available.

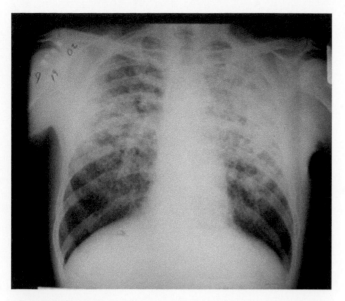

• Fig. 93.2 Chest x-ray of the patient showing bilateral patchy infiltrates.

Further Reading

1. Blumberg L, Enria D, Bausch DG. Viral haemorrhagic fevers. In: Farrar J, editor. Manson's Tropical Diseases. 23rd ed London: Elsevier; 2013 [chapter 16].
2. Monath TP, Vasconcelos PFC. Yellow fever. J Clin Virol 2015; 64:160–73.
3. Quaresma JAS, Pagliari C, Medeiros DBA, et al. Immunity and immune response, pathology and pathologic changes: progress and challenges in the immunopathology of yellow fever. Rev Med Virol 2013;23(5):305–18.
4. Visser LG. Fractional-dose yellow fever vaccination: how much can we do less? Curr Opin Infect Dis 2019;32(5):390–93.
5. Reno E, Quan NG, Franco-Paredes C, et al. Prevention of Yellow Fever in travellers: an update. Lancet Infect Dis 2020;20(6): e129–37.

SUMMARY BOX

Yellow Fever

Yellow fever is and arboviral infection caused by a flavivirus and transmitted by Aedes and Haemagogus mosquitoes. It is endemic in South and Central America and in Africa. There is no yellow fever in Asia.

The incubation period of yellow fever is usually 3 to 6 days. Most cases are subclinical or show mild and non-specific symptoms. After an acute febrile illness with headache and myalgia without a rash that likely represents the peak viraemia, there may be a period of remission, as seen in other flaviviral infections. Fever may then resume joined by back pain, nausea, vomiting and altered mental status progressing to the severe clinical syndrome described above. Haematemesis is commonly described. In fatal cases, death usually occurs 7 to 10 days into the illness.

Yellow fever causes an infection of hepatocytes and Kupffer cells. There is mid-zonal hepatocellular necrosis with a minimal inflammatory response. Councilman bodies and microvesicular fatty changes are seen. The sudden and marked decrease of hepatic transaminases in our patient just before death likely represented near total destruction of functioning hepatocytes and acute hepatic disintegration.

As with other flaviviruses there is no specific treatment for yellow fever, making prevention by use of the 17D live yellow fever vaccine imperative. Vaccine efficacy in immunocompetent persons is at nearly 100%. While most individuals in endemic areas (Amazon basin and sub-Saharan Africa) have poor access to vaccines and there are regular shortages during yellow fever epidemics there is dramatic under-use of the vaccination by travellers and expatriates. Data indicates that the number of unvaccinated travellers visiting risk areas is substantial. Each year, deaths in unvaccinated travellers to yellow fever endemic areas are reported.

94

A 20-Year-Old Woman from the Democratic Republic of the Congo With Fever and a Vesiculopustular Skin Rash

JOHANNES BLUM AND ANDREAS NEUMAYR

Clinical Presentation

History

A 20-year-old woman presents to her local hospital in a rural area of the Democratic Republic of the Congo with a history of fever, malaise, headache, dry cough, swelling of the neck and a disseminated skin rash, which appeared 2 days after the symptoms began. The skin lesions first appeared on the face and then spread centrifugally over her body, including the palms and soles of her feet as well as the oral mucosa. The lesions have developed from initial macules to papules, then to vesicles and finally to pustules. The oral mucosal lesions are painful and make drinking and eating difficult.

The patient resides in a village, where people live from agriculture, she has no relevant past medical history and is the mother of three children.

Clinical Findings

Vital signs: temperature 38°C (100.4°F), pulse 110 beats per minute, blood pressure 105/82 mmHg. Disseminated uniform umbilicated vesiculopustular skin lesions, ranging from 0.5 to 1 cm in diameter, all over the body with a predilection for the face, the hands and the feet (Fig. 94.1). Generalized lymphadenopathy with prominent swelling of the cervical lymph nodes. The examination of the lungs, heart, abdomen and the CNS is unremarkable.

Laboratory Results See Table 94.1

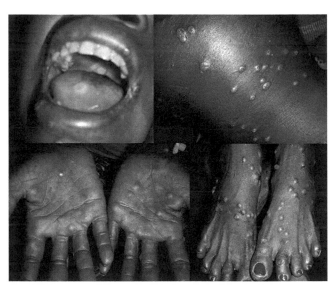

• **Fig. 94.1** Vesiculopustular skin rash seen at hospital admission

TABLE 94.1	Laboratory Results at Presentation		
Parameter		Patient	Reference
WBC (× 10⁹/L) (neutrophils: lymphocytes)		4.4 (73%:21%)	4–10
Haemoglobin (g/dL)		12.3	12–16
ESR		75 mm/h	<20 mm/h

Questions

1. What are your differential diagnoses?
2. What are the main criteria to distinguish these differential diagnoses from each other?

Discussion

A 20-year-old woman from a rural region of the Democratic Republic of the Congo presents with an acute febrile illness which is accompanied by a disseminated uniform vesiculopustular skin rash including the palms and soles of the feet as well as the oral mucosa and a prominent cervical lymphadenopathy.

Answer to Question 1

What Are Your Differential Diagnoses?

The clinical manifestation suggests a viral infection and the morphology and evolution of the skin lesions is characteristic for a poxvirus. Although smallpox was eradicated in 1979 and no cases have occurred since, a zoonotic poxvirus would be the primary suspicion, particularly monkeypox, which is endemic in rural regions of Central Africa. Varicella, caused by the varicella zoster virus, is another febrile illness associated with a vesicular rash that is often confused with monkeypox, but several features help distinguish the two illnesses (discussed below).

Cowpox usually presents with a single lesion (unless the patient is immunosuppressed); fever and lymphadenopathy are uncommon, therefore this seems to be less likely.

Answer to Question 2

What Are the Main Criteria to Distinguish These Differential Diagnoses from Each Other?

Important criteria to distinguish the main viral infections presenting with a vesiculopapular rash include the distribution of the skin lesions, the stage of the respective lesion(s), involvement of palms and soles, and the presence of fever and lymphadenopathy (Table 94.2).

The Case Continued...

Currently, no specific vaccine or treatment for monkeypox is available and clinical management is exclusively supportive. Persons who have been vaccinated against smallpox in the past appear to have some cross-protection against monkeypox; and if they get infected, develop milder symptoms than unvaccinated persons. Our patient is 20 years old, and was thus born after the worldwide smallpox vaccination

TABLE 94.2	Clinical Characteristics of Viral Infections Presenting With a Vesicular Rash (McCollum, 2014)[2]			
	Monkeypox	Smallpox	Cowpox	Varicella
Incubation period (days)	6–16	12–14	7–14	14–17
Fever (°C)	38.5–40.5	>40	Rare	<38.8
Rash	disseminated, uniform	disseminated, uniform	localized singular lesion(s) (rarely disseminated)	disseminated, non-uniform
Lesion distribution	centrifugal	centrifugal	-	centripetal
Lesion progression	homogenous rash (lesions are mostly in one stage of development); slow progression with each stage lasting 1–2 days	homogenous rash (lesions are mostly in one stage of development); slow progression with each stage lasting 1–2 days	-	heterogeneous rash (lesions are often in multiple stages of development on the body; fast progression
Frequency of lesions on palms or soles of feet	common	common	-	rare
Rash period (from the appearance of lesions to desquamation) (days)	14–21	14–21	21–56	10–21
Lymphadenopathy	yes	yes	rare	no
Case fatality rate	1%–10%	10%–50%	1%–3%	0.13%

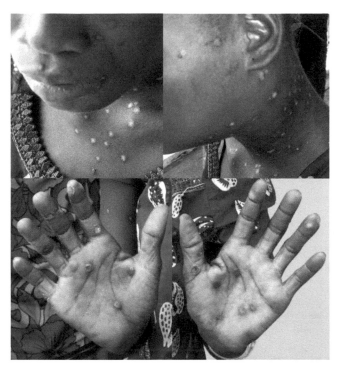

• **Fig. 94.2** Healing skin lesions at discharge from the hospital

programmes were stopped in the early 1980s. She made an uneventful recovery; however, with scarring from the skin lesions (Fig. 94.2).

SUMMARY BOX

Human Monkeypox

Human monkeypox is a sporadic smallpox-like zoonotic viral exanthematous disease. It occurs in the rain forests of Central and West Africa. The virus was first identified in 1958 in laboratory monkeys. Human monkeypox was not recognized as a distinct infection in humans until 1970. Then, during efforts to eradicate smallpox, the virus was isolated from a patient with suspected smallpox infection in Zaire (now the Democratic Republic of the Congo). Although the natural animal reservoir of monkeypox remains unknown, several lines of evidence point to rodents as a likely reservoir. The sporadically observed human cases and small outbreaks are confined to remote villages and believed to result from close contact between humans and wild animals. However,

the precise exposure is often difficult to pinpoint in areas where contact with animals through household rodent infestations and hunting or preparation of bushmeat from a variety of species is common. Outside endemic areas, there was an outbreak of monkeypox in the United States in 2003 associated with infected prairie dogs sold as pets.

Although considerably less infective than smallpox, monkeypox can also spread from human to human through the respiratory route or by contact with an infected person's bodily fluids. Transmission is believed to occur through saliva and respiratory secretions or contact with exudate or crust material from the skin lesions. Risk factors for transmission include sharing a bed or room or using the same utensils as an infected person.

The clinical picture of monkeypox is similar to smallpox but shows a considerably milder course with a case fatality rate of ≤10%. It is believed that the rising number of reported human cases in recent years is largely attributable to the waning herd immunity after the suspension of smallpox vaccination in the early 1980s.

In endemic regions, the fairly distinct rash of monkeypox is primarily a clinical diagnosis because neither commercial assays nor the required laboratory infrastructure are usually readily available. The definitive diagnosis is established by PCR, culture, immunohistochemistry or electron microscopy but demands biosafety level 2 laboratory facilities. Optimal diagnostic specimens for PCR are lesion exudate on a swab or crust specimens (stored in a dry, sterile tube without any transport media and kept cold). Interpretation of serological tests can be hampered by cross-reactivity with other orthopoxviruses including previous smallpox vaccination.

Further Reading

1. Blumberg L, Enria D, Bausch DG. Viral haemorrhagic fevers. In: Farrar J, editor. Manson's Tropical Diseases. 23rd ed London: Elsevier; 2013 [chapter 16].
2. McCollum AM, Damon IK. Human monkeypox. Clin Infect Dis 2014;58(2):260–7.
3. Sklenovská N, Van Ranst M. Emergence of Monkeypox as the Most Important Orthopoxvirus Infection in Humans. Front Public Health 2018;6:241.
4. Reed KD, Melski JW, Graham MB, et al. The Detection of Monkeypox in Humans in the Western Hemisphere. N Engl J Med 2004;350:342–50.

95

A 42-Year-Old Male Refugee from the Democratic Republic of the Congo With Progressive Depression

MICHAEL LIBMAN

Clinical Presentation

History

A 42-year-old man presents with recent insomnia, difficulty concentrating, and emotional disturbance. He had been a professor in a university in Kinshasa, Democratic Republic of the Congo. As a result of civil unrest, he had been arrested and tortured, eventually crossing the country overland over a period of a year. He settled in a refugee camp in Tanzania, and finally emigrated to Canada. In Canada, he continued to be under significant stress, with financial and employment difficulties. After 15 months in Canada, he presents with labile affect, delusions and hallucinations. His delusions were of a depressive nature, consisting mostly of feelings of persecution and conspiracy by locals with agents of his home country. His hallucinations were mainly auditory; he perceived people talking about him.

Clinical Findings

His general examination on initial presentation was unremarkable, other than a flat affect and intermittent somnolence. He underwent psychiatric care, was given a diagnosis of depression and received a series of medical treatments. Nevertheless, he continued to deteriorate with progressive fatigue and symptoms of depression. His only other significant complaint was severe low back pain after a relatively minor injury. Over the following year, he began having falls, developed bilateral posterior cervical adenopathy and intermittent fevers.

Laboratory Results

His basic laboratory investigations were normal, other than a mild normochromic normocytic anaemia. HIV serology was negative.

Questions

1. What are the most likely diagnoses which could account for progressive mental status changes in this individual?
2. Which tests are most likely to help make the diagnosis?

Discussion

A 42-year-old male refugee from the Democratic Republic of the Congo presents with a slowly progressive depressive illness, with features of somnolence. There is no response to the usual medical treatments for depression. Gradually, evidence of a systemic illness appears, including anaemia, adenopathy, and intermittent fevers.

Answer to Question 1

What Are the Most Likely Diagnoses Which Could Account for Progressive Mental Status Changes in This Individual?

There are several illnesses which may present with subacute or sometimes chronic psychiatric symptoms. The differential could include cryptococcal meningitis, although this would be rare in an HIV-negative, otherwise healthy individual, and the course is usually more rapid than this. Tuberculous meningitis has to be considered; but again, the slow progression would be atypical. Cerebral toxoplasmosis may present with psychiatric symptoms depending on the location of the lesion, which should be seen on brain imaging, and is also unlikely in the absence of advanced HIV or other immunosuppressive condition. Neurocysticercosis could present with neuropsychiatric symptoms related to hydrocephalus or complex seizures. Imaging, again, should provide a diagnosis. Neurosyphilis should always be considered. Rare psychiatric syndromes have been described with illness including malaria and typhoid of unclear pathophysiology, but the presentation is typically more acute than is seen in this case.

Although depression would not be unusual in any refugee, the very indolent but relentlessly progressive symptoms in someone from West Africa, and particularly the Congo, should trigger investigations for West African trypanosomiasis, caused by *Trypanosoma brucei gambiense*.

Answer to Question 2

Which Tests Are Most Likely to Help Make the Diagnosis?

Several tests which are non-specific may give clues to the diagnosis of African Sleeping Sickness. There is often evidence of general inflammation, and chronic immune stimulation. This includes high erythrocyte sedimentation rate (ESR) and c-reactive protein level (CRP). There are usually very high levels of polyclonal IgG and IgM in serum as well as various non-specific autoantibodies such as antinuclear antibodies. Traditional specific tests include looking for trypanosomes in thick and thin blood films and aspirates of enlarged lymph nodes. Serology, typically using a simple card agglutination test, is considered very sensitive for West African disease, although of moderate specificity. Most importantly, testing the CSF for pleocytosis and organisms is needed to rule out CNS involvement. In higher resource settings, molecular testing of blood and CSF has replaced the less sensitive microscopic analysis.

The Case Continued...

MRI of the brain revealed non-specific midbrain abnormalities, with focal hyperintensity lesions seen on a FLAIR sequence (Fig. 95.1). His lumbar puncture revealed 219 red cells and 342 white cells, mostly lymphocytes, per microlitre. Protein was very high, glucose mildly low, and CSF IgG and IgM were very elevated and polyclonal in nature. Morula cells were seen in the CSF. Morula cells (or Mott cells) are thought to be abnormal plasma cells containing cytoplasmic vacuoles filled with immunoglobulins which have not been released.

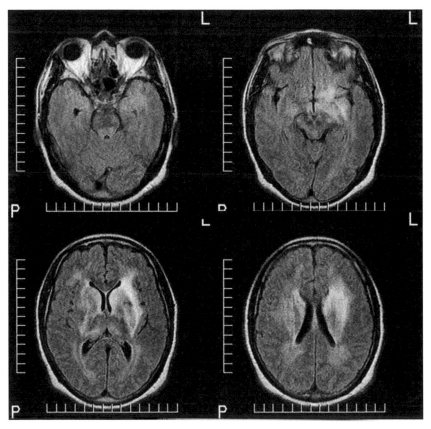

• **Fig. 95.1** MRI of the brain, with midbrain abnormalities seen on FLAIR sequences.

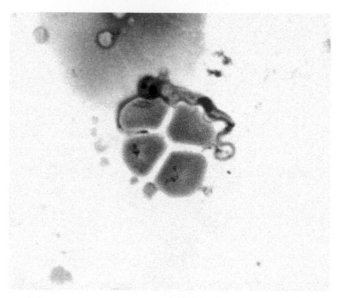

• **Fig. 95.2** Trypanosome seen on Giemsa staining of concentrated CSF specimen.

Serology was highly positive on the card agglutination test, and *Trypanosoma brucei* species were detected by CSF smear (Fig. 95.2). CSF PCR confirmed *T. brucei gambiense.* In contrast, blood smears and blood PCR were repeatedly negative. Treatment was initiated with eflornithine for 2 weeks, with a very slow but nearly complete clinical response over 1 year.

SUMMARY BOX

West African Trypanosomiasis

West African trypanosomiasis had been well controlled and almost eliminated in the region of the former Belgian Congo soon after independence in 1960. This was primarily achieved by vector control and through active case finding and treatment, since humans are the only reservoir for this parasite. Unfortunately, because of prolonged civil unrest, control programs have diminished and there has been a resurgence of disease.

The great bulk of cases currently originate from the Democratic Republic of the Congo, although Chad, Uganda, and a few other countries have smaller foci of disease activity. Diagnosis is not that difficult when appropriate testing is done, although there is little familiarity with presentation or testing strategies outside of endemic areas. Disease that does not involve the CNS can be treated relatively easily with pentamidine. Neurological involvement was revolutionized by the discovery that the antineoplastic agent eflornithine was highly effective and far less toxic than the previously used arsenicals. Currently, the standard regimen used in endemic areas combines eflornithine with oral nifurtimox (NECT). Compared with eflornithine monotherapy, NECT has higher cure rates (95–98%), lower fatality rates (<1%), it is easier to administer and has fewer side effects. An oral agent, fexinidazole, is in advanced development and looks very promising.

Further Reading

1. Burri C, Chappuis F, Brun R. Human African Trypanosomiasis. In: Farrar J, editor. Manson's Tropical Diseases. 23rd ed. London: Elsevier; 2014 [chapter 45].
2. Bottieau E, Clerinx J. Human African trypanosomiasis: progress and stagnation. Infect Dis Clin North Am 2019;33(1):61–77.
3. Chappuis F. Oral fexinidazole for human African trypanosomiasis. Lancet 2018;391(10116):100–2.
4. Franco JR, Simarro PP, Diarra A, et al. Epidemiology of human African trypanosomiasis. Clin Epidemiol 2014;6:257–75.
5. Michelsen SJ, Buscher P, Hoepelman AI, et al. Human African trypanosomiasis: a review of non-endemic cases in the past 20 years. Int J Infect Dis 2011;15(8); 2011 e517–24.

96

A 19-Year-Old Boy from India With Drooping, Diplopia and Dysphagia

PRISCILLA RUPALI

Clinical Presentation

History

A 19-year-old boy from India presents to the local hospital with drooping of eyelids, double vision and difficulty swallowing for the past 2 days. He also had low-grade fever with throat pain in the preceding week. He belongs to a nomadic tribe living in the jungle. He is the eldest of four siblings and immunization history is not available.

Clinical Findings

He is dyspnoeic and his vitals are: temperature 37.8°C (100°F), pulse rate 60 beats per minute, respiratory rate 24 breath cycles per minute and blood pressure 90/50 mmHg. The oral examination shows bilateral white membranes over the tonsils (Fig. 96.1). He also has diffuse submandibular swelling but only discrete lymph node swelling. The central nervous system examination shows bilateral ptosis (Fig. 96.2), sluggish extraocular and palatal movements with no obvious motor or sensory deficit.

Laboratory Results

Laboratory results on admission are shown in Table 96.1.

Bilirubin, total serum protein and albumin were normal. Blood cultures and throat culture showed no growth. HIV serology was negative and so was HBs antigen and anti-HCV.

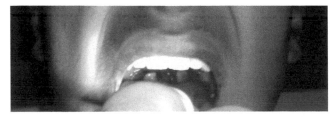
• **Fig. 96.1** Oral examination showing bilateral pseudomembrane over the tonsils.

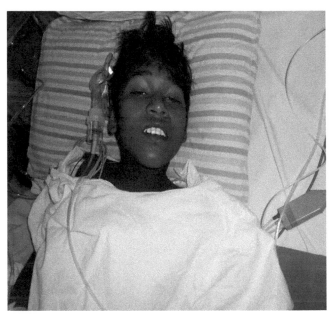
• **Fig. 96.2** Bilateral ptosis seen in the patient.

ECG

His ECG is showing a complete heart block.

Questions

1. What is the most likely diagnosis and what is the differential diagnosis?
2. What could in this kind of case scenario be given as post exposure prophylaxis for the contacts?

Discussion

A 19-year-old nomadic boy, probably unimmunized in childhood, presents to the hospital with ptosis, diplopia and dysphagia preceded by a week of low-grade fever and throat pain.

TABLE 96.1 Laboratory Results on Admission

Investigation	Result	Reference
Haemoglobin (g/dL)	13.7	11–15
White Blood Cells ($\times\ 10^9$/L)	21.2	4–12
Platelets ($\times\ 10^9$/L)	39	150–300
Creatinine (mg/dL)	1.42	0.5–1.4
Trop T (pg/mL)	766	<14
AST/ SGOT (U/L)	53	8–40
ALT/ SGPT (U/L)	35	5–35
Alkaline Phosphatase (U/L)	96	40–125
Sodium (mmol/L)	138	135–145
Potassium (mmol/L)	3.9	3.2–4.7
Magnesium (mmol/L)	2.09	1.8–2.4

Answer to Question 1

What Is the Most Likely Diagnosis and What Is the Differential Diagnosis?

A probably unimmunized boy presenting with ptosis, diplopia and dysphagia along with white pseudo-membranes over the tonsils and submandibular swelling should raise the possibility of diphtheritic neuropathy.

The other possibility is krait snake bite which is common in India. It also manifests with neurological deficits including drooping of eyelids, diplopia and dysphagia without obvious fang marks, and living in the jungle increases the probability. However, submandibular swelling along with membranes over the tonsils makes it less likely.

Botulism can be a possibility because the patient has cranial nerve involvement, but there is no progressive descending paralysis, again, rendering this a less likely differential diagnosis.

Early disseminated Lyme disease is another differential to keep in mind because the patient also has both neurological and cardiac involvement with heart block; however, Lyme disease is so far rarely seen in India.

Answer to Question 2

What Could in This Kind of Case Scenario Be Given as Post-Exposure Prophylaxis for the Contacts?

Because the most important diagnosis in this case is diphtheria, close contacts and medical personnel taking care of the patient should receive antimicrobial prophylaxis with erythromycin 500 QID for 7 to 10 days. Their immunization statuses should be current; if not, they can each receive a TdaP booster.

The Case Continued…

The PCR for *Corynebacterium diphtheriae* from a throat swab was positive confirming the diagnosis. The patient was treated with amoxicillin/clavulanic acid and diphtheria antitoxin 100 000 units. He was put on a temporary pacemaker because he developed complete heart block. However, he subsequently developed ventricular tachycardia with hypotension. He got cardioverted, intubated and mechanically ventilated because he went into cardiorespiratory failure. The patient's condition worsened further, and thus family members wanted to take him home against medical advice.

SUMMARY BOX

Diphtheria

Diphtheria is caused by the Gram-positive bacillus *C. diphtheriae*. The incidence of diphtheria has steadily declined over the past decades as a result of successful vaccination programmes and improvement of hygiene and living conditions. Nevertheless, the infection continues to affect vulnerable populations, such as refugees and indigenous peoples, as well as those living in areas of political or civil unrest and infrastructure failure, who suffer from reduced vaccination coverage.

C. diphtheriae has four biotypes—gravis, intermedius, mitis and belfanti. All strains can produce a toxin which is encoded by a lysogenic β–phage and causes severe disease. Humans are the only known reservoir. *C. diphtheriae* is usually transmitted through droplets, secretion or direct contact. Both symptomatic individuals and asymptomatic carriers can transmit diphtheria. The common primary sites of infection are the upper respiratory tract and the skin. The incubation period is 2 to 5 days. The most common presentations of respiratory diphtheria are a low-grade fever, sore throat, malaise and cervical lymphadenopathy. Local necroses lead to formation of grey and white pseudomembranes on the mucosa of the upper respiratory tract, quite adherent to the underlying tissue, which bleeds on scraping. In some patients, it may produce extensive swelling of tonsils, uvula, cervical lymph nodes, submandibular region and anterior neck known as bull neck. The severity of systemic complications is directly proportional to the extent of local disease and includes myocarditis and neuritis. Myocarditis may present as arrythmias including complex heart blocks, cardiac failure and cardiogenic shock. Neuropathies include paralysis of the soft palate and posterior pharyngeal wall, followed by cranial neuropathies and late onset peripheral neuritis. Cutaneous diphtheria may often present as a shallow ulcerative lesion with a grey-white membrane. The definite diagnosis requires isolation and culture of the organism from the lesion with a positive toxin assay, relevant clinical symptoms and epidemiological risk factors. The management includes airway protection and treatment with antibiotics; and in severe cases, diphtheria antitoxin.

The latter should be administered promptly, because it only neutralises circulating and not intracellular toxin. Its effectiveness therefore decreases over time in relation to symptom onset. The antibiotics used are erythromycin or procaine penicillin for 14 days. Close contacts, especially household contacts, should each receive an age-appropriate booster vaccine if not currently immunised, along with a single dose of benzathine penicillin or 7 to 10 days of oral erythromycin.

Further Reading

1. Hien TT, White NJ. Diphtheria. In: Farrar J, editor. Manson's Tropical Diseases. 23rd ed London: Elsevier; 2013 [chapter 35].
2. Truelove SA, Keegan LT, Moss WJ, et al. Clinical and epidemiological aspects of diphtheria: a systematic review and pooled analysis. Clin Infect Dis 2019; https://doi.org/10.1093/cid/ciz808.
3. Sanghi V. Neurologic manifestations of diphtheria and pertussis. Handb Clin Neurol 2014;121:1355–9.
4. Rahman MR, Ilsam K. Massive diptheria outbreak amoing Rohingya refugees: lessons learnt. J Trav Med 2019;26(1):1–3. https://doi.org/10.1093/jtm/tay122.

97

An 87-Year-Old Japanese Man With a Serpiginous Erythema on the Right Thigh

HARUHIKO MARUYAMA, HIROKO TAKAMATSU, YOON KONG AND YUKIFUMI NAWA

Clinical Presentation

History

An 87-year-old Japanese man from Kyushu district in the south-western part of Japan presents to a local dermatology clinic with a serpiginous erythema on his right anterior thigh. There is no pain, no tenderness or itching sensation and he is not febrile. The local clinic refers him to a tertiary hospital for further work-up.

Clinical Findings

There is a U-shaped serpiginous skin lesion on the anterior thigh just beneath the inguinal region (Fig. 97.1A). Although the upper part of the lesion has a brownish red tint, the lower part has bright red colour and shows marked swelling.

Laboratory Results

Differential count is normal apart from a slight anaemia (Hb 13.1 g/dL; (reference: 13.5–17.5 g/dL)). Eosinophil count and total IgE level are within normal range. CRP is not elevated.

Liver function tests, creatinine, BUN and LDH are normal.

Questions

1. What kinds of diseases should be considered in your differential diagnosis?
2. What additional information should you obtain from the patient?

Discussion

An elderly Japanese man from Kyushu presents with a serpiginous lesion on his thigh, which has developed over several weeks. He is otherwise in good health. Laboratory results are normal apart from slight anaemia.

Answer to Question 1

What Kinds of Diseases Should Be Considered in Your Differential Diagnosis?

A serpiginous erythema ("creeping eruption") is most commonly caused by the migration of larvae or juveniles of parasitic helminths. There are several parasites which should be considered in the differential diagnosis: with fine winding erythematous tracks, most commonly located on the lower extremities, the most likely diagnosis is cutaneous larva migrans (CLM) caused by animal hookworms. CLM may present with multiple tracks and may cause severe itch. CLM is a clinical diagnosis and there are no additional tests to confirm it.

Gnathostoma species may cause erythematous tracks wider in diameter than CLM, very much like the finding seen in this patient. A serpiginous erythema on the chest or abdominal wall is a typical clinical feature of gnathostomiasis, which can be diagnosed with the aid of serological tests available at specialist laboratories.

Additional differential diagnoses to consider are sparganosis, paragonimiasis and fascioliasis, which are caused by migration of larval stages of animal tapeworms or flukes, respectively. Usually, cutaneous sparganosis presents as a slowly moving solitary swelling without signs of acute inflammation such as pain and redness. Peripheral eosinophilia is less common than in skin lesions caused by other

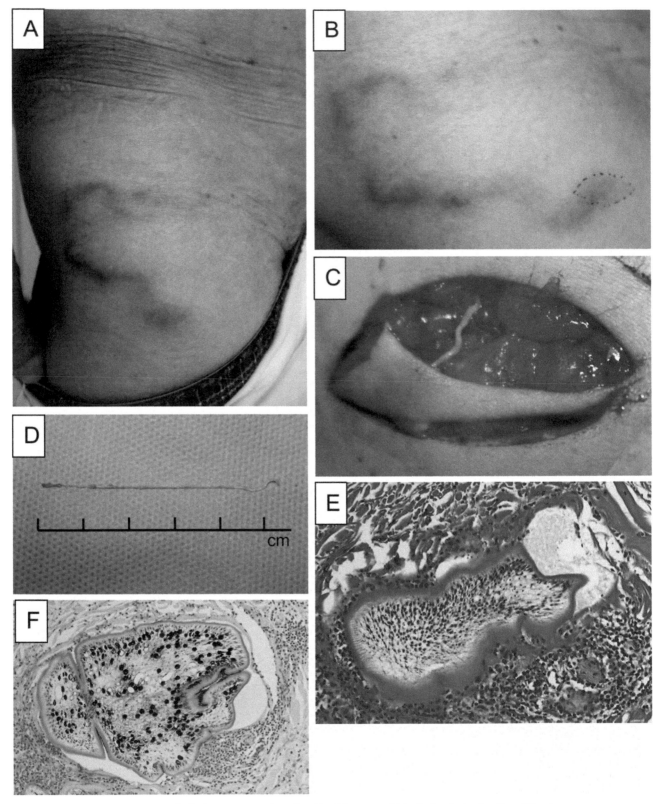

• **Fig. 97.1** A and B: Erythematous track on the skin of the upper thigh; C: Surgical extirpation of the plerocercoid larva ("sparganum"); D: The extirpated plerocercoid larva; E: Histopathological examination with H&E staining; F: Kossa's staining showing calcareous corpuscles, rounded masses of 7- to 35-micron diameter composed of concentric layers of calcium carbonate, characteristic of tapeworm tissues.

helminth species. It is of practical importance to distinguish between gnathostomiasis and sparganosis, because surgical treatment is generally useful in sparganosis but not quite successful in gnathostomiasis.

Answer to Question 2

What Additional Information Should You Obtain from the Patient?

When seeing a patient with a serpiginous erythema, it is important to obtain a thorough travel history and find out about food consumption habits (especially of fresh, uncooked, or undercooked food), and find out if the patient has drunk any untreated water in rural areas.

The Case Continued...

The skin lesion was suspected to be caused by a helminth infection, and serum was therefore sent to the reference laboratory for serological testing.

The patient had never been overseas and had no history of eating raw meat of frogs, freshwater fish, snakes, chicken or other birds, or mammals. He denied drinking untreated natural water.

Nevertheless, serology for *Spirometra erinaceieuropaei* came back positive, and sparganosis was suspected. The patient received surgical resection under local anaesthesia as shown in Fig 97.1B and 1C. A white ribbon-like worm, about 5 cm long and 1 mm wide, was removed from the subcutaneous connective tissue (Fig. 97.1D), confirming the diagnosis. Histopathological examination revealed numerous calcareous corpuscles by Kossa's stain (Fig. 97.1E and 97F). After surgery, the patient received praziquantel 3600 mg once daily for 3 days to clear possible residual infection.

SUMMARY BOX

Sparganosis

Sparganosis is a major food-borne zoonosis in Asia, especially in China, Korea, Japan and Thailand. In addition, cases have been reported from the USA, South America and several African countries. Recently, sporadic indigenous cases have been reported from Europe.

Sparganosis is caused by the migration of larvae ("spargana") of the genus *Spirometra*, which are zoonotic tapeworms.

In Asia, *S. erinaceieuropaei* is the causative species, whereas in the USA, *S. mansonoides* is the main pathogen. Recently, *S. decipiens* was added as a new species in Korea. Molecular identification is required for the precise species identification of the causative pathogen.

The definitive hosts of *Spirometra* species are wild and domesticated carnivores; the hermaphroditic spirometra adults live in the small intestine of the host animals. When ova are shed into water, the life cycle may continue: cyclops (freshwater crustaceans) act as first intermediate hosts, and fish, reptiles and amphibians act as second intermediate hosts.

Humans get infected mainly by eating raw or undercooked frogs or snakes. Undercooked free-range or backyard chicken meat and meat from some wild rodent species is also considered a source of infection. In addition, infection can occur by drinking or accidentally ingesting untreated water in rural areas containing infested copepods. Sparganosis can also be acquired when raw flesh of infested snakes and frogs is directly applied on the human body, e.g. on wounds or onto sore eyes, as poultice during traditional healing practices. In such cases, larvae can directly penetrate the human skin or mucous membranes.

After being ingested, the spargana penetrate the human intestinal wall and migrate into the subcutis (as seen in our case) and potentially any other tissues (e.g. eye, brain or spinal cord) and body cavity.

Generally, sparganosis is recognized as slowly moving erythema of the deep subcutis to form subcutaneous nodules or tumour-like lesions. A serpiginous erythema as seen in this case is rather uncommon. Larvae may also invade the eye and cause a wide variety of symptoms; ocular sparganosis may even lead to blindness. When in the CNS, spargana can cause symptoms like any space occupying lesion such as seizures and palsies.

Surgical removal is the most effective treatment for sparganosis. If untreated, the larvae can live for up to 20 years. Care should be taken to remove the entire parasite, because a remaining scolex will allow the larva to regrow and lead to a relapse. Repeat serological tests showing a decline in titres can help confirm cure. If the sparganum is surgically inaccessible, high doses of praziquantel are recommended (e.g. 40–60 mg/kg per day in three divided dose for 2 days).

Further Reading

1. Baily G, García H. H. Other cestode infections: Intestinal Cestodes, Cysticercosis, other larval cestode infections. In: Farrar J, editor. Manson's Tropical diseases, 23rd ed, Lndon, Elsevier; 2013 (chapter 57).
2. Liu Q, Li MW, Wang ZD, et al. Human sparganosis, a neglected food borne zoonosis. Lancet Infect Dis 2015;15(10):1226–35. https://doi.org/10.1016/S1473-3099(15)00133-4.
3. Kim JG, Ahn CS, Sohn WM, et al. Human sparganosis in Korea. J Korean Med Sci 2018;33(44):e273. https://doi.org/10.3346/jkms.2018.33.e273.
4. Czyżewska J, Namiot A, Koziołkiewicz K, et al. The first case of human sparganosis in Poland and a review of the cases in Europe. Parasitol Int 2019;70:89–91. https://doi.org/10.1016/j.parint.2019.02.005.

98

A 17-Year-Old Boy from South India With a Fever and a Reduced Level of Consciousness

ALICE MATHURAM

Clinical Presentation

History

A 17-year-old boy from South India presents to a large local tertiary care hospital with a high-grade fever, vomiting and headache of 3 days' duration. His relatives also noted irritability and decreased verbalization for 1 day. The day before the onset of illness the boy had been on a picnic to a nearby hill resort along with a group of friends, where he had a swim.

Clinical Findings

In the emergency department, he is febrile with a temperature of 38.8°C (101.8°F). He is tachycardic and tachypnoeic. His Glasgow Coma Scale (GCS) on admission is 10/15. He has marked neck stiffness, bilateral brisk reflexes and positive extensor plantar response. However, there are no focal deficits or cranial nerve abnormalities.

His sensorium drops further within an hour and he is intubated to protect his airways.

Laboratory Results

CSF analysis is done after administering mannitol. CSF is cloudy, cell counts are 24800 cells/mm³ with 97% neutrophils. CSF protein is very high at 931 mg/dL (reference: 15–45 mg/dL), and glucose is very low at 2 mg/dL (reference: approx. 45–60 mg/dL). CSF Gram stain does not reveal any bacteria. The wet mount preparation for free-living amoebae is negative.

Imaging

The CT scan of his brain is shown in Fig. 98.1.

Questions

1. What aetiological agents should be considered in this patient as a likely cause of acute meningitis?
2. What additional methods can be employed to identify the pathogen given that the wet mount preparation is negative?

Discussion

A 17-year old Indian boy presents with an acute meningoencephalitis. There is a history of recent swimming in a fresh water pool in the middle of summer in South India.

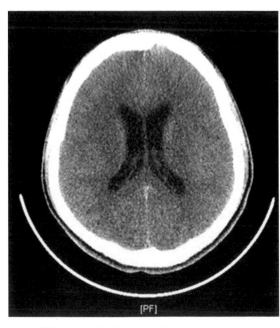

• **Fig. 98.1** CT scan of the brain showing cerebral oedema and mild prominence of the lateral ventricle.

He has features of pyogenic meningitis on CSF examination with neutrophil-predominant leukocytosis but Gram stain is negative.

Answer to Question 1

What Aetiological Agents Should Be Considered in This Patient as a Likely Cause of Acute Meningitis?

Streptococcus pneumoniae, Neisseria meningitidis and *Hemophilus influenza* are the most common pathogens to cause acute bacterial meningitis. Listeria meningitis is rare in immunocompetent adolescents.

Given his exposure to fresh water, free-living amoebae that cause acute meningoencephalitis also have to be included in the differential diagnosis.

Answer to Question 2

What Additional Methods Can Be Employed to Identify the Pathogen Given That the Wet Mount Preparation Is Negative?

Additional methods include CSF bacterial cultures and PCR for pneumococci and meningococci.

To identify *Naegleria fowleri,* which causes primary amoebic encephalitis, Gram stain is not useful and CSF should be stained with Giemsa or Wright's stain. PCR assays for *N. fowleri* have also been developed.

Culture of CSF in non-nutrient agar or agar with low levels of nutrient in which non-mucoid strains of *Klebsiella, E. coli* or *Enterobacter* have been grown as a source of food for the amoebae has been used to cultivate free-living amoebae.

The Case Continued...

Treatment was initiated with ceftriaxone 2 g IV every 12 hours and dexamethasone 10 mg every 6 hours; in addition, IV amphotericin B 1.5 mg/kg per day and rifampicin 600 mg once a day were given to cover for possible primary amoebic meningoencephalitis. The boy was admitted to the medical ICU and was initiated on cerebral protective measures with mannitol and 3% sodium chloride. His hemodynamics rapidly deteriorated requiring multiple inotropes. Arterial blood gas analysis showed severe metabolic acidosis. He went into acute kidney injury, his GCS dropped to 3/15, and he developed anisocoria. CT done at this point revealed gross cerebral oedema with sulcal effacement, hydrocephalus and a foramen magnum herniation. He subsequently developed diabetes insipidus. He had a severe refractory hyperkalemia of 7.9 mmol/L with several runs of ventricular tachycardia. Hemodialysis could not be done because of hemodynamic instability. He succumbed to his illness on the third day of admission.

A day after his death, CSF amoebic cultures revealed motile trophozoites and the flagellate forms of the parasite confirming the diagnosis of primary amoebic meningoencephalitis caused by *N. fowleri* (Fig. 98.2).

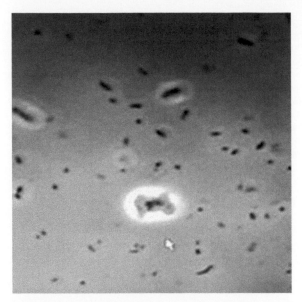

• **Fig. 98.2** The trophozoite form of the organism isolated from CSF.

SUMMARY BOX

Primary Amoebic Meningoencephalitis (PAM)

PAM is caused by the pathogenic free-living amoeba *N. fowleri* ("Brain-eating amoeba"). It is found in warm fresh water bodies (lakes, rivers, hot springs), inadequately chlorinated swimming pools and in contaminated tap water. *N. fowleri* is a thermophilic parasite which can grow in temperatures up to 45°C. Infection occurs by direct invasion of the central nervous system through the cribriform plate and olfactory neuroepithelium after aspiration or inhalation of contaminated water. This results in an acute and fulminant meningoencephalitis with very high lethality (about 95%). The usual cause of death is cerebral herniation secondary to raised intracranial pressure. Mainly children and young adults are affected.

N. fowleri is the only species in the *Naegleria* genus that causes human infection. It occurs worldwide and exists in 3 forms: trophozoite, flagellate and cystic forms. The trophozoite form is the invasive form of *N. fowleri*. It is also the reproductive stage of the parasite and replicates by binary fission. *N. fowleri* trophozoites move by extending a blunt pseudopodium and destroy tissue they come into contact with. They feed on Gram-negative bacteria. On entry into the CSF, the trophozoites convert themselves into the flagellated form, which neither feeds nor divides. The trophozoite converts into a cyst once food is lacking or the environment dries up.

Exposure to *N. fowleri* is common, as evidenced by serology; however, only a few develop infection (there are an estimated 2.6 cases per million exposures). The clinical presentation of PAM is very similar to acute bacterial meningitis. A high index of clinical suspicion and a history of exposure to possible sources of infection is required to make the diagnosis.

CSF wet mount (positive in 14%–16% only) may demonstrate actively motile trophozoites and will aid an early diagnosis. *N. fowleri* can be cultivated in non-nutrient agar with the presence of Gram-negative bacilli (a source of food to the parasite). *Naegleria* species are distinguished from other species of free-living amoebae by enflagellation: amoebae grown on a culture plate or taken directly from a clinical specimen are suspended in 1 ml of distilled water, and within an hour flagellae develop in a considerable proportion of trophozoites. This form has 2 anterior flagellae, is rapidly motile and may spontaneously revert to the trophozoite stage.

PAM is almost invariably fatal and treatment recommendations are based on case reports of the few documented survivors because clinical trials are lacking. The treatment of choice seems to be amphotericin B. Other drugs such as rifampicin, fluconazole, voriconazole and azithromycin have in vitro activity against *N. fowleri* and may be used in combination with amphotericin B for synergy. There is documentation of survivors among those treated with miltefosine, a drug used to treat leishmaniasis.

Further Reading

1. Visvesvara GS. Pathogenic and opportunistic Free-living amoebae: agents of human and animal disease. In: Farrar J, editor. Manson's Tropical Diseases. 23rd ed. London: Elsevier; 2013 [chapter 50].

2. Gautam PL, Sharma S, Puri S, Kumar R, Midha V, Bansal R. A rare case of survival from primary amebic meningoencephalitis. Indian J Crit Care Med 2012;16(1):34–6.

3. Wellings FM. Amoebic meningoencephalitis. J Fla Med Assoc 1977;64(5):327–8.

4. Visvesvara GS, Moura H, Schuster FL. Pathogenic and opportunistic free-living amoebae: Acanthamoeba spp., Balamuthia mandrillaris, Naegleria fowleri, and Sappinia diploidea. FEMS Immunol Med Microbiol 2007;50:1–26.

5. Cope JR, Conrad DA, Cohen N, et al. Use of the novel therapeutic agent miltefosine for the treatment of primary amebic meningoencephalitis: report of 1 fatal and 1 surviving case. Clin Infect Dis 2016;62(6):774–6.

99

A 43-Year-Old Male Traveller Returning from the Australian Outback with Fever, Joint Pains and a Rash

ANDREAS NEUMAYR

Clinical Presentation

History

A 43-year-old Swiss traveller presents to clinic 6 days after returning from a 3-week trekking tour through the outback in Queensland, Australia. Directly after his arrival back home, he developed acute fever of 38°C (100.4°F) accompanied by headache, malaise, mild dry cough, myalgias, as well as progressive symmetrical polyarthralgias of the small peripheral joints (especially affecting the hands and feet).

Clinical Findings

On physical examination the patient shows symmetrical bilateral cervical and axillary lymphadenopathy and a maculopapular rash (trunk > extremities; see Fig. 99.1). The painful peripheral small joints were neither swollen nor warm nor did they show any signs of inflammation. A

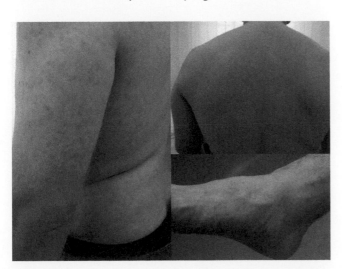

• **Fig. 99.1** Disseminated Maculopapular Rash in a Traveller Returning from Australia With Fever and Symmetrical Joint Pains

closer assessment revealed symmetrical dermal hypersensitivity of both legs, and on palpation symmetrical painful tendons/ligaments of the soles and ankles, suggestive of enthesitis.

Laboratory Results

His differential blood count was normal apart from mild lymphocytosis (71%, range 20%–40%). CRP was not elevated. ALT and GGT were mildly raised. AST (SGOT) and creatinine were normal.

Questions

1. What are your differential diagnoses?
2. What diagnostic test would you perform?

Discussion

After a 3-week trekking tour through the outback of Australia, a 43-year-old Swiss traveller presents with an acute febrile illness and severe musculoskeletal complaints including symmetrical polyarthralgias primarily affecting the small peripheral joints and signs of enthesitis, generalized lymphadenopathy, and a disseminated maculopapular skin rash.

Answer to Question 1
What Are Your Differential Diagnoses?

The acute clinical presentation of "fever and rash" is highly suggestive of a viral infection and the pronounced musculoskeletal symptoms strongly point towards an alphavirus infection. Three alphaviruses are endemic in Australia: Ross River, Barmah Forest and Sindbis (Table 99.1). Besides the endemic alphaviral infections, chikungunya has to be considered. It happens to occur in outbreaks, therefore the current epidemiological situation in the place travelled to is of key importance.

TABLE 99.1 Characteristics of Human Pathogenic Alphaviruses Endemic in Australia

Virus	Epidemiology and endemic regions	Occurrence and number of reported cases	Frequency of main symptoms (%)
Ross River	Australia, Papua New Guinea, West Papua	~5000 cases per year in Australia; in 1979–1980 an epidemic with >60000 cases hit some pacific islands (New Caledonia, Fiji, Samoa, Cook Islands)	Fever: 20–60 Rash: 40–60 Myalgia: 40–80 Arthralgia/arthritis: 80–100
Barmah Forest	Australia	~2000 cases/year	Fever: 50 Rash: 40–60 Myalgia: 50–80 Arthralgia or arthritis: 70–95
Sindbis virus group	Eurasia, Africa, Australia, Oceania; primarily reported from West Russia ("Karelian fever"), Finland ("Pogosta disease"), and Sweden ("Ockelbo disease")	Geographically most widely distributed alphavirus (lack of data on human cases) Karelian fever: rare (no data) Pogosta disease: ~140 cases (range 1–1282)/year Ockelbo disease: ~30 cases/year	Fever: 15–40 Rash: 90 Myalgia: 50 Arthralgia/arthritis: 95

In addition, the patient's history of outdoor activities includes other endemic arboviral as well as rickettsial diseases in the differential diagnosis of "fever and rash".

There have been endemic cases of dengue fever in the past in Queensland, however rarely. Additionally, in Australia, Kunjin virus, a strain of West Nile virus, and Murray Valley virus are endemic. Although both viruses primarily cause encephalitis, non-encephalitic courses may occur and present as a flu-like acute febrile illness with headache, arthralgia, myalgia, fatigue and rash. Five rickettsial diseases are reported from Australia: Queensland Tick Typhus *(Rickettsia australis)*, Flinders Island Spotted Fever *(R. honei)*, Australian Spotted Fever *(R. honei marmionii)*, Murine Typhus *(R. typhi, R. felis)* and, in the tropical northern part of Australia, Scrub Typhus *(Orientia tsutsugamushi)*.

Answer to Question 2
What Diagnostic Test Would You Perform?

The pronounced musculoskeletal symptoms strongly suggested an alphavirus infection as the most likely differential diagnosis, and a Ross River virus infection was suspected based on the epidemiological likelihood. During the first few days of the acute infection, detection of viral RNA in the blood by PCR can confirm the diagnosis. After the virus is cleared from blood towards the end of the acute phase, serological detection of specific IgM and IgG antibodies is the diagnostic method of choice.

The Case Continued…

Given that PCR testing was not readily available and the patient was already symptomatic for 6 days, serological testing was performed, which confirmed the suspected diagnosis of a Ross River infection (Table 99.2). Serologies for Rickettsial infections were negative.

Under symptomatic treatment with ibuprofen, the polyarthralgias subsided slowly over the subsequent weeks before finally disappearing after about 6 weeks.

TABLE 99.2 Results of the Serological Testing for Arboviral Infections Performed in Our Case

Virus	Serology Result		Interpretation
	IgM-IFA*	IgG-IFA*	
Ross River	1:1640	1:160	positive
Barmah Forest	<20	<20	negative
Sindbis	<20	<20	negative
West Nile	<20	<20	negative
Murray Valley	<20	<20	negative

*IFA: indirect immunofluorescence assay

SUMMARY BOX

Ross River Fever

Ross River virus is an arbovirus maintained in nature by a transmission cycle between susceptible vertebrate host reservoirs, such as large marsupial mammals, and various mosquito species. The virus was first isolated from mosquitos in 1963 near the Ross River in northern Queensland and has repeatedly caused large outbreaks in the region, giving rise to the term *epidemic polyarthritis*. Today, Ross River virus disease is the most common mosquito-borne disease in Australia.

Ross River infections typically present as acute febrile illness accompanied by fatigue, myalgia, a maculopapular rash (lasting 5–10 days) and debilitating symmetrical polyarthritis primarily affecting peripheral joints including the wrists, fingers, ankles and knees. Similar to other alphaviral infections, the polyarthralgias characteristically persist for several weeks to months beyond the acute phase of the infection. This phenomenon is suspected to arise from the inflammatory immune response stimulated by the prolonged virus persistence in joint tissues. Treatment is exclusively supportive with non-steroidal drugs; physiotherapy has also been shown to be beneficial in some cases. Symptoms mostly subside slowly over several weeks to months. However, some patients remain symptomatic for more than a year. Long-term sequelae or permanent damage of the affected joints are not reported.

Further Reading

1. Blumberg L, Enria D, Bausch DG. Viral haemorrhagic fevers. In: Farrar J, editor. Manson's Tropical Diseases. 23rd ed. London: Elsevier; 2014 [chapter 16].
2. Suhrbier A, Jaffar-Bandjee MC, Gasque P. Arthritogenic alphaviruses-an overview. Nat Rev Rheumatol 2012;8(7):420–9.
3. Liu X, Tharmarajah K, Taylor A. Ross River virus disease clinical presentation, pathogenesis and current therapeutic strategies. Microbes Infect 2017;19(11):496–504.

100

A 25-Year-Old Man from Ethiopia With a Nodular Rash

SABA M. LAMBERT AND STEPHEN L. WALKER

Clinical Presentation

History

A 25-year-old man who lives in Addis Ababa, Ethiopia attends your clinic complaining of a progressive skin eruption of the body and limbs for 1 year. The rash is not itchy or painful. He has had no previous skin problems and no contact with a similarly affected person. Additionally, his friends have noted a change in his appearance over the preceding 12 months.

Clinical Findings

There is a papular and nodular eruption on the extensor aspects of the forearms, arms, thighs and trunk (Fig. 100.1). Furthermore, there is a diffuse infiltration of the skin of the face and nodules on the pinnae (Fig. 100.2), with madarosis (loss of eyebrows and eyelashes). There is no loss of sensation within the skin lesions and no sensory or motor loss in the hands or feet.

Questions

1. What other clinical sign would you attempt to elicit?
2. Which investigations would you use to confirm the diagnosis?

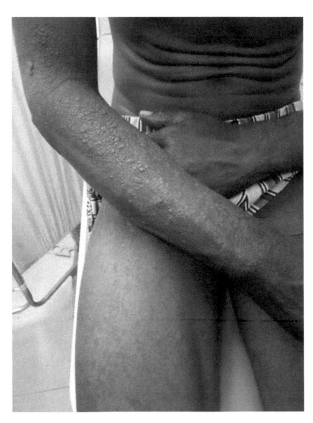

• **Fig. 100.1** Papular and nodular eruption on the extensor aspects of the forearms; thighs and trunk were also involved.

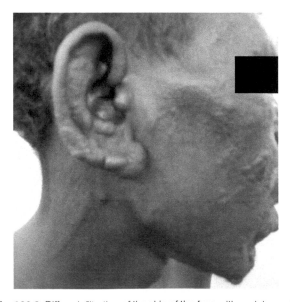

• **Fig. 100.2** Diffuse infiltration of the skin of the face with nodules on the pinnae. Visibly thickened greater auricular nerve.

Discussion

A 25-year old man from Ethiopia presents with nodular and papular skin changes and madarosis, which have evolved over the previous year. There is no loss of sensation associated with the skin lesions and no sign of neuropathy.

Answer to Question 1

What Other Clinical Sign Would You Attempt to Elicit?

In a leprosy-endemic country or in a migrant from a leprosy-endemic country, it is important to consider the diagnosis of leprosy in any individual with a nodular and/or infiltrative process affecting the skin.

The cardinal signs of leprosy are hypopigmented skin lesions, which have reduced sensation and thickened peripheral or cutaneous nerves. It is therefore important to assess the patient's peripheral nerves to determine whether they are thickened. Note the thickened greater auricular nerve in Fig. 100.2.

Answer to Question 2

Which Investigations Would You Use to Confirm the Diagnosis?

Slit-skin smears taken from the earlobes, supra-orbital ridges and skin lesions stained with Wade-Fite stain are likely to demonstrate acid- and alcohol-fast bacilli in this patient. A skin biopsy would show an infiltrate of foamy macrophages with haematoxylin and eosin (H&E) stain and acid-fast bacilli with Wade-Fite stain. An HIV test should be performed in any individual with an unexplained skin complaints.

The Case Continued...

His HIV serology was negative. The patient had thickened peripheral nerves and a nodular eruption in keeping with lepromatous leprosy. He was started on World Health Organization multi-bacillary multi-drug therapy, which he took for 12 months with resolution of the skin nodules and infiltration. Monthly assessment of his nerve function did not reveal any deficit.

Three months after completing multi-drug therapy he developed fever, painful erythematous subcutaneous nodules (Fig. 100.3) on the limbs and trunk and pain in both testes.

He was diagnosed with erythema nodosum leprosum and commenced on prednisolone 40 mg daily which controlled the fever and discomfort and resulted in resolution of the skin lesions. However, on reduction of the prednisolone dose the symptoms recurred. Prednisolone was again increased and he required oral prednisolone for 3 years and developed hypertension and osteoporosis.

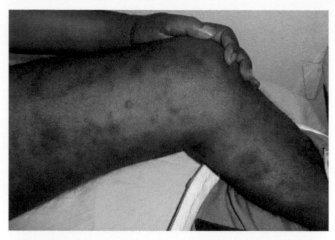

• **Fig. 100.3** The same patient 3 months after completing multi-drug therapy with painful erythematous subcutaneous nodules on the limbs.

SUMMARY BOX

Leprosy Reactions

Leprosy is complicated by immune-mediated inflammatory episodes called "reactions". Reactions are a significant risk factor for the development of nerve-function impairment, which leads to disability. Reactions may occur before, during or after successful completion of multi-drug therapy. Reactions are more common in patients with multi-bacillary leprosy and patients who have high bacterial loads.

There are two types of leprosy reactions, both of which require immunomodulatory therapy: Type 1 reactions predominantly occur in the borderline forms of leprosy and typically affect pre-existing skin lesions and nerves. They are often associated with oedema of the hands, feet and face. They require prolonged courses of oral corticosteroids which are usually tapered over 20 to 24 weeks. Type 2 reactions or erythema nodosum leprosum (ENL) are painful complications of borderline lepromatous leprosy and lepromatous leprosy, particularly in individuals with a bacterial index greater than 4 (>10 bacilli in every field of microscopy). ENL is characterised by fever, tender nodular skin lesions and may be accompanied by arthritis, neuritis, dactylitis, peripheral oedema and orchitis in men. Thalidomide is usually effective but is not available in many leprosy-endemic countries because of teratogenicity. ENL patients are therefore often treated with prolonged courses of high-dose oral corticosteroids. Adverse effects are common with both thalidomide and oral corticosteroids and the latter is associated with fatalities in patients with ENL. Other drugs such as clofazimine, azathioprine, ciclosporin, methotrexate, apremilast and anti-tumour necrosis factor blockers have been used in chronic ENL.

Further Reading

1. Walker SL, Withington SJ, Lockwood DNG. Leprosy. In: Farrar J, editor. Manson's Tropical Diseases. 23rd ed. London: Elsevier; 2013 [chapter 41].
2. International Textbook of Leprosy. 30 October 2019. Available from: https://internationaltextbookofleprosy.org/.

3. Walker SL, Lebas E, Doni SN, et al. The mortality associated with erythema nodosum leprosum in Ethiopia: a retrospective hospital-based study. PLoS Negl Trop Dis 2014;8(3):e2690.

4. Lambert SM, Nigusse SD, Alembo DT, et al. Comparison of Efficacy and Safety of Ciclosporin to Prednisolone in the Treatment of Erythema Nodosum Leprosum: Two Randomised, Double Blind, Controlled Pilot Studies in Ethiopia. PLoS Negl Trop Dis 2016; 10(2):e0004149.

5. Wagenaar I, Post E, Brandsma W, et al. Effectiveness of 32 versus 20 weeks of prednisolone in leprosy patients with recent nerve function impairment: a randomized controlled trial. PLoS Negl Trop Dis 2017;11(10):e0005952.

101

A 46-Year-Old Male Traveller with Chronic Cough After a Trip to South America

ESTHER KUENZLI AND ANDREAS NEUMAYR

Clinical Presentation

History

A 46-year-old male Swiss traveller spent a 2-week holiday in the border region of Argentine and Brazil. Two weeks after his return, he developed flu-like symptoms and exertional dyspnoea. Ten days after the onset of symptoms, the patient presented at his general practitioner with fever and a pronounced frontal headache. Physical examination did not reveal any abnormalities. The differential blood count was unremarkable and C-reactive protein was only mildly elevated. After ruling out sinusitis by x-ray and dengue fever by serology, the provisional diagnosis of an unspecified viral infection was made.

Over the following 10 days, the patient developed a nonproductive dry cough. Chest x-ray revealed an infiltrative process in the right upper lung field (Fig. 101.1). A CT scan of the chest showed a 2 × 4 cm consolidation in the right upper lobe with ipsilateral mediastinal and hilar lymphadenopathy, a discrete right-sided pleural effusion and multiple pulmonary micronodules in both lungs (Fig. 101.2) (100.0°F).

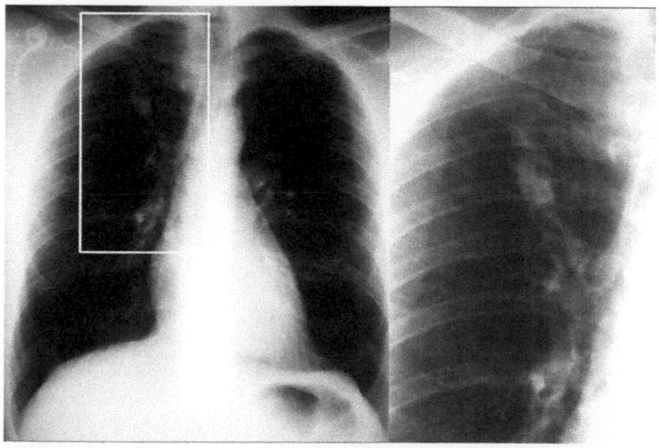

Clinical Findings

Except for a temperature of 37.8°C (100.0°F), the clinical examination was unremarkable.

Laboratory Results

His differential blood count was again normal. Liver function tests (AST, ALT, GGT, AP) and creatinine were normal. CRP was slightly elevated (10 mg/L, normal <5mg/L), ESR was 26 mm/h.

• **Fig. 101.1** Chest x-ray showing an infiltrative process in the right upper lung field.

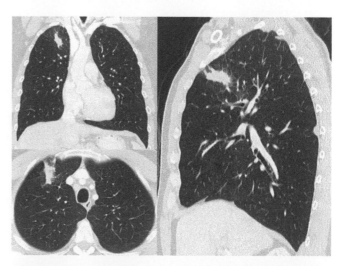

• **Fig. 101.2** CT scan of the chest showing consolidation in the right upper field, mediastinal and hilar lymphadenopathy, a discrete right-sided pleural effusion and multiple pulmonary micronodules in both lungs.

283

Questions

1. What is your suspected diagnosis and what additional tests would you carry out next?
2. What other differential diagnoses would you suspect?

Discussion

A 46-year-old Swiss traveller develops flu-like symptoms with fever, headache, progressive exertional dyspnea and a dry cough 2 weeks after returning from a 2-week holiday in the border region of Argentine and Brazil. Three weeks after the onset of symptoms, the man returns to his general practitioner with persisting complaints. Apart from a low-grade fever, physical examination is unremarkable. Laboratory results are normal, besides slightly elevated inflammatory markers. Radiological imaging reveals a consolidation in the right upper lobe with right mediastinal and hilar lymphadenopathy, a discrete right-sided pleural effusion and multiple pulmonary micronodules in both lungs (suggestive of a granulomatous process).

Answer to Question 1

What Would Be Your Primary Diagnosis and What Additional Tests Would You Carry Out Next?

The history of chronic pulmonary symptoms and the imaging results were interpreted as highly suggestive of pulmonary tuberculosis and prompted the further diagnostic steps:

An interferon-gamma release assay (IGRA) turned out negative. Bronchoscopy revealed normal endobronchial findings, the cytological investigations of the bronchoalveolar lavage as well as the brush biopsy were unremarkable, and the *Mycobacterium tuberculosis* complex PCR performed on the lavage fluid was negative.

Answer to Question 2

What Other Differential Diagnoses Would You Suspect?

Community-acquired pneumonia should be considered, involving both "typical" (e.g. *S. pneumoniae*) and "atypical" pathogens (*Mycoplasma* species, *Chlamydia* species, *Legionella* species). Q-fever (*Coxiella burnetii*) should also be considered.

Given the history of travel to South America, endemic mycoses (in particular paracoccidioidomycosis and histoplasmosis) should also be on the list of differentials. Pulmonary blastomycosis is limited to North America; rarely, cases are reported from Africa and India. Coccidioidomycosis is also more common in North America but may occur in South America in small geographical pockets.

The Case Continued...

After the negative evaluation for pulmonary tuberculosis, community-acquired pneumonia was suspected. Empirical clarithromycin treatment covering for atypical pathogens was

TABLE 101.1 **Overview of Clinical Manifestations of Pulmonary Histoplasmosis**

Clinical manifestation	Risk Factor	Clinical Time-Course	Chest Imaging	Indication for Treatment	Treatment
Acute Pulmonary Histoplasmosis	High inoculum exposure	1–2 weeks	Diffuse infiltrates	Only in case of moderate or severe disease or in immunosuppressed patients	(Severe: Amphotericin followed by Itraconazole [12 weeks])
Sub-acute Pulmonary Histoplasmosis	Low inoculum exposure	Weeks to months	Focal infiltrates	If symptoms last >1 month or in immunosuppressed patients	Itraconazole [6–12 weeks]
Chronic Pulmonary Histoplasmosis	Underlying lung disease, smoking	Months to years	Cavities, fibrosis	Always	Itraconazole [~1–2 years]
Progressive Disseminated Histoplasmosis	Immunosuppression	1–2 weeks	Diffuse reticulo-nodular infiltrates	Always	Amphotericin B followed by Itraconazole [1 year] followed by secondary prophylaxis until immune recovery

Adapted from Azar and Hage (2017)[2].

started. When after 1 week neither the symptoms nor the follow-up x-ray showed any improvement and all serological investigations for atypical bacterial pathogens (*Chlamydia pneumonia, Chlamydia psittaci, Mycoplasma pneumonia, Legionella pneumophilia, C. burnetii*) came back negative, the empirical treatment was changed to levofloxacin. Despite levofloxacin treatment over the next 3 weeks, the dry cough and the febrile temperatures persisted. The patient complained about drenching night sweats and the follow-up CT scan did not show any improvement. At this point, the patient was referred to a tropical medicine clinic to evaluate the possibility of a travel-related infection.

After reviewing the patient's travel history (revealing, on inquiry, a visit to an aviary), the symptoms and the radiological findings, the differential diagnosis of an endemic mycosis, especially histoplasmosis, was considered. This was finally confirmed by positive *Histoplasma capsulatum* serology (immunodiffusion test, complement fixation test, and western blot). Additional serological tests for *Paracoccidioides brasiliensis, Coccidioides immitis, Blastomyces dermatitidis,* and *Cryptococcus neoformans* were negative. As a result of the prolonged symptoms without improvement for more than 7 weeks, it was decided to initiate antifungal therapy with oral itraconazole. At follow-up 2 months later, the patient's symptoms had markedly improved and the CT scan showed 90% reduction of the pulmonary lesions.

SUMMARY BOX

Histoplasmosis

H. capsulatum, the aetiological agent of histoplasmosis, is an environmental dimorphic fungus associated with bird and bat guano. Although human *H. capsulatum* infections have been reported from many regions around the world, most cases are reported from endemic foci in North, Central and South America.

Histoplasmosis can present in distinct clinical syndromes that vary by clinical course, severity, disease extent, radiographic findings and indication for treatment. Symptomatic acute pulmonary histoplasmosis occurs in approximately 10% of exposed persons after inhalation of fungal spores. Factors that increase the likelihood for symptomatic disease include being at the extremes of age, immunosuppression, and exposure to a large inoculum. The most common symptoms reported include cough, dyspnoea, malaise, fever and chills. Symptoms are self-limiting, usually lasting less than 2 weeks and are often misdiagnosed as bacterial pneumonia or viral respiratory illness. Exposure to smaller inocula of *H. capsulatum* may lead to the development of subacute pulmonary histoplasmosis, a slowly progressive infection over several weeks to months. Like in our case, the subacute form is characterized by milder but more persistent respiratory and constitutional symptoms. On chest imaging, focal opacities predominate and mediastinal and hilar adenopathy are common findings. The diagnosis can be established by serology, detection of antigen (serum, urine, bronchoalveolar lavage), or cytopathology and culture (sputum, bronchoalveolar lavage). Sporadic cases or clusters of pulmonary histoplasmosis in immunocompetent travellers are mostly linked to exploration of caves and visiting endemic regions in the Americas.

Further Reading

1. Blumberg L, Enria D, Bausch DG. Viral haemorrhagic fevers. In: Farrar J, editor. Manson's Tropical Diseases. 23rd ed. London: Elsevier; 2014 [chapter 16].
2. Azar MM, Hage CA. Clinical perspectives in the diagnosis and management of Histoplasmosis. Clin Chest Med 2017;38(3): 403–15.
3. Staffolani S, Buonfrate D, Angheben A, et al. Acute histoplasmosis in immunocompetent travelers: a systematic review of literature. BMC Infect Dis 2018;18(1):673.
4. Denning DW, Chakrabarti A. Pulmonary and sinus fungal diseases in non-immunocompromised patients. Lancet Infect Dis 2017; 17:e357–66.

102

A 16-Year-Old Male Refugee from Somalia With High Fever and Slurred Speech

JOHANNES JOCHUM

Clinical Presentation

History

A 16-year-old male refugee from Somalia presents to the emergency department of a hospital in Germany with high fever, chills, headache and generalised body pain for 1 day.

Eight months prior, he left his hometown in northern Somalia and migrated to Libya, where he lived for about 6 months. He often stayed in overcrowded locations and had to sleep on the ground. Seventeen days before the onset of symptoms, he had crossed the Mediterranean Sea from Libya to Italy by rubber boat together with 150 other migrants. From there, he reached Germany by car.

He noticed pruritus while in Italy, which he believed to be some kind of food allergy. Since leaving Somalia he has lost a lot of weight. He had always been healthy before. In particular, he does not recall any previous episodes of malaria.

Clinical Findings

The patient appears sick and dehydrated. His temperature is 39.5°C (103.1°F), his heart rate is 125 beats per minute. He is awake and fully oriented, but his speech appears slurred and he is slow to respond. He is slightly jaundiced and shows conjunctival injections. There is no rash and no skin lesions. The examination of the chest and of the abdomen is unremarkable.

Laboratory Results

His laboratory results are shown in Table 102.1.

Questions

1. What is the differential diagnosis?
2. Which investigations would you perform (in order of priority) and how do they affect treatment?

TABLE 102.1 Laboratory Results on Admission

Parameter	Patient	Reference
WBC (× 10⁹/L), (neutrophils: lymphocytes)	11.2 (90%:10%)	3.8–11.0
Haemoglobin (g/dL)	13.7	14.0–17.5
Thrombocytes (× 10⁹/L)	118	150–400
AST (IU/L)	24	10–50
ALT (IU/L)	24	10–50
Total bilirubin (mg/dL)	2.3	<1.0
Lactate dehydrogenase (IU/L)	300	87–241
C-reactive protein (mg/L)	298	<5
Malaria rapid diagnostic test	negative	negative

Discussion

A 16-year-old male Somalian refugee presents with fever and headache. Eighteen days before, he arrived in Italy from Libya. On examination, he is febrile, tachycardic and slightly jaundiced. He is fully oriented, but his speech is slurred. Laboratory results show moderate neutrophil leukocytosis, thrombocytopenia and markedly elevated C-reactive protein.

Answer to Question 1
What Is the Differential Diagnosis?

The leading differential diagnosis is malaria, even if the rapid diagnostic test is negative and the neutrophil leukocytosis is not typical. Because the patient originates from the Horn of Africa, both falciparum and non-falciparum malaria have to be considered. *Plasmodium vivax* malaria is particularly commonly seen among refugees from the region arriving in Europe. Some of them report antimalarial treatment during their journey, but most probably they have only received drugs for the acute episode and no "radical cure" to get rid of the hypnozoites. Both drugs currently used for the latter purpose, primaquine and – more recently – tafenoquine, require Glucose-6-Phosphate Dehydrogenase deficiency to be ruled out, which is unlikely to have been done at health posts on their way.

Malaria rapid diagnostic tests have a lower sensitivity for non-falciparum species compared with *Plasmodium falciparum*.

Considering possible exposures during migration, leptospirosis, relapsing fever (caused by *Borrelia species*), Trench Fever *(Bartonella quintana)*, and rickettsial infections also match both clinical picture and laboratory abnormalities.

Of the rickettsial infections, spotted-fever group infections such as Mediterranean tick-bite fever (e.g. *Rickettsia conorii*) are possible. The characteristic eschar may be missing or remain undetected.

Given the precarious living conditions during his journey, louse-borne (epidemic) typhus *(Rickettsia prowazekii)* and flea-borne (endemic) typhus *(Rickettsia typhi)* also have to be considered.

Bacterial sepsis can also explain all findings, and bacterial meningitis should be excluded as a focus even in absence of nuchal rigidity.

Enteric fever, brucellosis and tuberculosis appear less likely because of the rapid onset of the illness. Viral diseases are unlikely because of the marked elevation of C-reactive protein shortly after the onset of symptoms. Viral haemorrhagic fevers are highly unlikely because the patient has not been in an endemic region during the past 3 weeks. In theory, human-to-human transmission for some VHF appears possible, but no index case was reported at that time.

Answer to Question 2

Which Investigations Would You Perform (In Order of Priority) and How Do They Affect Treatment?

The most important diagnostic test in this patient is microscopy of thick and thin blood films. It allows prompt diagnosis of both malaria and relapsing fever. If positive, specific pathogen-directed treatment is possible. Asymptomatic malaria parasitaemia can be misleading in semi-immune patients from highly endemic countries: parasitaemia may be mistaken for clinical malaria and the actual diagnosis may be missed.

Blood cultures should be taken even if malaria parasites have been found, because malaria may be associated with Gram-negative sepsis.

Should blood films turn out negative, lumbar puncture and imaging (ultrasonography and chest x-ray) should be performed and urinalysis should be done to investigate for pyelonephritis. *Leptospira* species, at this early stage of illness,

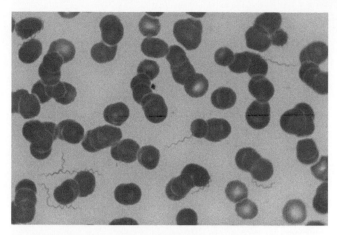

• **Fig. 102.1** Thin blood film showing extracellular loosely coiled spiral-shaped *Borrelia* species (Pappenheim stain, × 1000).

may be found in peripheral blood and CSF by molecular methods.

If focus and aetiology of the disease remain uncertain, empirical antimicrobial therapy should be started. Given the spectrum of differential diagnoses, the combination of a third-generation cephalosporin with doxycycline seems to be a reasonable choice.

The Case Continued...

In the emergency room, bacterial sepsis was suspected and the patient was started on antibiotic treatment with cefotaxime.

Blood microscopy revealed numerous extracellular loosely coiled spiral-shaped bacteria with a length of around 20 μm (Fig. 102.1). A diagnosis of relapsing fever was made. Antimicrobial therapy was continued unchanged, because the bacterium is usually susceptible to third-generation cephalosporins in vitro. However, fever and tachycardia persisted, and the platelet count further dropped to 32×10^9/L. On the third day, treatment was therefore switched to doxycycline 200 mg daily, leading to a full recovery of all clinical and laboratory abnormalities. There were no signs of Jarisch-Herxheimer reaction (see Summary Box). PCR analysis of a blood sample confirmed the diagnosis of louse-borne relapsing fever.

SUMMARY BOX

Louse-borne Relapsing Fever

Louse-borne relapsing fever is a neglected and almost forgotten infection caused by *Borrelia recurrentis*. Its vector is the human body louse, *Pediculus humanus humanus*. Through the spread of lice in congested conditions, large outbreaks can occur. Once a widespread disease of poverty, war and detention, the current endemicity is thought to be largely limited to the highlands of the Horn of Africa where in cold, wet weather, poor people with louse-infested clothes crowd together for warmth and shelter. However, in 2015 almost 100 East African asylum seekers fell sick with louse-borne relapsing fever (LBRF) shortly after arrival in Europe.

The usual incubation period is 2 to 15 days. Clinical symptoms are caused by the presence of borreliae in the bloodstream. Disease onset is typically sudden with high fever, rigors, headache, neck stiffness, conjunctival injection, dry cough and gastrointestinal symptoms. Coma, myocarditis and haemorrhages may occur. After 5 to 7 days of fever, borreliae are cleared from the bloodstream by the host immune system, leading to a brisk defervescence with profuse sweating, bradycardia, and arterial hypotension. In the absence of antibiotic therapy, bacteria change their surface antigens and re-appear within 3 weeks in the bloodstream, eliciting another episode of clinical illness (hence the name *relapsing fever*). Case fatality rate is 10% to 30% if untreated and 2% to 6% with adequate treatment.

During the episodes of fever, borreliae are readily detectable in the blood by microscopy. Treatment consists of tetracyclines, penicillin, or macrolides. Tetracyclines (Tetracyclin or Doxycyclin) are most effective and a single dose is sufficient for cure. Usually, therapy is given for a longer period because louse-borne relapsing fever is in the abscence of PCR-based diagnostic methods difficult to distinguish from tick-borne relapsing fever for which 10 days of treatment are required.

The most feared side effect of antimicrobial treatment is the development of the Jarisch-Herxheimer reaction (JHR), a cytokine-triggered hyperpyrexia with arterial hypotension secondary to rapid disintegration of spirochetes. Patients can progress into a state of shock, unresponsive to volume replacement and requiring vasopressor therapy. Risk of JHR in one study was higher with tetracycline treatment compared with beta lactam antibiotics; this however remains disputed. Deaths despite treatment are mainly attributable to this complication.

Lice have to be removed by changing or washing clothes and bed linen, additional pediculicide treatment is usually not necessary.

Further Reading

1. Warrell DA. Louse-borne relapsing fever (Borrelia recurrentis infection). Epidemiol Infect 2019 Jan;147:e106.
2. Osthoff M, Schibli A, Fadini D, et al. Louse-borne relapsing fever - report of four cases in Switzerland, June-December 2015. BMC Infect Dis 2016 17 May;16:210.
3. Hoch M, Wieser A, Löscher T, Margos T, Pürner F, et al. Louse-borne relapsing fever (Borrelia recurrentis) diagnoses in 15 refugees from northeast Africa: epidemiology and preventive control measures, Bavaria, Germany, July to October 2015.
4. Lucchini A, Lipani F, Costa C, Scarvaglieri M, Balbiano R. Louse-borne relapsing fever among East African refugees. EID 2016; 22(2):298–301.
5. Reboxa T, Rahlenbeck SI. Treatment of louse-borne relapsing fever with low dose penicillin or tetracycline: a clinical trial. Scand J Infect Dis 1995;27(1):29–31.

103

A 43-Year-Old Man from Peru With a Chronic Fistulating Foot Lesion

PEDRO LEGUA AND CARLOS SEAS

Clinical Presentation

History

A 43-year-old man is transferred from the Peruvian Cancer Institute after a negative work-up of a painful non-healing ulcerative lesion on the left foot. His illness began 3 years earlier; and after 1 year, the patient noticed progressive swelling on the sole that extended to the whole left foot in a matter of 6 months and has since significantly impaired his normal activities. Multiple papular lesions have developed that started to drain initially dark brown material and more recently yellow purulent material. The patient reports that he squeezed very small white grains from the lesions of his foot. The patient has received oral antibiotics with no improvement. No fever, lymphadenopathy, or systemic symptoms. No relevant past medical history. He was born and still lives in Nazca, a desert area south of Lima. He is a farmer, harvests corn and potato and works mainly barefoot. No travel history.

Clinical Findings

His vital signs are normal. There is marked swelling of the left foot involving the sole and dorsal aspects of the foot with multiple draining orifices (Fig. 103.1). Normal sensation; no lymphadenopathy; the rest of the examination is normal.

Laboratory Results

His full blood count is normal, and there are normal results for glucose, creatinine and electrolytes. Urinalysis is normal. X-ray shows mild osteomyelitis of the fifth metatarsal bone of the left foot. Serologies for HIV and HTLV-1 are negative.

Questions

1. What is your differential diagnosis?
2. What tests would you do to establish the diagnosis?

Discussion

A male farmer from the Peruvian coast presents with a chronic painful foot lesion with formation of sinus tracts that drain white grains.

Answer to Question 1

What Is Your Differential Diagnosis?

The differential diagnosis of subcutaneous conditions producing sinus tracts and granules includes mycetoma, which can be produced by bacteria or fungi, actinomycosis, and

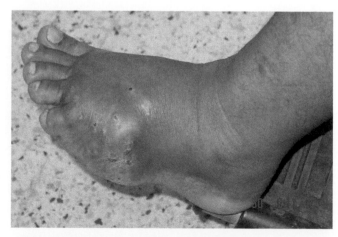

• **Fig. 103.1** Tumour and marked swelling of the dorsal and lateral aspects of the left foot with multiple draining orifices.

botryomycosis, a chronic staphylococcal infection. Conditions producing sinus tracts but without drainage of grains include chronic bacterial osteomyelitis, especially that caused by *Mycobacterium tuberculosis;* sporotrichosis; other fungal infections and syphilis. Finally, malignancy can also have a similar clinical picture.

Answer to Question 2

What Tests Would You Do to Establish the Diagnosis?

The diagnostic test of choice would be a biopsy of the lesion, which should be sent for cultures for bacteria (aerobic and anaerobic), mycobacteria and fungi, and for pathological examination.

The Case Continued…

Biopsy of the foot showed an inflammatory reaction surrounding a grain, with filamentous structures inside the grain (Fig. 103.2). Gram stain of an expressed white grain showed tiny branching Gram-positive filamentous bacteria consistent with actinomycetoma; culture grew *Nocardia* species. The granules of an actinomycete can be differentiated from a eumycetoma (caused by a fungal infection) based on the width of its filaments (0.5–1 μm in actinomycetoma), whereas in eumycetoma these are several microns wider (2–6 μm). Direct microscopy (KOH) and culture for fungi were negative. Fine-needle aspirations were negative for conventional or possibly super-infecting bacteria.

Knowing that the most likely cause of actinomycetoma in this case was *Nocardia* species, the patient was started on two drugs, cotrimoxazole (8 mg/kg per day) and amikacin (15 mg/kg per day once daily) given in four to five cycles of 5 weeks each. During the first 3 weeks the two drugs were combined, and during the remaining 2 weeks cotrimoxazole was used alone. (The number of cycles is determined by the clinical evolution. Cotrimoxazole as a monotherapy is continued for at least 1 year.)

Our patient received five cycles, after the first two cycles improvement was noticed: the swelling of his leg was reduced, all sinus tracts were closed, and no more grains could be obtained. He was cured with no relapses after 4 years.

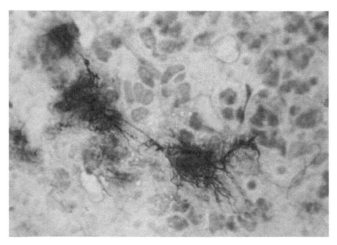

• **Fig. 103.2** Gram stain of an expressed white grain from a sinus tract showed tiny branching Gram-positive filamentous bacteria.

SUMMARY BOX

Mycetoma

Mycetoma (Madura foot) is a chronic subcutaneous infection with actinomycetes or fungi, which leads to the development of draining sinus tracts, discharging grains. The grains represent aggregated organisms. The colour of the grain may represent the aetiological agent. The term *actinomycetoma* refers to a mycetoma with a bacterial cause, usually attributable to *Nocardia* (white grains), *Streptomyces* (white/yellow grains) or *Actinomadura* (red grains).

Mycetoma is seen in the tropics and subtropics, more commonly in dry areas. The main areas affected are Mexico, Central America and the northern parts of South America, the Middle East, parts of Africa and India. It was first described in Madurai, India, hence the name "Madura foot".

The infection is acquired from the environment secondary to a penetrating injury. Actinomycetoma is frequent in farm workers because of greater exposure to minor skin trauma by *Acacia* thorns and splinters present in the soil. Its greatest incidence is between the fourth and fifth decades of life. The legs are the most commonly affected site, but actinomycetoma can potentially be present in most regions of the body. In Mexico, the second most frequently affected parts of the body are the back and the chest, probably because of the habit of carrying wood and lying on the ground.

The main and very important differential diagnosis in this case is eumycetoma, a mycetoma of fungal aetiology that produces black grains. This common subcutaneous mycosis in the tropics, and by far the most common cause of this clinical presentation in Perú, may be caused by a wide variety of fungal organisms but is usually caused by *Madurella mycetomatis*. Clinical diagnosis is thus not sufficient in these cases and an exact agent must be ascertained. Osteomyelitis from eumycetoma, however, would be more unusual and takes much longer to develop. Both eumycetoma and, as in this case, actinomycetoma, appear to be localized phenomena caused by local inoculation without any potential for widespread dissemination. Diagnosis is established by microscopic demonstration of the organisms within the grains or by culture of the grains on special media. Treatment depends on knowing if the causative organism is a bacterium or a fungus. Treatment of actinomycetoma requires a combination of antimicrobial drugs for many months, as described above. In contrast, eumycetomas are poorly responsive to medical therapy with antifungal agents such as azoles and may require aggressive surgery or amputation.

Further Reading

1. Hay RJ. Fungal Infections. In: Farrar J, editor. Manson's Tropical Diseases, 23rd ed. London: Elsevier; 2013 (chapter 38).

2. Welsh O, Vera-Cabrera L, Welsh E, et al. Actinomycetoma and advances in its treatment. Clin Dermatol 2012;30(4):372–81.

3. Zijlstra EE, van de Sande WWJ, Welsh O, et al. Mycetoma: a unique neglected tropical disease. Lancet Infect Dis 2016;16: 100–12.

4. Ahmed AA, van de Sande W, Fahal AH. Mycetoma laboratory diagnosis: review article. PLoS Negl Trop Dis 2017;11(8): e0005638.

5. Suleiman SH, Wadaella el S, Fahal AH. The surgical treatment of mycetoma. PLoS Negl Trop Dis 2016;10(6):e0004690.

Index

Note: Page numbers followed by *f* indicate figures and *t* indicate tables.